DATE DUE

A Few Months to Live

to Live

Different Paths to Life's End

Jana Staton

Roger Shuy

Ira Byock

Georgetown University Press / Washington, D.C.

Georgetown University Press, Washington, D.C.
© 2001 by Georgetown University Press. All rights reserved.
Printed in Canada

10 9 8 7 6 5 4 3 2 1   2001

This volume is printed on acid-free offset book paper.

Library of Congress Cataloging-in-Publication Data

Staton, Jana.
  A few months to live: different paths to life's end / Jana Staton, Roger Shuy, Ira Byock.
    p. cm.
  Includes bibliographical references and index.
  ISBN 0-87840-840-1 (cloth: alk. paper)—ISBN 0-87840-841-X (pbk.: alk. paper)
    1. Death—Social aspects—Montana—Missoula—Case studies. 2. Death—Montana—
  Missoula—Psychological aspects—Case studies. 3. Terminally ill—Montana—Missoula—
  Case studies. 4. Terminally ill—Home care—Montana—Missoula—Case studies.
  5. Caregivers—Montana—Missoula—Case studies. I. Shuy, Roger W. II. Byock, Ira. III. Title.

  HQ1073.5.U62 M577 2001
  306.9'09786'85—dc21

                                                    00-047671

Table of Contents

Acknowledgments

This book would not have been possible without the generosity of the people who permitted us to share a critical time in their lives. During the course of our research, people who were living with terminal illnesses allowed us to become their friends, rather than merely researchers. We cannot begin to express the depth of our gratitude for this privilege. The families and caregivers for these people earned our gratitude as well. It would have been far easier for them to have simply dismissed us. Instead, they became our collaborators, and, in the course of this work, they too became our friends.

We are grateful to the Kornfeld Foundation for its support of this research. Without the Foundation leadership's vision and belief in us, this study might well not have been possible.

The research on which this book is based is a component of the research program of the Missoula Demonstration Project, Inc. (MDP), with core support from the Nathan Cummings Foundation, the Project on Death in America of the Open Society Foundation, the Mayday Fund, and the Robert Wood Johnson Foundation.

We are grateful to the MDP staff, including co-founder Barbara Spring and Research Manager Kaye Norris, as well as members of the MDP Research Committee. We wish to extend special thanks to Linda Torma, Pat Blandford, and Helen Lee—with whom we often discussed various aspects of our work. We also received valuable advice and encouragement from the MDP's International Research Advisors, especially Myra Bluebond-Langner, Phyllis Silverman, Joan Teno, and Robert Kastenbaum. Colleagues who read early drafts of the manuscript and offered valuable comments include Muriel Friedman, Colleen Nicholson, and Stan Nicholson (from the MDP Board of Directors).

Finally, we appreciate Georgetown University Press's anonymous reviewers, whose ideas and thoughtful suggestions pointed us in the direction of clarifying the book's multiple audiences and helped steer us away from verbal obscurity and disorganization.

Preface

A Few Months to Live reports the findings of a unique study of the last months of nine terminally ill people. It looks beyond the usual categories of facts and figures of death and dying. By offering detailed observations and numerous direct quotes, it provides a glimpse of the real-life experience of people who are living through their dying along with the family members who are caring for and living through it with them. The title—*A Few Months to Live*—accurately captures the focus on participants' everyday life: what was going well for them, what they enjoyed, and what was difficult, not simply about dying and death but about living with advanced, incurable illness.

This book examines how particular dying persons deal with their diminished power and control, their degrees of discomfort and pain, the drains on their economic security, their decreasing mobility, and their shrinking social networks, as well as the extent to which they manage to maintain hope and dignity. Unblinkingly, it shows their struggle to maintain a sense of continuity and connection with life and their strivings to make meaning and to grow even as they die. We believe that these factors are crucial to understanding people's efforts to remain part of the world of the living at a time when these aspects of life and self-image are being eroded by the terminal illness.

The participants in our study were nine people living in Missoula, Montana, during 1997—along with those who cared for them (mostly at home). We visited the study participants wherever they were living. We collected data by talking with participants informally in conversations that we tape recorded for later analysis. The visits continued until their deaths and memorial services and included at least one after-death visit with each family. We had access to participants' home care settings and to their families' perspectives for periods ranging from two months to more than ten months. This book provides extensive quotations in the participants' own words. It is our belief that the feelings, concerns, and general everyday existence of people can be represented by their own language better than ours.

This study, which was funded principally by the Kornfeld Foundation, is part of the Missoula Demonstration Project: The Quality of Life's End (MDP). The MDP was created to study end-of-life experiences and convene the Missoula community in efforts to improve end-of-life care. Our study was one of several baseline research projects in this Northwest mountain community. Our intention and hope is that this book and the findings it reports will be used by students and colleagues from a broad range of fields, spanning the social and clinical sciences, and that it will find application across a range of health care and public policy issues.

A Tour Guide to A Few Months to Live

Our goal is to provide a continuous record of the lived experience of dying and caregiving. We want to convey the texture and tone of the experience of living with life-limiting illness and disability, the giving and receiving of care, the myriad of subtle and not-so-subtle adaptations to illness, disability and the ever-present awareness of limited time as we observed them. Negotiations and compromises are revealed—externally, between caregiver and recipient, and internally, between each individual's expectations and the reality of the demands and limitations that life imposes. We witnessed participants' struggles to make sense, and make meaning, during what can seem a senseless, meaningless, and personal assault. Each chapter of *A Few Months to Live* focuses on a specific aspect of the lived experience of dying, caring, death, and grief.

Recognizing that this book will be of interest to readers from different fields and with a range of primary concerns, we hope that the following "tour guide" may prove helpful. *A Few Months to Live* is organized from the framework of the participants' experience and from our first encounters with them, beginning with their accounts of the time they first heard the announcement of "bad news," planning (or not planning) for their care, understanding their illness, coping with symptoms and daily life, searching for meaning or spiritual growth and striving for closure, the experiences of patients and families during the final days of life, and memorial services or funerals when these occurred.

We hope that the entirety of the participants' experiences will capture the interest of general readers, including professional clinicians and health care providers, families, and academics of various specializations. Not all readers will be concerned with every aspect of the participants' experiences or the details of the study, however. The Introduction, which describes the current crisis in end-of-life care in America and the framework of this study within the MDP research program, may be of special interest and usefulness to policymakers, researchers, and physicians. (More information about the research is provided in the two appendices.) Chapter 1 introduces the nine individuals in the study and their immediate families, summarizing in one place pertinent information about their diagnoses, disease trajectories, functional capacity, and caregiving arrangements. This chapter is intended to provide a handy reference for all readers to the circumstances, illnesses, and family structures that we encounter or refer to in other chapters; in particular, the first chapter will provide sufficient clinical data to allow health professionals to make comparisons with their own patients.

Readers with particular interest in communication issues—including ethicists, linguists, and medical educators—will find in chapter 2 a record of how these participants talked about their own dying and death, and in chapter 4 an account of how they talked about their professional care and health providers.

Sociologists and social workers may be more concerned with how participants planned for this crucial period of their lives; they will find this perspective in chapter 3, which describes the end-of-life decisions our study participants made. Medical practitioners may find chapter 5 of particular interest because it describes in the patients' own words how they viewed their illness and dealt with their symptoms (especially pain).

Medical professionals seldom see the mundane, everyday activities that absorb the lives of terminally ill patients who are dying at home—which chapter 6 describes in detail. Those who must plan for home health care and physicians and nurses whose patients may be cared for at home may be especially interested in this chapter. Chapters 7 and 8 are devoted to the experience of the family caregivers—a critical but often overlooked part of terminal illness that social workers and psychologists may appreciate. Theologians and philosophers may be particularly interested in chapter 9, which describes how these participants sought to make meaning and their sources of psychological and spiritual strength during this period. Chapter 10 describes how these participants spent their final days of life, and chapter 11 focuses particularly on the personal symbols and rituals families created to mark the death of their loved ones. Chapter 12 discusses the implications of the study findings and suggests some directions for both community efforts and research to improve the end of life.

Appendix A provides technical information about the research design of MDP's baseline Community Profile and summarizes the initial demonstration efforts that have begun to emerge from the project. Appendix B discusses our study methodology and approach to analysis, which may be of interest primarily to researchers who may want to conduct similar community-based research. Appendix B also contains statistical and demographic information on the Missoula community.

We hope that the voice of the people directly affected by terminal illness can be heard in this book. If we have succeeded in this endeavor, *A Few Months to Live* may contribute to academic efforts to understand the nature of end-of-life experience and care—and to public efforts to respond to the critical national challenge of caring for one another through the end of life.

Jana Staton
Roger Shuy
Ira Byock
Missoula, Montana

Introduction

This book describes the experience of having only a few months to live from the perspective of terminally ill patients and their caregivers. As much as possible, their stories are told in their own words. We introduce nine patients dying of chronic obstructive pulmonary disease, heart disease, and cancer who were living or receiving care in the small western city of Missoula, Montana, during 1997. They differ in age, diagnosis, and ethnicity. How they think and talk about their impending death, plan and conduct their daily lives, deal with pain, and make meaning out of their situation frames most of the book. We also present the experience of their caregivers and support systems (or lack thereof) and what spending most of one's waking hours with a loved one who is dying is like.

A National Crisis: The Context of Dying and End-of-Life Care in America

One can tell a lot about a society by the way it deals with death and cares for people who are nearing life's end. The issues include the needs of those who are dying and the needs of their families and friends who may be providing, or want to provide, a large portion of their care. The context in which the Missoula Demonstration Project (MDP) and this particular study arose is a true national crisis that surrounds end-of-life experience and care.

A large body of research has documented serious deficiencies in basic medical care, communication, comfort, and adherence to people's stated preferences. The National Institute of Medicine's report, *Approaching Death* (Field and Cassell 1997), details the severity and pervasive nature of the crisis and highlights inadequacies in medical education, financing, cultural attitudes, and clinical practice. SUPPORT, a major study of end-of-life care in prestigious teaching hospitals (Knaus, Lynn, and Teno 1995) found that even within otherwise excellent medical institutions, pain and physical suffering among dying patients remain inadequately treated—or even assessed. In study after study, up to 40 percent of patients with advanced, incurable illness are reported to have received grossly inadequate analgesia (Field and Cassell 1997; Knaus, Lynn, and Teno 1995; Cleeland, Gorin, and Hatfield 1994; Bernabei et al. 1998; Breitbart, Rosenfeld, and Passik 1996). Being of minority ethnicity, older than eighty, or having dementia can seriously increase the risk of having one's pain untreated (Bernabei et al. 1998; Cleeland 1997; Todd et al. 1993). In addition, most Americans still die in clinical settings; approximately 60 percent in hospitals and 20–25 percent in nursing homes. This book, which focuses on dying at home, is intended to provide a complement to the predominance of studies that focus on institutional dying.

Studies report that patients' preferences for care often are not honored, even when those choices are clearly conveyed (Danis et al. 1996). As if that were not bad enough, the American health care system routinely pauperizes people and their families for being chronically ill and not dying quickly enough. In the large SUPPORT study, one-third of the families of dying patients reported losing most or all of the family's major source of income; one-third reported losing the family's life savings, and one-fifth said that a family member had to move or delay their own medical care, education, or career to meet the basic needs of their dying loved one (Covinsky et al. 1994). Dying patients and their families have known for years about these errors of omission and commission and the tears in the fabric of social support during times of serious illness and need for care. Being chronically ill or disabled or trying to care for a loved one who is dying provides an opportunity few can escape to learn first-hand about the discontinuity, poor communication, confusion, inattention to comfort, and lapses in care that too often typify dying in America.

The roots of this crisis extend far deeper than lapses of clinical competence or structural flaws in the current health care system. Cultural denial marks the confused and conflicted way our society approaches life's end. Research and public opinion surveys demonstrate that Americans do not fear death so much as the process of dying. We are terrified of becoming ill, being in pain, or becoming physically dependent. We worry most about becoming a burden to others (American Health Decisions 1997).

Most people say they want control over the way they live and the way their lives end, but few do anything about it. Only a small percentage—30 percent or less of adults in most surveys—have filled out a living will or durable power of attorney for health care (Gallup 1997). Even many people living with advanced illness refuse to talk about cardiopulmonary resuscitation or mechanical ventilation with their doctors (Hofmann 1997). In strict psychological terms, this resistance is not truly the defense mechanism of denial. People simply do not want to talk about the subject. Most people say they would prefer that their families make decisions for them if they become unable to speak for themselves (Hines et al. 1999), although only a few of these people tell their families what kind of care they would want.

The Burden of Family Caregiving

The other face of the crisis is the burden that inadequate formal systems of care and support services places on families. Family caregiving or informal caregiving by relatives and close friends represents the unrecognized backbone of care in America. Family or informal caregiving—provided free of charge and motivated by love, commitment, personal responsibility, or a sense of mutual self-interest—is an enormous resource that deserves close public attention. The economic impact of such care is extraordinary, amounting to $196 billion dollars per year—dwarfing the costs of home health care ($32 billion) and nursing home care ($83 billion) combined (Arno et al. 1999).

Family caregiving is not easy. Chief among the challenges that caregivers face is the unceasing and intensive nature of the care that their ill loved ones require. A recent study by the National Alliance for Caregiving (NAC) and the American Association of Retired Persons (AARP) found that caregivers—mostly women—devoted an average of 4.6 years to caregiving; many spent 10 years or more (NAC/AARP 1997). Other studies show that home caregivers have major needs for help with transportation, homemaking services, nursing care, and personal care (Emanuel et al. 1999). Significant physical and emotional stress were reported by 15 percent of all caregivers and by 31 percent of those who provided the highest levels of care (NAC/AARP 1997). A study conducted by the Administration on Aging of women providing or anticipating long-term care for a relative found that the common thread was the pressing need for much more information about what such caregiving would be like and about their options. The study concluded that without information on which to base corrective action, many older American women will continue to experience stress, frustration, and physical and mental strain (Greenwald 2000).

The unmet needs of nonprofessional caregivers add another dimension to the crisis of care. Insufficient support for family caregiving predictably leads to a breakdown of care at home—where a consistent predominance of study subjects and survey respondents say they want to be—and leads to institutionalization, which most people say they want to avoid. The stress of unmet needs can take a toll on families, leaving them feeling frustrated and even guilty, and often results in higher use of health resources for stress-related illness (Levine 1999; Meshefedjian et al. 1998; Schulz et al. 1995).

The current depth of this crisis, and the need for change, is masked by the relatively small number of persons who are living out an extended dying period. As America grays with the aging of the "baby boom" population, however, persons who require care for chronic illness through the end of life will mushroom in proportion to the total population. At the same time, social trends such as reduced birthrates, an increased proportion of women working outside the home, and geographic mobility within American families are combining to constrict the pool of available private caregivers within individual networks of relatives and close friends who have traditionally provided care to chronically ill and frail elderly persons.

Signs of Hope

There are signs of hope for the twenty-first century. The expansion of hospice and the rapid development of palliative medicine are providing excellent clinical models on which the caring professions can draw as the new century begins. In response, major medical organizations and certifying boards—including the American Society of Clinical Oncology, the American Board of Internal Medicine, and the American Medical Association's Educating Physicians in End-of-life Care (EPEC) program—are beginning to integrate palliative medicine principles into clinical practice, standards, curricula, and examinations. All of these efforts are emblematic of the serious resolve with which organized medicine is meeting the challenge of caring for society's dying members.

Another notable professional effort that has emerged as part of the national shift in attention is Last Acts. This coalition of provider institutions and professional associations was formed to influence every relevant sector of society—from managed care to long-term care, from mass media to medical textbooks, from professional training to public schooling, from the workplace to places of worship.

One set of hopeful examples is provided by a national grant and technical assistance program of the Robert Wood Johnson Foundation, Promoting Excellence in End-of-Life Care. This national program supports the development of programmatic best practices that target contexts of care and special populations of dying patients. These contexts include systems of care such as large managed care organizations, regional comprehensive cancer centers, and Veterans Administration medical centers, as well as difficult environments of care such as isolated Alaska Native frontier villages, poor inner-city communities, and maximum security prisons. Challenging special populations of patients with advanced illness being targeted include children; people with serious, persistent mental illness; those who have diseases such as Alzheimer's dementia; and those receiving kidney dialysis for end-stage renal failure.

There also are state-based initiatives in more than twenty states, many supported by another Robert Wood Johnson Foundation program, Community-State Partnerships to Improve End-of-Life Care. These initiatives often have a dual purpose of correcting regulatory barriers to effective pain management and effective use of advance directives while raising professional and public expectations for end-of-life care.

In addition to these efforts, several promising social innovations in care for the most ill, elderly, and frail among us dot the country. Some of the most exciting of these efforts meld clinical care with the humanities, including artistic and spiritual activities and nurturing environments. The Eden Alternative and its derivatives represent an important movement toward the "greening" of nursing homes and assisted long-term care facilities, especially for dementia care (Thomas 1996). In Eden nursing homes, there is a strong emphasis on "greening" the environment with plants and pets. Eden facilities also foster intergenerational activities between seniors and young children and pleasurable human interaction. The impact of "Edenizing" nursing homes for patients with dementia can be profound. People who have been withdrawn often brighten when they interact with a colorful bird, an affectionate dog, or a cooing baby. Even having responsibility for a plant has a notable impact on a person's health.

Other initiatives springing up include parish nursing, block nursing, and careteam networks, which provide critical support to caregivers. In a handful of cities and Veterans Administration hospitals, volunteers from the "Twilight Brigade"—a project of Compassion in Action—offer company and personal attention to people who might otherwise face life's end alone. Auntie Helen's Fluff and Fold in San Diego and Auntie Bea's in Los Angeles are dedicated to making sure that people living with HIV disease have clean pajamas and bed linens. In rural Nebraska, Telecare pairs elderly people who are at risk for isolation and depression with fifth graders who call and visit by phone every school day. Some projects are loosely affiliated with religious congregations or are otherwise "faith-based," (e.g., Stephen's Ministry and Parish Nursing).

Limitations of Current Research on End-of-Life Care

As valuable as research has been in documenting the crisis and illuminating its components, most prevailing studies reflect some of the same shortcomings and limitations as the caregiving being studied—such as an overemphasis on the clinical perspective and medical concerns and a focus on the individual, distinct from family, friends, and community. To date, most studies of end-of-life experience and care, even those focused on ethics or communication, have been conducted within a medical framework and perspective. Typically, the person who is dying is viewed as a patient, often in relationship to clinicians or the health system. Dying is regarded as a constellation of problems, comprising the ravages of disease on physical comfort, function (especially independence), and the financial and social assaults that accompany illness and treatment. Clinical and health service research generally have approached dying as a discrete period of time and as a distinct event or set of events, rather than as a continuum of experience. Within this prevailing conceptual framework, decision making is analyzed as a medical process, with assumed goals of better symptom management and better communication between clinicians and patients and/or families regarding their preferences and respect for their rights.

All of this is well and good, but many important realms of end-of-life experience are not encompassed by these assumptions or by standard medical or health service approaches to research. Dying is more than a set of medical problems that confront the ill person and his or her family. Although the symptoms and disability of illness and injury obviously affect the experience of dying, they do not independently determine the quality of a person's life. Nor do the stresses and struggles with illness completely define a family's experience of caregiving and grief. Ultimately, dying is a time of living and must be understood within a continuum of lived experience of the ill person and the friends and relatives who constitute the person's "family."

Doctors, nurses, and other clinicians who care for people with advanced illness can benefit from an awareness of what dying patients and their personal family caregivers in similar circumstances have learned: what is important to them, what they fear, and what they hope for during their physical dependence and frailty. The kind of sociological, linguistic, and ethnographic research methods used in this study and other research (Bluebond-Langner 1996; Silverman 1999; Davies et al. 1995) can inform clinical practice by revealing what patients and families are likely to consider helpful in dealing with symptoms, physical dependence, and frailty during this waning phase of life. This information can enable clinicians, family caregivers, and members of the ill person's family and community to better communicate with, care for, and support people during these difficult times.

Understanding the important effects of dying and death on the immediate community requires research approaches that are more sociological or ethnographic than medical. Although such studies are unlikely to be published in medical journals, they are relevant to broader efforts to improve the quality of end-of-life and bereavement care. There is value, for instance, in understanding how the psychological and social effects on work colleagues that follow a co-worker's sudden death compare with those following a death that comes after months of progressive illness. Knowing more about the needs of people in acute grief and about receptivity over time to various forms of support from co-workers can assist in developing effective programs and systems of support. Likewise, various types and settings of terminal care—from hospital-based care to long-term, nursing home-based care to home health and hospice care—may affect the family and immediate community in ways that are not captured by standard approaches of clinical health systems or health service research but have important implications for health and social policy.

By incorporating the family's perspective, this book provides some balance to the predominant focus in end-of-life research on the individual alone. Studies of populations or large patient cohorts, such as the SUPPORT study, almost invariably have focused on patient experiences and deemphasized or excluded family or community experiences. Although there is little disagreement that the dying person is the most dramatically affected by his or her illness and impending demise, the relatives and close friends whom patients identify as "family" are intimately—and often profoundly—affected by the patient's advanced illness. The events that surround the death of an individual and the time of grieving are part of the lived experience of close relatives or friends of the deceased. In this book, the caregiver's experience is holistically interwoven with that of the dying participant's to focus sharply on this often invisible aspect of dying.

The Missoula Demonstration Project

This book arose from the baseline research efforts of the Missoula Demonstration Project: The Quality of Life's End (MDP), a collaborative, community-wide effort to study and transform end-of-life experience and care. The MDP was founded in 1996 to research the experience of dying and the determinants of the quality of individual experiences and care related to life's end and to demonstrate that a community-based approach of excellent physical, psychosocial, and spiritual care improves the quality of life for dying persons and their families. The community setting for the project is Missoula County, Montana. This area in the mountains of western Montana, near the Idaho border, is home to nearly 90,000 residents. The community includes the University of Montana, which has 10,000 students and serves as a regional medical center for a population of about 350,000.

The early stages of this fifteen- to twenty-year project have concentrated on building a researched baseline of understanding about the community's attitudes, actions, and values regarding dying and death. In particular, *A Few Months to Live* was designed to capture the aforementioned issues and concerns—symptoms and pain relief, communication, quality of life, family caregiving, functional ability and enjoyment, impact on family finances—from the perspective of dying persons and their family members who are active in caregiving.

This study represents one part of the MDP's innovative, community-based approach to end-of-life research and community-based effort to improve the quality of life's end. We do not assert that the findings of this study or our experience as a community will be generalizable to all people, places, or times. Indeed, this work is a study of particularity. Every one of the people we studied was living or receiving or providing care in Missoula during the late 1990s. Neither does this study purport to exhaustively describe the state of dying or caregiving in Missoula. *A Few Months to Live* describes a single component of a much larger, long-term study that attempts to comprehensively describe end-of-life experiences and care in this small, western American city at the end of the twentieth century.

This book reports in detail on critical aspects of the experiences of dying, caregiving, and grieving that otherwise might remain hidden from view. It documents aspects of end-of-life experience that typically are not discussed—because they are considered too personal or unpleasant or simply too mundane for most scientific inquiry. In fact, these details and the perspectives of the people they convey can be compelling. Without them, no understanding of dying, caregiving, or grieving could be complete.

The MDP's focus on documenting and describing the community itself comes from an understanding that the level and quality of clinical and support services available to people during times of individual need also influence the collective quality of each community's life. Therefore, studying end-of-life experience and care in community settings is essential if we are to fully understand the social impact and cultural implications of end-of-life policies and various modes of care. Recent research reinforces this conclusion, with indications that problems related to symptom management, use of advance directives, and the tendency to use aggressive, life-prolonging care in the days before death may be less severe outside urban, tertiary hospital settings (Hanson et al. 1999).

In constructing a platform for ongoing research, the MDP built on the experience of the Framingham Heart Study, a longitudinal set of studies of the effects of lifestyle on cardiovascular health, disease, and morbidity (Gresham et al. 1998; Wilson et al. 1998; Voelker 1998). The Framingham Heart Study demonstrates the rich potential for long-term, community-based research. Beginning with a modest database in 1948 in the town of Framingham, Massachusetts, the Framingham Heart Study has been examining the relationship of lifestyle, medications, and personal habits to cardiovascular health over individual lifetimes. Unlike the Framingham studies, however, in which enrolled patients could be followed for many years, the very nature of the dying and caregiving experience dictates that another methodology is needed for this study. The MDP settled on sequential, cross-sectional studies to be repeated over a period of 15–20 years. The initial baseline research included the study into the perspectives of persons living with terminal illness, caregiving, and grieving—which provides the data for this book.

Studying the End of Life in Missoula

Surprisingly, authors who write about geriatric medicine rarely deal with matters of death. Likewise, writers of thanatology seldom consider the experience of aging when they discuss issues of death (Seale 1998, 44). This situation leaves an important transition area—the end of life, when it is acknowledged that an illness will be terminal, even if the patient is not yet actively dying—largely ignored.

There are several ways to study this end-of-life experience. One can examine this experience from the perspectives of the medical profession, other health caregivers, patients' families, or patients themselves. One can study this experience in medical settings such as hospitals, nursing homes, hospice houses, or the homes of patients and their families. One can do long-term or short-term studies. One can do experimental or qualitative research. One can have systematic representative samples of the population to be studied or proceed on a case-study basis. One can carry out structured interviews or simply engage in conversations that permit patients and their families to narrate however they see fit.

This book provides texture to the diversity of the death and dying experience in Missoula in 1997. The analyses highlight the contrasts among the participants: Some know everything about their disease, some nothing; some families find closure and peace, other are at war before and after the death; some people are able to find meaning despite pain and impending death, others have difficulty. It emphasizes the range of different experiences, the contrasts rather than "central tendencies" or trends. It describes the complexity and ambiguity of the experience in some cases, as well as its simplicity in others. Confronted with the mystery of death, our study participants were not able to "solve it" in any single way. As one of the caregivers in our study commented, "I still have lots of questions."

Most research operates under time constraints of some type, and this study is no different. Because terminally ill people traditionally are considered to have between six months and one year to live, one year of research provided our time frame. For the type of study that the MDP envisioned and commissioned, qualitative research using ethnographic methods seemed most salient, humane, and practical.

An Ethnographic Approach

Ethnographic research consists of the systematic description of a human culture. This study can be described as ethnographic because it is inductive, exploratory, observational, and designed to identify themes, problems, and gaps in our basic understanding of how the end of life happens within the context of individual experience, looking outward from the ill person's perspective. The goal is to provide descriptive evidence of how the vitally important event of dying happened in Missoula (circa 1997) when patients were diagnosed as terminally ill.

This ethnographic study attempts to be holistic, painting an overall picture as completely as possible to make sense of small scenes that are captured in detail. It attempts to set findings in context, at least as much as is ethically and physically possible. It attempts to capture the insider's perspective (anthropologists and linguists use the term "emic" to refer to this perspective) of each participant's reality. Such perspectives may not always conform to those of others involved in patients' lives, including professionals or other family caregivers. Therefore, this study compels recognition and acceptance of multiple realities.

The current trend in medicine to be "patient centered" provides a strong motivation for capturing, in the words of the terminally ill and their caregivers and with as much rich detail as practical, what they do, what they know, and what they believe as a life nears its physical end. In talking with people about what they know and experience, we made use of Spradley's (1979) insights about what distinguishes a friendly conversation from a formal interview:

It is best to think of ethnographic interviews as a series of friendly conversations into which the researcher slowly introduces new elements to assist informants to respond as informants. Exclusive use of these new *ethnographic elements,* or introducing them too quickly, will make interviews become like a formal interrogation. Rapport will evaporate, and informants may discontinue their cooperation. At any time during an interview it is possible to shift back to a friendly conversation. A few minutes of easygoing talk interspersed here and there throughout will pay enormous dividends in rapport (59).

After establishing rapport and stating the purpose and direction of the study and letting people self-generate whatever topics they wished, we probed with follow-up questions to expand and clarify these topics, much as one would do in normal everyday conversation.

Study Participants

This study is built around conversations with nine terminally ill people in Missoula County in 1997, along with family members (or in one case close friends) who participated in their care. As the study progressed, conversations with family members assumed more and more importance as a means of understanding the experience from a holistic or ethnographic perspective. For this reason, we refer to patients and family members as "participants," to indicate their status as persons, rather than medical patients. (In some cases, *participants* refers to the terminally ill patients, as the context will make clear.)

Among the nine patients in the study, two suffered from emphysema, two from metastatic breast cancer, two from other types of cancer, and two from heart disease. Another patient suffered from a disease that has not, to this point, been identified to us by the patient, her friends who provided care, or her physician, except as "old age." At the time the research was completed (December 1998), the only participants remaining alive were the two who had breast cancer.

This study began with several visits with the individuals who were terminally ill. We also spent considerable time, separately, with caregivers to learn about their perspectives and experiences. In most cases, caregivers felt free to speak more openly when we met with them alone. In all cases in which family caregivers participated, they also signed the consent form (see Appendix B).

Occasionally other visitors were present during all or part of our meetings with patients and caregivers. Because our research took place in customary or natural settings, we felt that including them as well (with their permission) was important and natural. In some cases, we sought out nonfamily caregivers to help us understand some of the things that we did not understand fully from our visits with patients. Such people included friends, additional family members who were helping with caregiving, and ordained clergy and other faith community leaders.

Confidentiality

We have given all of the participants and primary caregivers in this study first-name pseudonyms to ensure their privacy and confidentiality. We have deleted all other names and identifying characteristics. Where other individuals are referred to in the conversation, we have inserted general descriptors—"our hospice nurse," or "Sharon's doctor"—except when the physician was referred to on a first-name basis (as is common in Missoula). In those cases, to reflect this common informality in Missoula, we created first-name pseudonyms for the physicians as well.

Format of Visits

The data gathered in this study can be best called conversations between the researchers and the participants. We believe that a conversational format is less intimidating that the conventional question-answer interview. For the participants, such a procedure has the advantage of naturalness and comfort. We believe that accommodating the comfort of participants—patients and caregivers—is important, even though this process makes analysis more difficult and complex for the researcher.

Our visits began like any normal conversation would: We got to know the person—chatting about mutual experiences and interests, people we both knew, the weather, or whatever came naturally. We answered their questions about our purpose, the MDP, and what we hoped to accomplish. During the course of our visits, participants began to tell us about themselves—their feelings, comforts, discomforts, views of life, attitudes toward death, and many other things. We elicited demographic information naturally rather than formally, as with written forms. We let participants introduce topics as they wished, saving our questions as follow-ups to their personal agendas.

This is not to say that the researchers asked no questions, for questions are natural in all conversations (see Appendix B for a list of the topics we discussed in our follow-up queries). Nor is it the case that the researchers had no agenda of their own. Before the study began, we created a "conversational guide" to help shape our visits; this guide included all of the major concerns and topics that we thought might be relevant. We memorized it and used it as a mental guide to help us bring up topics that might not have come up or to probe more deeply into a topic—especially during later visits, after we had allowed participants to establish their own concerns. The conversational guide appears in Appendix B.

Obviously we wanted to learn about participants' problems, things that were helpful to them, what they would like most to do during their last few months of life, what they were learning from this experience, what fears they had, how they felt about their current and past care, what they wish they had done differently, what hopes they had, and the degree to which they were aware of the fact that they were terminally ill. Yet we wanted to learn these and other things in a manner that did not take the form of an interview. We believed that by letting the other person bring up his or her own topics and agendas, we could learn about what concerns him or her most. In short, our role was more like that of a new friend than a clinical researcher.

Understanding the Subculture of Terminally Ill People

Culture has been defined in many ways. Usually, however, the definition connects a shared system of behavioral and ideational patterns associated with particular groups of people, including their customs or way of life (Harris 1968, 16). We usually think of a culture as a group on whose membership insiders and outsiders agree.

The shared system of meaning called *culture* "is learned, revised, maintained, and defined in the context of people interacting" (Spradley 1979, 56). Spradley suggests that it may be useful to think of culture as a cognitive map that serves as a guide for acting and interpreting experience. Such a map does not compel us to follow a particular route, however. Frake (1977) describes this culture map as follows:

> People are not just map readers; they are map-makers. People are cast out into imperfectly charted, continually shifting seas of everyday life. Culture does not provide a cognitive map, but rather a set of principles for map making and navigation. Different cultures are like different schools of navigation designed to cope with different terrains and seas (607).

Different groups of people who seem to differ greatly regarding the things that are important to them are said to have different cultures. But there are many routes on this map of culture, and different route-taking does not necessarily signify the existence of a different culture. When certain clear but relatively minor differences exist within an otherwise homogeneous group of people, such differences may be the basis for considering those people a subculture.

For example, most adults from Missoula share many things in common and may, for all intents and purposes, be considered members of the same American culture. Within this group, however, are smaller groups of Native Americans from various tribes, Hmong refugees, and a smattering of people from Eastern Europe and other parts of the world. To the extent that some aspects of their beliefs, values, rituals, and attitudes differ from those of the majority, such groups may be considered subcultures of the larger majority culture in this area. Another subculture, from an ethnographic perspective, is the one that comprises people who have a terminal illness. They perceive and experience themselves—and are perceived and experienced by others—as differing from the continuously living majority who make up the general culture.

Any effort to describe the subculture of terminally ill persons should consider "insider" and "outsider" points of view. The ethnographic perspective is "to grasp the native's point of view" (Malinowski 1922, 25). Physical deterioration in a person's body provides evidence of that person's new status to outsiders—that is, the medical profession that, in turn, defines patients as terminally ill. The way medical professionals view such patients is not the subject of this study. The way the insiders—that is, the patients and their caregivers—view this designation and what they choose to do about it may differ quite markedly, however, from the outsider perspective. Following Frake, the subculture of the terminally ill does not provide exact routes but sets of principles for navigation. The participants in this study, having been assigned to the subculture of the terminally ill, do not always take the same routes—nor do their caregivers. These different routes form the basis for the analysis that follows. We begin with the principles or characteristics that define the subculture and describe how the participants take approaches and make decisions.

In some ways, the subculture of terminally ill people is similar to a minority group that lacks social, cultural, or economic power. Like other minority groups, people who are terminally ill differ from the majority who are continuously living. In many respects, terminally ill persons share some similarities with other American minorities that are based on race, nationality, gender, or age. Unlike these other minorities, however, dying people were members of the larger culture until recent events caused them to migrate to the subculture of those about to die. This reassignment is not of their own choosing, and it carries with it few of the advantages that the larger culture offers. Unlike other subcultures, terminally ill persons know that their membership in this new subculture will last only for a very short time—and that there is no way to return to their previous status.

Many characteristics of majority cultures—such as power, comfort, control, economic security, mobility, continuity, wide social networks, hope, growth, and dignity—are less available or are available in different ways to the subculture of the dying. For example, there is a predictable diminishing of control that occurs when one's body fails. Hope often diminishes, naturally, with the discovery that the end of life is near. The intellectual, spiritual, and emotional growth that characterizes most of life to this point takes a back burner to other, more pressing, matters or takes on new directions. The sense of continuity can be disrupted. The comforts of life take on new dimensions and significance. Financial stresses often increase with rising medical expenses. Formerly wide social networks can be reduced by isolation-inducing medical treatment, by the lowering of a sense of dignity, and as peers die or move away. Formerly mobile people now find that getting around is physically difficult; this restricted mobility affects their sense of control, hopefulness, continuous human growth, sense of continuity, social networks, comfort, dignity, and financial status. Some terminally ill persons or their families refuse psychologically to "join" this subculture, avoiding the plain evidence of death's nearness.

Some of the participants in this study laid careful plans for the inevitable changes in economics and comfort that their new medical condition brought about. Often, however, there was little or nothing they could do about the changes in power, control, and mobility. The ways in which they handled the hopelessness of being told they were terminal, managed to grow in mind and spirit, identified a sense of continuity in their lives, and sought self-recognition while dying turned out to be their most powerful stories. The extent to which they faced these issues and did something about them reflects the differences among the participants, and it frames the different routes navigated by the participants and their caregivers on the map of terminal illness.

Frank (1995) notes that patients' narratives are told *through* rather than *about* the body. He describes three forms of narratives: restitution, chaos, and quest. All three types appear in this book. At first, the narratives of two of our participants, Dennis and Barbara, focused on hopes for restitution—premised on the heroic hope for a cure; later, however, their conversations showed more similarity to quest narratives as they began to depict their illness as a journey with a departure and spiritual return. Two other participants, Ralph and Sharon, were past the stage of considering restitution but held on to the same promise of the quest. Walt's narrative reflected simple acceptance of his condition, with little restitution or quest involved. The chaos narratives of Mabel showed her despair and loss of control and hope. The narratives of Kitty and Roberta, although increasingly less clear to us from their growing dementia, suggested the existence of a quest narrative at some earlier point in their life trajectories.

Seale (1998, 29) observes, "Participation in ritual, in conventional anthropological usage, affirms membership in the collectivity." The chapters that follow describe some of the rituals of the dominant culture that these terminally ill people fought to preserve or, in some cases, failed to preserve. Such rituals include meals, bathing, receiving visitors, experiencing a sense of time, physical activities, reading, celebrating special events, getting outside, enjoying pets, and being entertained. The participants also describe their beliefs, values, and attitudes—such as their willingness or ability to plan, their attitudes toward pain and dying itself, their reactions to getting the "bad news," their relationships with professional and home caregivers, their openness in talking about their own death, and their search for meaning in their lives.

Debilitating diseases promote failure to maintain such rituals, beliefs, values, and attitudes, at least in the way they are found in the dominant culture. Seale (1998, 170) describes death as "a final fall from culture," noting as well that those who die "have usually experienced a social death which preceded their biological death." These Missoula participants do not all "fall from culture" or experience a "social death;" they choose instead to hang on to whatever dignity they can and, in some cases, chart their own good deaths.

Conclusion

At the dawn of the third millennium across most of America, discussions of life's end have been dominated by the issue of physician-assisted suicide. A private conversation about end-of-life care typically begins with the question, "What do you think about Kevorkian?" This peculiar perspective has captured and may continue to frame America's view of life's end—but not in Missoula.

Missoula is no utopia. What is different here, however, is that we have not allowed ourselves to be confined by the suffering-or-suicide dichotomy or mesmerized by the promise of a quick fix. Instead, Missoulians are taking a hard look at dying and grief and taking steps to improve the quality of life's end. With the help of the MDP, Missoula is gaining a broader perspective and a sensitivity to the needs of people who are dying, as well as their caregivers and grieving family. We do not have all the answers, but we are asking critical questions: What individual and collective responsibility—and "response-ability"—do we have toward people who are dying: family members, friends, neighbors? What value is there in the last phase of life? Can there be any value in the process of dying? Missoulians are investigating the meaning of living in a community with one another in ways that integrate dying and caregiving within the continuum of human life.

Perhaps, not too many years from now, wherever people are discussing dying and end-of-life care, someone will ask, "Have you heard what they're doing in Missoula?" If the answer is "yes" and the discussion that follows reflects a heightened awareness of the positive potential for caregiving and quality at life's end, our efforts will have been worthwhile. We hope that readers everywhere can learn, as we have, from the individuals and families who have generously shared with us their lives, insights and perspectives, struggles and successes. It is in this spirit that we offer *A Few Months to Live.*

Chapter 1

Study Participants

Nine individuals and their families participated intensively in our study and are profiled here. The profiles provide a frame of reference and summary in one place; they include diagnoses, medical treatments, and living situations. Each profile follows the same format:

- Disease, diagnosis, trajectory
- Treatment, professional care, and advance directives
- Functioning at time of study
- Family constellation
- Family involvement in care
- Changes during the study
- Death

The following summary describes the general characteristics of the nine participants for whom we were able to complete sufficient information. Profiles of individual participants follow.

Participants

Enrollment:	9 enrolled participants: 3 men, 6 women
Age:	2 were in late thirties to forties
	7 were age sixty to late eighties
Ethnicity:	1 Native American
	1 with Native American ancestry
	7 mainstream Caucasian backgrounds
Settings:	All received medical care in Missoula County
	1 lived in a small town outside Missoula County
	1 moved to Missoula from a rural area for care
	7 were long-time Missoula residents
Illness:	4 with cancer: breast (metastasized), ovarian/lung, lymphoma
	2 with emphysema (congestive obstructive pulmonary disease)
	2 with congestive heart failure
	1 diagnosed as "old age," poor circulation
Date of terminal diagnosis:	12 months to 4 weeks prior to referral and first visit; most diagnosed in spring 1997
Care:	8 cared for at home for most of final year of life
	6 on home care, served by local hospice
	2 had home health care services
	1 was at Hospice House, then at board and care home, then returned to Hospice House
Family context:	1 lived alone, had no children, spouse, or siblings; church friends provided assistance
	2 had spouses providing primary care
	1 cared for by mother
	2 cared for by daughters in the daughter's home
	1 cared for by sister

1 cared for by spouse and then by sister for last 3 weeks

1 at board and care home; two daughters lived close

Economic status: All were from working or middle class backgrounds

Dennis

Dennis was a husky thirty-nine-year-old former high school baseball star in the Montana city where he grew up. After he graduated from high school, he married, had two children, and eventually became a golf pro in a small town about an hour's drive from Missoula. He had stopped working more than a year before his death as his condition worsened. He was divorced, but he had preserved a "good" though distant relationship with his ex-wife and children. His parents lived in a nearby small town.

Disease, Diagnosis, Trajectory

Dennis had been diagnosed with peripheral T-cell lymphoma, a rare form of cancer, seven years earlier. The original diagnosis was accompanied by a clear statement that his cancer was incurable and terminal, though with hope for a ten-year remission before the symptoms worsened. Within the first year, available treatments failed to produce remission. A variety of experimental treatments followed during the next six years, in Missoula and at regional medical centers in Boise and Seattle. When Dennis entered this study, in July 1997, he had been seriously ill for a year as cancerous lesions erupted all over his body.

Treatment and Professional Care

Although Dennis lived in a rural area outside Missoula County, he received his medical treatment in Missoula. At the time of the study, he was making a weekly trip to Missoula for palliative chemotherapy, with the hope of living through the summer. Because of constant severe pain, he used a self-administered pain pump with Fentanyl. In his final months, other symptoms included fatigue, depression, anxiety, and shortness of breath. Although the severity of his symptoms could have qualified him for hospital care, he insisted on home care, and he remained at home as he was dying. Dennis had a signed Comfort One order instructing emergency medical personnel not to resuscitate him and had executed a living will.

Functioning at Time of Study

Dennis was able to get up from his chair or bed to use the bathroom; on good days, he was able to get outside for limited recreation. He was able to play a round of golf with his parents several times over the summer. Other trips outside his home were limited to weekly visits to Missoula for medical treatment. His mind was alert until the last two weeks, despite his reports of some euphoria from pain medications. He had a very detailed understanding of his medical condition and treatment, and his conversation remained intelligent and rational.

Family Constellation

Dennis's immediate family consisted of his mother, Carrie; his father; an older sister living with her family in Idaho; and a younger brother living in California. His father lived thirty miles away on the family ranch. Dennis had two children, ages nine and eleven, who lived with his ex-wife 160 miles away in another Montana city. The children saw him only irregularly because of the distance and the illness.

Family Involvement in Care

In fall 1996, Dennis's mother moved into his house to provide the twenty-four-hour care he needed to remain at home. Throughout the last year of Dennis's illness, his mother was his major caregiver, with minimal assistance from a home health nurse and intermittent housekeeping help. There was no consistent back-up support or respite help available to Dennis's mother because of the high level of constant assistance Dennis required for comfort, which his mother had mastered, and because of their rural location. Dennis's father was limited by his emphysema; he offered companionship relief to Dennis and his mother but was unable to provide any physical care. During the summers, Dennis's sister came several times to relieve her mother, who was simultaneously involved with the care of her own ninety-two-year-old mother in a nursing care facility 100 miles distant. Two months before Dennis's death, his brother moved back home to help his father and to be a support to his mother and Dennis.

Changes during the Study

Dennis's participation in the study was brief, primarily because his condition worsened dramatically in August—to the extent that having visitors was impossible. He remained conscious and cognizant until his last week of life, when his breathing became difficult and oxygen was needed, and he gradually slipped into a coma.

Death

Dennis died in early October 1997—at home, as he wished—with both of his parents present. They had professional assistance during the last week from a home health nurse. Just before he died, plans were being made to move him to his parent's ranch, where other family members could be constantly present, but he died before this could happen. Before his death, he planned much of his own funeral with his sister.

Barbara

Barbara was a strong, vibrant, forty-six-year-old woman of Native American heritage who came to Missoula in 1991 to take a position at the university. She was forty at that time; she had advanced degrees and a national reputation as a leader in her field and in Native American education. She had two children and had recently remarried.

Disease, Diagnosis, Trajectory

Barbara was diagnosed with ovarian cancer in 1991. After an operation, the cancer remained in remission from 1992 to fall 1994, when it metastasized to her lungs. After two years of treatment, remission, and then more treatment during 1995 and 1996, she underwent a lung removal in April 1997 in Missoula. At that time, the cancer was found to have spread to other major organ systems. Chemotherapy provided a few months of remission through the summer and early fall.

Treatment and Professional Care

All of Barbara's chemotherapy and radiation treatments over the preceding six years had been with the same oncologist in Missoula. During her last year, that physician left the area, and she was transferred to another oncologist in Missoula. After her lung operation in 1997, when the cancer was found to have metastasized, she underwent chemotherapy and received blood transfusions on an outpatient basis. She had home health care nurses to help maintain her central venous line and administer fluids and intravenous (IV) medications. She remained on oral pain medication throughout the summer; she had some difficulty keeping it down at times. She had increasing shortness of breath as well. After a month-long hospital stay in October, she was discharged to her sister's home for the last three weeks of her life.

Barbara had signed a living will, and her doctor had written a Do Not Resuscitate (DNR) order at the time of her lung operation in the spring of 1997.

Functioning at Time of Study

Barbara continued her professional work throughout her illness; she worked at home with a computer connection when she did not feel well enough to go into her office. Her work was largely administrative, so it continued year-round but could be performed at home. She was able to have dinner with family and friends, and she took several short trips during the summer: to visit friends in South Dakota and to the Oregon Coast to see the ocean one last time.

Family Constellation

Barbara's children from an earlier marriage were a daughter, age nineteen, and a son, age fourteen. She had remarried and at the time of the study lived with her son and her husband, Dan, in the family home. Her daughter had moved away the year before but moved back to Missoula during the summer of 1997 to be near her mother and begin college. Barbara came from a large, close-knit family; she had five brothers and three sisters. During her last year, one sister was living in Missoula. Her parents, who were in their seventies, still lived on the reservation.

Family Involvement in Care

At Barbara's request, her sister Irene moved to Missoula from an eastern university to be near her in her last year of life. Barbara's daily care, however, was largely in her own hands and those of her husband until her last hospitalization in fall 1997. At that point, disagreements within the family over the best course of treatment resulted in Barbara's decision to stay with her sister after she left the hospital. Her sister was able to provide round-the-clock care with the assistance of a home health service and numerous relatives and friends who brought food and supported both women.

Changes during the Study

At the beginning of the summer, Barbara had begun chemotherapy and had a brief remission. She was often fatigued, but she felt she was getting stronger and had plans to go into her office at least weekly at the beginning of the fall semester. Instead, she was admitted to the hospital in Missoula twice—once in September and again for a month in October—because of dehydration and difficulty with nutrition.

Death

Barbara's last three weeks at her sister's home in Missoula were a time for family and friends to visit and nurture her. She was able to get up and cook for her children. Her sister cooked special foods, played classical music, read traditional Native American tales and the Bible to her, and burned sweetgrass for a smudge to help her spirit pass over. Friends and tribal elders made the long journey from the reservation to visit her for the last time in this world.

When her family was sure her death was very near, they decided to take her to Hospice House. She was admitted in the early afternoon and died close to midnight of the same day, surrounded by her parents, daughter, sisters, aunt, and brothers.

Ralph

Ralph was a seventy-year-old retired builder of log homes. He had been a medic in the Army during the Korean conflict. Until his last two years, he had lived on his family's homestead in a rural area outside Missoula, with his longtime companion and mate, Sandy. He had no children of his own but had a large extended family.

Disease, Diagnosis, Trajectory

Ralph had chronic obstructive pulmonary disease (COPD). His awareness of his serious medical condition began almost the day he retired, seven years before he entered the study, when he contracted pneumonia and was treated at the Veterans Hospital in Helena, Montana. There he was first diagnosed with COPD and osteoporosis. A year before his death, he spent several months in the hospital with a lung infection. After the infection was controlled, he was sent to a Missoula nursing home for physical therapy for about a month. This therapy helped him recover sufficiently to return to his rural home, but the Veterans Administration insisted that he get a doctor from Missoula for continuing outpatient care. The one he chose recommended hospice care. Ralph and Sandy agreed that this approach would be best, even though it required them to move to Missoula.

Treatment and Professional Care

During Ralph's last year of life in Missoula, he had continuous weekly care from the same hospice nurse, a bath aide, and a therapist twice a week for ultrasound treatment for his osteoporosis, along with regular visits from a hospice volunteer about his own age and a Reiki provider. The hospice physician also made house calls. Ralph was on oxygen and taking Roxanol during this last year. His major complaint was shortness of breath. He received all of his caregiving at home until his last four days, when he was transferred to Hospice House to die. Ralph had executed a Comfort One order (the Montana DNR for emergency medical technicians), a living will, and a durable power of attorney for health care (DPOA) that named Sandy.

Functioning at Time of Study

Ralph was able to walk short distances with the support of a walker but otherwise used a wheelchair. He enjoyed the view of trees and the river from his apartment; on good days, he could take a short walk along the river with Sandy's help. About a month before Ralph's death, Sandy drove Ralph back to his rural homestead through the fall foliage for dinner with his brother—an exhausting trip, but a high point for him. Until the last week or so of his life, Ralph was always friendly and talkative with any visitors.

Family Constellation

Sandy and Ralph had never married, but they had a committed relationship that was recognized by their families and friends. Ralph and Sandy had met twenty years previously after she moved nearby; they had been together ever since. Sandy had three children by a previous marriage, all of whom lived in other states and visited Montana only rarely. Besides Sandy, who was his primary caregiver, Ralph had an older brother (also ill with emphysema) who lived on his own part of the family homestead, a younger sister who lived with her husband just down the road, and a stepdaughter from Ralph's first marriage who lived nearby with her family.

Family Involvement in Care

Sandy provided Ralph's day-to-day care, with substantial help from hospice. The move to Missoula meant that there could be little or no physical help from Ralph's family. Ralph's brother was eighty years old and also suffered from emphysema. His brother, sister, and sister-in-law came down weekly during Ralph's last few months for brief visits, as did their children and grandchildren, but all of the caregiving fell on Sandy's shoulders.

Changes during the Study

Ralph's physical condition did not change significantly during most of his last six months of life. During his last month he was housebound, unable to take even a short walk outside, and considered another car trip to the homestead too exhausting to attempt. Two weeks before Ralph died, he was experiencing more and more difficulty choosing the words he wanted to use and remembering recent events. Even his favorite topics of conversation— conservation and nature—became difficult for him to articulate. During his last week he was delirious at times. He slipped into a coma five days before his death.

Death

Ralph died sixteen months after he moved to Missoula and was referred to hospice—far longer than predicted for his end-stage emphysema condition. Ralph's condition in his last week became overwhelming for Sandy to handle alone, even with hospice help; Sandy herself suffered from degenerative arthritic disease. She transferred him to Hospice House in late November, where he died within four days. Sandy spent some time with him that day, and he had a few lucid moments when he recognized her. When Ralph died, the hospice chaplain called her and drove her back to Hospice House for a final goodbye.

Sharon

Sharon was a vibrant, intellectually adventurous woman of seventy-four who had moved to Missoula from a rural area after her husband's death in 1982. She had found Missoula exciting and interesting and had made a new life and new friends for herself before her illness.

Disease, Diagnosis, Trajectory

Sharon had been ill with emphysema for many years. Two years before her death, living alone in an apartment with stairs became impossible for her, and she moved in with her sister Connie. Sharon also had osteoporosis and began experiencing painful compression fractures. During the six months before her death, she began to experience increasing short-term memory loss, possibly caused by side effects of medications and oxygen deprivation. Her other major symptom was fatigue with any exertion.

Treatment and Professional Care

Sharon was admitted to hospice care in June 1997, after her physician suggested that it was time. A major inducement was that the Medicare hospice benefit would cover all medications. Sharon began twenty-four-hour oxygen about this time and started on oral morphine to breathe more easily. Her major pain was from the compression fractures. Through hospice, she had the services of a weekly "bath lady," a volunteer, and visits from a social worker and the chaplain.

Sharon had a living will and a DNR order in place. She and her sister had discussed but never completed a DPOA for health care.

Functioning at Time of Study

During the last six months of her life, Sharon awakened very early, struggling for breath until late morning. When she could get up, she stayed in a recliner in the dining room in front of the television, with her books and tapes close by. She could not be left alone, even briefly. She talked with visitors and ate in her chair as well. For most of the time prior to her death, she was still able to sleep through the night. She no longer had energy to go for rides or leave the house, but she enjoyed a continual stream of visitors: children and grandchildren; nieces; and some friends, especially from her spiritual community. Six weeks before Sharon died, her sister Connie organized a birthday party and invited family and friends to come in small groups to see her and have cake.

Family Constellation

Sharon was a widow with three adult children. Two sons worked and lived in the greater Missoula area; her daughter had recently moved away from Missoula to a nearby state, but came back monthly for a long weekend or week to stay with her mother. Sharon had two teenage granddaughters. In addition to her sister Connie (also a widow), Sharon had another sister who lived with her husband in California.

Family Involvement in Care

During Sharon's last six months, Connie provided all of Sharon's nursing care, including administering her frequent medications, supported by a weekly visit from the hospice nurse. Each of Sharon's sons came to stay with her one afternoon a week. A cousin who lived nearby was able to come any time Connie needed someone to stay with Sharon so that she could go out. Sharon's daughter came back frequently on weekends to stay with her; in August, when Sharon was very ill with an infection, her daughter stayed for a week. Sharon's sister from California visited for a week at the beginning of the summer and again at the end of summer. All three sisters openly viewed these visits as their last times together.

Changes during the Study

Sharon developed an infection in August and became very weak, with loss of appetite, more fatigue, and increasing memory and comprehension difficulties. She received antibiotic treatment for the infection; the treatment, along with her sister's second visit, helped her rally. She regained some memory, and her comprehension improved during the early fall, and she appeared to be doing well until November, when she took a sudden turn and died within three days.

Death

In mid-November, Sharon went to sleep after a weekend afternoon visit from one son and never fully awakened the next day. She remained comatose until her death. Hospice brought a hospital bed and other assistance on Monday. Her other son came to see her on Monday, but the suddenness of this turning point prevented her daughter from being able to reach home before Sharon died. Sharon's sister Connie and Connie's daughter were with Sharon when she died early on Tuesday morning at home. In keeping with Sharon's wishes, her family held a private dinner/memorial service for her family and friends rather than having a traditional funeral.

Sarah

Sarah was an eighty-year-old widow who was born near Missoula, where she got married and raised her own children. She also took in a large number of foster children, while she was raising her own children, as well as after they were grown; ran her church's day-care service, and otherwise spent her life helping people. Her husband had developed Alzheimer's disease and had died several years earlier.

Disease, Diagnosis, Trajectory

A diagnosis of breast cancer and surgery ten years earlier preceded Sarah's development of pain from bone metastases. At some point, she had back surgery related to the cancer. At the beginning of this study, she had been living at Hospice House for two months. Before moving to Hospice House, she lived briefly with her daughter, Karen, but was so confused by her medication that her daughter could no longer care for her. At Hospice House her medications were constantly monitored and she became less confused and disoriented. After four months, Sarah had to leave Hospice House because her condition was stable. Subsequently, she had a series of light strokes, but her pain remained under control.

Treatment and Professional Care

Sarah continued to see her long-time physician for monthly outpatient visits. While Sarah was at Hospice House she also saw the hospice doctor about once a week. While she was there, treatment of pain and other symptoms improved her general functioning greatly. Like many breast cancer patients, Sarah's deterioration was slow. In fact, hospice staff finally had to advise her that she was doing so well that she would need to find another place to stay. Sarah was upset, even though she was quite aware of this possibility. After Sarah left Hospice House, her daughter at first placed her in a nursing home, which proved unsatisfactory. Her daughter finally found a private board and care facility for Sarah, where she was living at the time this study ended. She did not have hospice care at that point. Sarah had signed a living will.

Functioning at Time of Study

At Hospice House, Sarah enjoyed the many visitors who came through to visit other patients. She used a walker to get around because she had a lingering problem with balance. Her complaints regarding pain varied from "all the time" to "just sometimes." She had considerable loss of vision, and her hands shook from what she described as light strokes. She was sometimes visited by friends from the senior citizens' center. Sarah's daughter Karen visited several times a week and took her home for meals, as well as to appointments with the doctor and for short drives. During the period at Hospice House, Sarah was mentally alert, pleasant, optimistic, and accepting of her condition. On our last visit with Sarah, in March 1998, she was functioning at about the same level as she had been when we first met her, seven months earlier.

Family Constellation

Sarah was a widow with three daughters, two of whom lived in the Missoula area. Her other daughter lived in another state. Sarah's husband had died years earlier, suffering from what was referred to as both Parkinson's disease and Alzheimer's. Sarah had taken sole care of her husband for four years at home before placing him in a nursing home.

Family Involvement in Care

Sarah's daughter Karen appeared to be the only family member who was involved regularly in Sarah's care. Karen had tried to care for Sarah in her own home, but Sarah's need for constant monitoring made this arrangement unsatisfactory. Karen kept in close contact with her mother through almost-daily visits and phone calls as Sarah went through the progression of Hospice House, nursing homes, and the board and care facility. The other daughter who lived in the Missoula area shared fiscal responsibility for Sarah's ongoing care and living situation.

Changes during the Study

Sarah had several small stroke episodes during the study period and showed some decline in energy but no dramatic changes. Her pain levels varied; often, leaving Hospice House and hospice care became more difficult to manage on an outpatient basis. Her mental awareness and positive attitude remained stable and intact.

Death

Sarah remained alive at the time the study was completed, twelve months after our first visit with her. She died in August 1999, more than two years after being diagnosed as terminally ill. She returned to Hospice House in her last months, when she again required skilled nursing care. Her daughter Karen and other family members were with her at her death, and friends and church members visited her until the end. Sarah's memorial service was held at the senior citizen's residence, so that her friends there, as well as her family and church friends, could be present.

Walt

Walt was an eighty-year-old retired plumber who lived with his wife, Dorothy, in Missoula. Although Walt was born and raised in an adjacent county, he had lived and worked most of his adult life in Missoula, after serving in World War II. Walt retired at age seventy when his health began to decline. His family was very close-knit; family members made frequent visits throughout Walt's last year of life and showed evidence of great concern and love for him.

Disease, Diagnosis, Trajectory

Walt suffered from advanced heart and lung disease. Eleven years earlier, Walt had a work-related accident; while he was in the hospital he was told for the first time that he had a bad heart. Later, he had an episode in which he collapsed at the dinner table with another attack. Then, in fall 1996, he was hospitalized again with a nearly fatal heart attack. After his most recent heart attack, the family decided on home care. Several years earlier, Walt had rejected having a pacemaker, after seeing his own parents live beyond their wishes with this device.

Treatment and Professional Care

Walt was bed-ridden and was taking 45 milligrams of long-acting morphine three times a day, with occasional immediate-release morphine (Roxanol) when the pain or breathlessness became severe. A year before his death, when he was hospitalized, it became clear that his condition was terminal. Walt's doctor referred him to hospice care. A hospice nurse came regularly, as did various hospice volunteers, including the "bath lady." Walt's wife, Dorothy, was particularly relieved that the hospice doctor came to the house because of the difficulty of having to take Walt to the doctor's office.

Walt had signed a living will and had a Comfort One order (the Montana DNR for emergency medical technicians), but we could not determine whether he had ever considered or signed a DPOA for health care.

Functioning at Time of Study

During his last month, Walt was able to get out of bed to use the bathroom, but he also was incontinent and wearing diapers. He usually had to be awakened for pain medication. He would then go back to sleep until he woke up to eat. Often he had too much nausea to eat anything. His activities were very limited. He did not care much for television, except for baseball games, and he described his life as pretty boring. He enjoyed visitors, especially family members, as long as they did not stay too long. Dorothy would wake him up when visitors arrived, believing that such visits were more important than his rest.

Family Constellation

Walt lived with his wife and small dog in a new duplex that was built by his children. His youngest daughter lived in the other half of the duplex with her husband and their children. Walt had five children, all but one of whom lived in Missoula or western Montana. The four children living locally were all very involved in planning for and participating in Walt's care.

Family Involvement in Care

When Walt and Dorothy decided to sell their family house because of Walt's declining health, the proceeds were placed in a family partnership that was guaranteed to take care of their needs as long as they lived, and their children built the duplex for their parents and youngest sister, doing much of the work themselves. Walt's wife set aside her various personal interests to give full attention to his care; his children also contributed in many ways. Up to six months before his death, the children took Walt out for rides, to the doctor, or to see whatever interested him. After that, Walt was too fatigued and short of breath to leave the house. The daughter who lived on the east coast called two or three times a week. The others made regular visits, kept in touch, and did what they could to relieve their mother.

Changes during the Study

Our first visit with Walt was just a little more than two months before his death—rather late in his disease trajectory. He was unable to leave his bed and spent more and more time sleeping. According to Dorothy's report, at the time this study began Walt had already passed though the most troublesome phase of care, when he was very frustrated and sometimes angry at his inability to function, causing her considerable stress. During the time we were able to observe him, there was little or no change—a phase his wife described as the "mellow" stage.

Death

In Walt's earlier hospitalizations, his children had encouraged him to hang on and survive. Dorothy believed that Walt did not die a year earlier because his children were not yet ready. Walt was surrounded by his family during his last days of life. He could not eat, his kidneys were not working, and he knew that he was dying. The family openly communicated about this situation with Walt. The whole family told him they were willing to let him go, which he did on a September afternoon.

Kitty

Kitty was eighty when we met her, five months before her death. She lived alone in her home of forty years, with a dog and two cats from the Humane Shelter for company. She had worked as a medical technician in Missoula after college and was deeply involved in the life of her local church. An only child, she had never married, and she had no close living relatives. Kitty represents the growing number of elderly persons in Missoula who are "orphans"—people who have no spouse, children, or siblings alive to care for them in their last years.

Disease, Diagnosis, Trajectory

Kitty's early retirement, twenty years earlier, came about because of her cancer, which was successfully treated at the time. She also had a degenerative muscle disease for many years, which caused uncontrollable diarrhea. More recently, she had developed high blood pressure and then symptoms of congestive heart failure, including low blood pressure and increasingly frequent blackouts. Her symptoms were ascribed by her physician to "old age," according to her friends.

Treatment and Professional Care

Three years before Kitty's death, she began to have transient blackouts during the course of the day, with memory loss and impaired judgment and decision making. In spring 1997, she was hospitalized briefly after a blackout and resulting automobile accident, and referred to Hospice House. She refused to go,

insisting on returning home. At that point, her church friends organized themselves to provide for financial management, regular home visits, and Meals
on Wheels.

During Kitty's months at home, she was on oral medications but did not require oxygen. A home health aide and friends from church tried to monitor her
functioning and medications through visits and phone calls. Two months before Kitty's death, she developed a serious foot infection, with severe pain, and
received daily IV antibiotic treatments as an outpatient for two weeks. When
the hospice nurse found her incoherent and incontinent in November after a
weekend alone, Kitty agreed to go to Hospice House for her remaining days.

Kitty had signed a living will and had given copies to her doctor, clergy, and
hospice staff. Her doctor had written a DNR order. She did not have a DPOA
for health care, and there were no relatives able to speak for her.

Functioning at Time of Study

Kitty was home alone all day, but she had daily visitors: Meals on Wheels,
church friends, a hospice nurse. She listened to classical music on the radio,
watched TV, and napped whenever she felt like it. Most days, she stayed in an
easy chair in the living room. She left the front door unlocked so that she would
not have to get up to let visitors in. She talked about trimming her roses in the
fall but was not able to go outside. She continued to go to breakfast once a week
with her group of church friends until a month before her death.

Kitty's major concern was the care of her animals, if it were determined that
she was not able to stay at home. Her dog, Beau, became visibly ill in late August and was found to have cancer. She had him put to sleep in early November, a month before her own death. His loss may have made it easier for her to
accept the need to move to Hospice House later that month.

Family Constellation

Kitty never married. She bought a home in Missoula in 1956, and her widowed
mother moved to Missoula to live with her. Her mother died in a fire at home,
alone, about twenty years prior to our study. Kitty's closest relatives lived in
eastern Canada; with her mother's death, Kitty's church community in Missoula became her only family.

Family Involvement in Caregiving

Kitty's friends and the priest from her local parish church, which had formed
the center of her life, tried to be her care managers during the last months of her
life; they also arranged for hospice. Church friends made daily visits or phone
calls during Kitty's last six months at home. They also brought communion

weekly, arranged for administration of her financial affairs, became executor of her will, took her to doctor's appointments, and visited her daily when she moved to Hospice House for the last three weeks of her life.

Changes during the Study

Five months before her death, Kitty was able to move from the front room to the kitchen and bedroom easily, as well as to care for her animals. She became increasingly feeble and less able to move or care for herself in the ensuing months. She encouraged visits but found taking part in conversation more difficult. As her mental functioning and judgment declined, she became less aware of her constant diarrhea and began having more episodes of incontinence.

Death

One Monday morning, the hospice nurse found Kitty on the floor, confused, incontinent, and unable to get to the bathroom. She had pulled the IV line out of the vein in her arm. Hospice insisted that Kitty go to Hospice House, and with no alternatives left, she agreed. Once there, with her classical music tapes, Kitty began to enjoy the comfort and care. For two weeks, she was able to eat in the dining room and spend her days in the recliner in the living room. The last week she was often comatose, but she was conscious enough to recognize the church friends and priests who came to visit. She died surrounded by friends at Hospice House in December 1997.

Roberta

Roberta, age eighty-five, was a Missoula native. She returned to Missoula from Washington, D.C. (where her husband worked for the federal government), after her retirement from the same agency. Her husband had died many years ago. She had three daughters living in Montana with their families. She had once been the state women's archery champion, and she retained her regal poise until her death.

Disease, Diagnosis, Trajectory

Roberta had a history of congestive heart problems and decreasing blood oxygen levels for about ten years and had a pacemaker put in four years before our study. In spring 1997, she blacked out and fell while still living alone in her own home. She was taken to the emergency room and then admitted to a local hospital. During the last six months of her life, Roberta experienced low blood pressure, low oxygen levels in her blood, and increasing need for oxygen and medications as her heart functioned less and less effectively.

Treatment and Professional Care

After the hospital stay, Roberta's physician recommended hospice care to her family and certified her as terminally ill. She was able to receive all of her care at home. She was on oxygen as needed, as well as medications to improve her heart function. Hospice provided weekly nursing care and monitoring, and Roberta enjoyed twice-weekly visits from the bath aide. Two months before her death, Roberta was readmitted to the hospital overnight because of dehydration; she was given IV treatment, and her medications were adjusted. Roberta had signed a living will ten years earlier and more recently had agreed to a DNR and a DPOA for health care, naming her daughter.

Functioning at Time of Study

Roberta had never sought out friends or belonged to social groups, clubs, or a church community, and she became more reclusive in her last years. She was content with the friendship of her daughters and their families. Roberta's self-image was that of a young, active woman. During her first months at her daughter's home, Roberta still enjoyed knitting and crocheting, watching some TV, doing jigsaw puzzles, and looking out the large picture window of her daughter's home. She was able to go out to dinner on her birthday in early August, three months before her death.

Family Constellation

Roberta's middle daughter, Debbie, lived in Missoula; her other daughters lived in other Montana cities. Some of her nine grandchildren and their families also lived in Missoula or close by, so there were always grandchildren and great-grandchildren coming in to see her. Roberta had been a devoted grandmother, particularly siding with some of her grandsons when they had problems and needed extra support. Debbie's sons all made special trips home during the summer to visit their grandmother.

Family Involvement in Care

Roberta had lived in her own home—with much family assistance with meals and a home health aide to supervise medications and do housekeeping—until six months before her death. After her fall and hospital stay in the spring, her physician said she could improve but would no longer be able to live alone. The family tried a nursing home, and at first she thrived, becoming more outgoing and happy. After a month, however, she was not eating, became withdrawn, and began crying much of the time. Her daughter Debbie, who had provided most of her care for the previous three years, decided that Roberta would come to live with her for the remainder of her life.

Debbie's husband, Joe, quit a part-time job he had taken after retirement so that he could be around the house in the daytime when Debbie was at work. In addition, Debbie's nineteen-year-old grandson, who lived with the family while he attended college, would sometimes fix Roberta's breakfast and always chatted with her when he came home for lunch.

Changes during the Study

By fall 1997, Roberta had become increasingly frail and less mobile and was less able to read or use her hands to do stitching and crocheting. Her short-term memory and comprehension of what was going on around her began to fail markedly. Her family reported that her mood changed (which they attributed to decreasing oxygen levels), and she became less aware and showed increasing signs of dementia. Until the last week of her life, however, Roberta insisted on getting up and putting on an elegant dressing gown for the day; she was not willing to remain in bed, even though she would have been more comfortable lying down. She remained able to use the bathroom or commode by herself until she suffered a hip fracture about a week before her death.

Death

The week of her death, Roberta got up in the middle of the night and then fell with a broken hip. She was taken to the hospital in severe pain. Because of the fracture, she could not move or sit up, and plans were made to operate. Her three daughters agreed to the operation, to make her more comfortable, despite the risk to her life because of her frailty and age. Roberta's own physician counseled waiting a day, however, to conduct more tests. Before the scheduled operation could take place, the tests showed that Roberta's kidneys had failed. The family decided to bring her back home in traction. She remained heavily sedated but comfortable and aware that she was being taken home, before she fell into a coma. The Chalice of Repose came the evening before her death, and she died the next evening, with two of her three daughters at her bedside, along with her sons-in-law, grandchildren, and great-grandchildren. The family called her third daughter and two grandsons so they could also say good-bye to her on the phone, even in her comatose state.

Mabel

Mabel, who was eighty-seven at the time of the study, had moved to Missoula to live near her daughter several years earlier. Mabel's father died just before she was born, and her mother died when she was sixteen. Mabel grew up in a rural county near Missoula, completing only six years of school. She had worked as a waitress briefly, then married and raised two daughters, living in various areas of the Pacific Northwest.

Disease, Diagnosis, Trajectory

Mabel was diagnosed with breast cancer at age eighty, just before hip replacement surgery, and had a mastectomy one month later. The two operations close together made her recovery difficult and left her uncertain about the cause of her continuing pains. Three years later, complaints of chronic bursitis led to a bone scan and discovery that the breast cancer had spread to her bones. A physician diagnosed her cancer as terminal and rapidly advancing in late 1996, and she was referred to hospice. During this period, she also suffered several small strokes, which caused some degree of cognitive impairment. Despite the spread of cancer throughout her body, Mabel was still living at the time the study ended and was discharged from hospice care.

Treatment and Professional Care

Mabel was treated by local hospitals and physicians throughout her illness. We could not determine whether she had a family physician, but she saw several cancer specialists. After her year of hospice care ended, she continued with a monthly nursing visit from a home health service. She had no insurance coverage for her extensive medications, and her daughter, Bernice, began to use her mother's small funeral savings to pay for her medicines. All of Mabel's home care was provided by her daughter, who lived with her. Mabel's major pain medication was a seventy-two-hour analgesic patch, which her daughter changed; she also had oral non-narcotic pain medications. She continued to complain about bursitis pain and received cortisone shots to alleviate the pain. When the breast cancer reoccurrence was discovered, Bernice had Mabel execute a DPOA for health care and a living will.

Functioning at Time of Study

Mabel had significant hearing loss as well as macular degeneration that limited her vision. She could walk by herself from the bed to the bathroom and to her padded wheelchair in the living room of the apartment she shared with her daughter. She was able to take care of her bathroom needs by herself; the apartment was new and had been built for handicapped accessibility. Mabel spent all day sitting in her chair with the television on (despite her vision and hearing difficulties); she sometimes listened to phonograph records, watched small animals outside the patio door, and talked on the phone. She occasionally lay down in the afternoon, especially on days when the pain patch was near the end and she became shaky and weak.

Mabel did not identify any clubs, hobbies, church affiliation, or other interests outside of her family. She occasionally had visits from grandchildren or one friend her age. She most enjoyed the evening television news and having her daughter read her local news from the paper.

Family Constellation

Mabel's husband had been a blue-collar worker in Idaho; he had died many years earlier. Mabel had lived in Missoula since her husband's death. Mabel's daughter Bernice, recently divorced, began living with Mabel six years before the study period. Her other daughter lived in Idaho and visited several times a year with her children and grandchildren. Bernice had two sons—one in Missoula, the other recently moved to Minnesota. Bernice's grandchildren were bright spots in Mabel's life. Mabel's only living sister was very ill and lived at home in another part of Missoula; neither were able to get out, so they talked on the phone instead.

Family Involvement in Care

Mabel's daughter Bernice, who was in her mid-fifties and was not employed at the time, provided all of her mother's care. Mabel's other daughter did not provide any financial or physical assistance during the study period. Bernice's son lived in the Missoula area with his wife and children, and visited with his family once or twice a month on Sundays. Both worked full time and did not appear to provide Bernice with regular assistance in caring for Mabel.

Changes during the Study

During our visits over a nine-month period, there was relatively little change in Mabel's condition, except for improvement in pain—apparently as a result of treatment for bursitis. At the end of the study period, she was on the same medications; according to Mabel and her daughter, her level of functioning was about the same, despite the cancer.

Death

Mabel died in November 1998, eight months after our last visit. She died at home, with hospice caring for her at the end. Her daughter reported that family members knew she was dying and were able to be with her throughout the last week and at the time of her death.

Chapter 2

Communicating about Death and Dying

Glaser and Strauss (1964, 1965) provide a typology of awareness contexts about death. One type is the "closed context," in which relatives and health care workers prevent patients from knowing that they are dying. In the "open awareness context," such pretense is avoided, and the patients' terminal condition is openly acknowledged by all.

The major advantage of the closed context is the capacity to continue life as normal, as though the terminal illness were only temporary. Advocates of this context say that it provides the opportunity to preserve an intact social bond. They claim that such acts of silence by relatives and medical personnel give them the opportunity to demonstrate their care and concern, while freeing the patient from the mental pain of realizing that they are really dying.

By contrast, in the open awareness context people can take control over the manner, place, and timing of their own deaths and imbue it with meaning. Reporting the results of a study of patients who died in England, Seale (1998, 173) observes, "In this struggle distinctions between allies and enemies were clarified and there was an opportunity to display great courage in the eventual facing of the final threat: death itself. The reward for those who completed this heroic task was the realization and enactment of intimate emotions, in which the social bond between the dying self and others was affirmed." Seale reports that persons who died in an open awareness context talked openly about their impending deaths; they were very self-aware and planned how it would happen. For example, 79 percent of them chose where to spend their final days.

How They Got the Bad News

One of the hardest tasks that medical professionals face is telling patients that they have an incurable illness—that they will surely die soon. The participants in this study experienced a variety of such announcements. We could not be present when the actual diagnosis was given by their doctors, but we can report the memories that the study participants had about how the bad news was presented to them.

Technical Medical Terminology: Dennis

Dennis, a younger cancer victim, used crisp medical terms to describe what his doctor had told him about his terminal status:

> The doctor told me that my body would not continue to respond to chemotherapy. Uh, it would lessen and lessen its response time and its effectiveness and that it would sooner, more than later, go to strictly pain medication, palliative treatment. And that my immune system would be so compromised that, uh, through the ulcerated lesions, infection would get in and blood sepsis would set in and they would not be able to do anything and my body parts would just start shutting down. And he said, "At that point we'll just make sure that your pain medication is adequate, and we'll make you as comfortable as possible, but I don't see really going beyond the summer." He said, "Dennis, you're doing very well on Isidabom, and I think we can get you through the summer." He will tell it as it is. And you can tell it's hard sometimes, but he's as gentle as he can be.

"It was a blur": Barbara

The announcement that Barbara's long struggle with advanced cancer was nearing an end was marked for her by a serious episode in April 1997, with an operation for lung cancer. She was readmitted to the hospital in May, when the cancer was found to have spread, and no further surgery was feasible. Barbara had difficulty recalling the sequence of events three months later:

> I can't even remember when I had the CAT scan. That's how much of a blur those two months were. The CAT scan showed that there was some tumor that was in the pelvic region. I was in pain, and

that's basically why I went in. Of course, I didn't really understand it at the time. . . .

My doctor seemed to want to be encouraging as opposed to discouraging. I think maybe he personally made the decision about whether I could handle that [knowledge]. A lot of that is a blur with what I was told. I know that I remember my husband coming in, and he was in so much despair. I was asking him to talk to me and tell me and that's when he started crying and saying, "I don't want to lose you. I don't know if I can handle this."

Barbara's husband had equal difficulty talking about learning that his wife's cancer had spread and was terminal:

Well, it's in the terminal, well, I don't want to say terminal stage, because she just had her test, and it was cut down to 50 percent. When it's low or goes down, things are getting better. And it's been going down. . . .

But in April, the doctor said that this is, you know, it's past the stage, it's terminal. We can't give it a time. She had ovarian cancer. Then it spread to her lungs, then the diaphragm, and then they went inside and said it's all over her intestines. They said it didn't look good. I can't remember exactly how they said it. They said the surgery was real tough on her, and when they went in, it was just, it was all in there. The CAT scan and everything else wasn't picking it up. They said her chances of recovering are slim. But she did recover from it.

Researcher: Did they use the word *terminal*?

Dan: I'm sure they did. I can't remember the exact word. But they say that, and then her tests are coming down. That means better. It's confusing, unless they're saying well, it's terminal, but maybe their thoughts were she could be around for half a year, or a year, or five years, you know. It's a hard thing.

"The doctor told us to use hospice": Ralph

Ralph, an older emphysema patient, was much less clear about the exact way that he was given the bad news. He could not recall exactly how the conversation went, but from Ralph's perspective, the doctor's recommendation to get on hospice care was equivalent to telling him that he was dying.

I first learned about my illness between six and seven years ago. I got a real bad case of pneumonia. I went into the Vet's hospital, and they said, "You've got pneumonia." And they put me right in bed. And they kept me over there and they got me cleared up. And they said, "You got emphysema, and you got that thing where your bones deteriorate. Within a year I broke my back twice to add to it. When they were looking at that they found these bones were all deteriorated, so here comes this emphysema. It's a-comin' along there all the time. And so that's the way that all was. It was the doctor that told us to use hospice.

At this point, Ralph's caregiver, Sandy, broke in and explained that the VA doctor sent Ralph to a nursing home in Missoula to get physical therapy after months of pneumonia that was difficult to control.

He had a massive infection, which is a typical trait of COPD. You've got to really watch it. And they sent him for physical therapy to get him back on his feet again, which they did. And the minute that they put him in there, the doctor called and talked to him about getting hospice.

"You'd be good for the people [at Hospice House]": Sarah

An older bone cancer patient, Sarah, had a different experience with getting the bad news. She described how she was told indirectly that her condition was terminal:

Well, I have bone cancer, and then I had surgery on my back. Three openings. It was calcium buildup. And they had to go in and chisel it out. I had a stroke at the same time, and I'm a little inclined to go to one side, so the walker takes care of that. The doctor called Hospice House and asked them if I could come here. He told me that I would be real good for the people here. I thought that was a nice way of saying that that's where I'm going. Well, I left the rest of it up to him.

"Is it time for hospice?": Sharon

Sharon, an older emphysema patient, reluctantly moved in with her sister Connie in 1995, when she could no longer care for herself in her own apartment. By late spring 1997, Sharon's sister was feeling overwhelmed with the burden and complexity of Sharon's care and asked the physician what else could be done to help her sister. Connie tells this story about how she and her sister came to understand that Sharon did not have much longer to live:

> I was having chest pains again. Before my husband died, I began to have chest pains . . . and they started again for me, before I had all this help [from Hospice]. They had started just from stress. [Laughing] I always call the doctor when we don't know what to do with her. And she was just having a really hard time breathing and I called Jane [Sharon's physician], and she shocked me with a question: "Is it time for Hospice?" And I said, "Oh no, we're not ready for that." I was shocked. At first I wasn't even going to mention it to Sharon. But as I thought about that a few days later, I decided if she's eligible for hospice, that's her decision, not mine, to make. Then I did talk to her about it, and I guess what we saw as the primary advantage was the fact that it would take over her medication. She doesn't have insurance for medication, so that was a real expense. . . . So that's how that came about. Then Jane came to the house and made the assessment, and then hospice people came out and discussed with us. Sharon was the one who made the decision. Hospice came and she made the decision. . . .
>
> Sharon's reaction was greater than I expected. Because I thought she believed she was near the end of her life anyway. She's given death a lot of thought, and didn't expect to live this long. But to be told, that is a little different. I guess she didn't show much outward reaction but I could see that. She began to act as though the end was imminent, any day now. She began to do some things right way that she wanted to take care of before she died. There was a friend she wanted to see. She had us have her over here for lunch. One day I said to her, "Sharon, I don't think you need to think every day and every breath is your last," and I think after that she kind of relaxed more.

Sharon did not discuss this experience with us. Her only recall of this time was that her doctor made a home visit: "She's wonderful . . . she's been here."

"I'm not ready for hospice yet": Kitty

Kitty marked the onset of her illness in the recent past—"five months ago," in spring 1997—when she had an accident in her car:

> I had a blackout, a seizure. I took out a dumpster at Malfunction Junction, and ended up with the front end of my car under the bed of a truck. I wasn't hurt, but they wouldn't let me drive. They can't guarantee it wouldn't happen again.

This accident apparently led to a hospital admission:

> When I got out of the hospital the first time, the doctor arranged, he wanted to send me out to Hospice. . . . They wanted to put me out at Hospice House, and I wouldn't go. So I said, no, I'm not going to, and he kept . . . I think he thought maybe getting a Hospice nurse in would convince me. [Laugh]

In refusing to go to Hospice House, Kitty appeared to believe that she could delay the fact of her approaching death. To Kitty, "going to Hospice" was the signal that she would have to accept her imminent death:

> They wanted me to go to Hospice House and then I didn't want to, right now, you know, so I didn't! [Laughs] I know that if I continue to have these blackout spells, that eventually I probably will end up there. And that's fine—when the time comes I'll be perfectly willing to go, but I'm not ready yet.

Kitty's perspective, which was limited by increasing dementia from her illness, was that she still had quite some time to live. She never discussed her diagnosis or prognosis with us, even when we brought it up, and she always insisted to us and to her closest friends that she was "doing fine" or "I think I'm getting better all the time." Whatever attempts had been made to make Kitty's situation an open awareness context apparently were denied by Kitty, who reconstructed it to a closed context as far as she was concerned. After her death, her friends told us a different story:

> Kitty was in the hospital, and Stu [her physician][1] had talked her into going to Hospice. And she was ready to go, because I think she

---

[1]First-name pseudonyms have been used whenever participants referred to their physicians by their first names to reflect the first-name basis in many doctor-patient relationships in Missoula.

was afraid she couldn't take care of herself anymore, and then she got a burst of energy that morning and said, "I'm not going." And her doctor and I got on the phone—"What should we do?"—and we told her, "You may die in some pretty miserable circumstances." And she said, "I don't care." And we said, "You may die and not be found for two days." "What difference will it make to me?" And so we said, "Somebody's got to see you every day." And she agreed to let the home health nurses do that.

Kitty's friends agreed that her physician was not able to give Kitty or her friends a clear diagnosis or prognosis of her exact closeness to death:

She doesn't know [what her illness is]. She never knew. Stu and I spoke six, eight times about her. I asked Stu straight out. He said, "She's older. She's having these spells." I said, "What are they?" and he said, "We're not sure." . . .

She took a friend in and said to Stu, "Whatever you want to tell me, tell her so somebody knows." And the friend got no more than I did.

"The doctor declared Mother hospice": Roberta

"Declaring mother hospice" was the formal way that this family knew their mother and grandmother would not live long. It was never clear how much Roberta understood. By the time we met Roberta—a very elderly woman with congestive heart failure—she was unable to describe her illness or remember much of its recent history. Her only recall of her major hospitalization in spring 1997, which resulted in her being unable to return to her own home, was as follows:

I was all alone and sick, and I guess the doctor put me in there, didn't he?

Later she said she remembered "having a cold" in April.

The nature of congestive heart failure is a long period of increasing failure, limitations, and more frequent symptoms, such as blackouts and fatigue, over five or ten years. So there may be no dramatic moment when an "announcement" can be made. Roberta's daughter recounts the event of being referred to hospice, which helped her family understand that their mother's life expectancy was now limited to months, rather than years:

For about three years we've been taking care of her at her home. We felt very strongly that the longer she could be independent the better off she would be. We made sure that we brought her meals every night and that there was day care there for her during the day to make sure she had her meds. Until she fell. The last couple of months before she fell, she had been sickened. She wasn't eating her meals at all, just kind of withdrawn. We took her to the emergency room, and they placed her in the hospital. The doctor said she could not stay alone any more, but she could recuperate from what was happening to her.

For this family as well, the doctor's announcement that Roberta would now qualify for hospice care became the sign of death's nearness.

The time she was in the hospital, in April, the doctor declared Mother hospice.

Being "declared hospice" signals a change of state from illness to nearing death. A clearly signaled change of state helped this family begin to reorganize its priorities and expectations—from simply providing care for a chronically ill elderly woman to making plans to actively say goodbye. After the declaration, Roberta's grandchildren and great-grandchildren made arrangements to visit over the summer, and her daughter was able to value the days she had with her mother in a new way:

We had a beautiful summer together. Our sons are seeing more now in Grandma than they did. They loved her dearly growing up but they were kind of in their own little world, and now they're seeing her in a different way, value. In fact, they've made special trips home. So there's been a chance for the family to stay in touch with her.

A Letter to the Estate of: Walt

Walt, our older heart patient, was told of his terminal condition quite gently. Walt had a series of hospitalizations for heart attacks over eleven years. About a year before his death, his doctor suggested hospice care:

I didn't choose it. The doctor recommended that I go on hospice.

Along with his physician's referral, Walt's wife, Dorothy, told us the family story of how Walt and the family had learned that his condition was terminal through an inadvertent letter sent by a specialist who saw him in the hospital during his last hospitalization a year earlier:

> The doctor had taken care of him all night. It was one of our episodes in the hospital where things were really bad and they didn't think he would live the night. And we had told them not to do anything. The children were all there. The doctor had come to us and said, "Now I don't think he is going to make the night. He will be gone by morning." And the next thing I got from the doctor's office was a bill from him to the estate of Walt. And I showed it to Walt and we had a good laugh over it, and so did the kids. So we laughed heartily over it, all of us. And we saved the bill because we just thought it was really funny. Next time I took Walt to the doctor he looked at us so startled as we said hello to him. But those things make life funny. After that the doctors suggested that hospice come out and they just came out and talked to us and let us decide if we wanted to go on it. And I said, "Yes."

"I don't have cancer": Mabel

Exactly how Mabel found out she was terminally ill, or how much she under-stood about it, remains less clear to us than for other participants. Mabel was not able to relate what she knew in a cogent way. Bernice certainly indicated that she understood that her mother was terminally ill, but she was reluctant to talk about it. Even her comments to us out of her mother's hearing range were less than explicit, suggesting that the two of them were in a silent pact of closed awareness.

Mabel and Bernice found out that Mabel's breast cancer had spread to her bones about two years before we met them, during treatment for Mabel's arthritis:

> The doctor injected the cortisone in her hip for the arthritis. Mom firmly believes in her heart, and I firmly believe, that he accidentally hit a nerve. They ran her through all the tests, did the bone scans and everything, and they did find the bone cancer in there. Mom didn't believe it because she couldn't focus beyond the point that she knew he hit a nerve.
>
> They had started her on the Tamoxifen when she was in the hospital, in '94. Well, Mom went off of it in three months. "I don't believe it. I know he hit a nerve, and that's all there is to it." And then in '96, she fractured [something]. Well, she told him, "I don't

have cancer." And she wouldn't let him treat her for it because she didn't believe she had it.

By the time we met Mabel, her daughter had been told that her mother "had cancer in every bone." Mabel had finally agreed to take the Tamoxifen again:

> She has cancer in every bone in her body. Nancy [Mabel's doctor] found a nodule here not too long ago. And she's got one here [points under the arm]. And the back of her head is hurting real bad, so I'm sure there's cancers up there.

As with many very elderly people, even with this diagnosis Mabel's physician had difficulty saying exactly how "terminal" Mabel was. Bernice told us what the doctor had just told them, on our first visit in summer 1997:

Bernice:	The doctor was here this last Sunday. Mom come right out and asked her, if she knew how long she was going to live. And Nancy [Mabel's doctor], she says, "I won't even attempt to answer that." She says, "You're just so remarkable."
Mabel:	What did you just say?
Bernice:	You asked her how long you thought you had to live and Nancy said she wouldn't even attempt to answer that because you were so remarkable.
Mabel:	Ah, heck. But I sure am getting skinny (pinches arm). I used to have some flesh on it.

When we first visited Mabel, her assertions that she "couldn't believe" she had cancer and her alternative explanations for her many pains seemed to us to be a sign of her cognitive difficulty and decline. A year later, as Mabel continued about the same—having just passed her eighty-eighth birthday—her disbelief in her imminent death seemed more justified.

Getting the Bad News in the Subculture of Terminally Ill Patients

The act of telling people that they are dying is equivalent to telling them that the aspects of the culture of those who are living will exist no more for them. They will soon have no power or control, no physical mobility, no growth in terms of normal life, no hope of living longer, and a disconnect with their physical continuity. Whatever economic security they might have is at risk of being depleted by medical costs. Against such losses, one can hold out the offer of as much comfort as possible, hope for (or belief in) an existence after death, the discovery of whatever sense of continuity one can find, and the remnants of whatever sense of dignity one can muster under such circumstances. Small wonder that physicians find this communication so difficult.

Language offers many ways to say things. One can be direct or indirect. One can be blunt or tactful. One can prepare the receiver of the message well in advance or drop it on them all at once. One can ask for an opinion or give one's own. One can order, or one can suggest or recommend. One can highlight what few positives there are—as one doctor in our study did.

We do not vouch for the accuracy of the memories of our patients and caregivers as they reconstructed for us the past event of being told that they were terminal. Memories often are imprecise, especially when the event being remembered is one that would best be forgotten. Barbara could not recall what she was told, noting that it was "a blur." Nor was the retelling of this event always consistent between patients and their caregivers. For example, Ralph reported that the "doctor told us to use hospice." Ralph's caregiver, however, says that the doctor simply "talked to him" about getting hospice.

Only Dennis gave what appeared to be a more exact description of the words used by his doctor: "I think we can get you through the summer." Note how the doctor stressed the positive here, telling Dennis what he *could* do, rather than what he could not.

For several of our more elderly participants, the announcement of bad news was made more indirectly, with some kind of suggestion about the possibility or need to use hospice services. For persons with a chronic illness, such as congestive heart failure or emphysema, there is no bright line between disease and dying— no test, no moment when the physician can make a dramatic announcement that the person has only so many months left to live. So a decline in functioning, a lack of mobility, difficult breathing, and increased fatigue often become the markers for both the physician and the participant that they are now closer to death.

Suggesting or referring a patient to hospice becomes a way to indicate to the patient and the family that the end really is near. Sharon's doctor brought up the subject by asking the caregiver a question: "Is it time for hospice?" The caregiver left the decision to Sharon herself to make. Kitty saw it differently, believing that she had little to say about the matter: "They *wanted me* to go to Hospice House." Roberta's daughter reported that the doctor *declared* her mother hospice, seeming to put the decision more in the hands of the physician than the family. In contrast, Walt saw his doctor as making a *recommendation*, not *wanting* or *declaring*. Perhaps the most gentle announcement of bad news, however, was provided by Sarah's doctor, who told her that she would be good for the other patients at Hospice House.

Obviously, making the bad news announcement in a way that gives patients a choice about how to spend their remaining days offers them a last smidgen of power in an otherwise powerless context. By insisting that Sharon make the decision about hospice, Carol offered her sister one last area of decision-making power. Nor was hope totally destroyed when Dennis was told, "I think we can get you through the summer": He could hope for this at least.

How Participants Talked about Death

Once the bad news has been given, there are many other occasions in which death and dying can be discussed. The participants in our study evidenced a spectrum of ways to talk about their impending deaths. The extent to which we can determine that the communication was one of open awareness or closed awareness is not limited to the way the participants recall how the bad news was given to them. In their casual conversations with us, with no prompting, some openly accepted the fact that they were dying and used terms relating to death. Others avoided talking about their imminent deaths and used more euphemistic expressions about dying (Table 2-1).

Neither age nor illness correlates with these different communicative approaches. Nor does gender appear to make any difference.

The first two categories share an implicit or explicit acceptance of the fact of death, of the finality of one's life and physical existence—the open or semi-open awareness of dying. The latter two approaches share an avoidance of the fact of one's dying, of the finality of one's existence—that is, they exhibit a closed awareness. (We use the phrase "finality of one's existence" to refer to the fact of the end of the physical life of the body; we do not refer to the continued existence, or nonexistence, of a self or soul after death.)

Table 2-1   Openness of Talk about Death

Uses term, accepts fact	Avoids term, accepts fact	Uses term, avoids fact	Avoids term, avoids fact
Dennis	Walt	Kitty	Mabel
Ralph	Sarah	Barbara	Roberta
Sharon			

Open Awareness: Using Terms for Death and Accepting the Fact of Death

"Death looming over me": Dennis

In our first visit with Dennis, he was absolutely clear that his illness was terminal:

> It's kind of a scary time, because of the finality of things as it's happening. Medically my disease is *nontreatable*. They can only put it into short-term remissions. And by that I mean a matter of weeks, a month maybe. And then I am *not expected to live* past the summer. [*Here and elsewhere in this section, we add emphasis to show how participants accepted impending death. Their speech itself did not reflect that emphasis.*]

≈ ≈ ≈

> What my doctor said was that my body would not continue to respond to chemotherapy. It's a *palliative* treatment. . . . And that my immune system would be compromised, that either through the ulcerated lesions, infection would get in and blood sepsis would set in, and they would not be able to do anything and my body parts would just start *shutting down*, but I don't see really going beyond the summer.

Nor did Dennis have any difficulty saying the words *die* and *death*:

> The latest statistic is 500 people per year in the United States will contract this disease, and they usually *die* of something else because of their age. . . .
>
> I have a pastor who likes to drop in . . . and we've had quite lengthy discussions on *dying*, etc. . . .
>
> I can talk to my family about just about anything. . . . Maybe it's that there is *death* looming over me that loosens my tongue.

Researcher: You couldn't live in a more beautiful place.

Dennis: Nor would I want to *die* in a more beautiful place. The tragedy of *death* is the suddenness and the unknown.

"It was a good life": Ralph

Ralph also was very clear with us from our very first visit that his illness was incurable:

> I'm in bad shape.
>
> In the shape I'm in, I don't think I'm going to be around very long. I'm in pretty bad shape.
>
> It's gettin' to the point where very little bit more and I'd be a lot better off, um, I suffer quite a bit.
>
> I just got a matter of a couple, a few days now.

Ralph had no problem saying the words *dying* and *die*.

> What concerns me most is *dying*.
>
> It gets a person to think, you know, you're *dying*.
>
> If we knew the day you're *dying*, you can face it.
>
> I'm about to *die*.
>
> I'm gonna *die* seein' that some things is better now.

Ralph also spoke of his life in the past tense, as though it were already over:

> Life *has gone* awfully fast.
>
> I *had* a real good life.
>
> It *was* a fun life.

Having a Party: Sharon

Sharon was not only quite aware that death was very near but also very comfortable using words such as *die* and *kick off*:

> I just didn't realize it was going to take so long for me to *die*.
>
> I hope it *doesn't go on* too long.

I'm *hanging on* entirely too long. If you think there's one more thing I need to tell that needs to be said, hurry up and get me to say it.

Often, Sharon's expression of death awareness even took on a light-hearted tone. On one visit, Sharon's hospice nurse was still with her when we arrived, and we were able to observe the following exchange:

Sharon:	I'm sure you're not going to sit here and watch me *die.*
Nurse:	Well, Sharon, I may be here to watch you die.
Sharon:	I hope you are.
Nurse:	Do you want to have a party right at the end? Balloons, streamers, a cake?
Sharon:	Angel food [cake].

After the nurse left, Sharon continued her thoughts on the party:

My children are having a birthday party, my children and Connie. I hope I stay alive that long. [Laughs] My 74th will be my last one. Maybe I should make a little poem: "74 and no more."

This conversation led to the topic of what Sharon had in mind for her own memorial service, with the following surprising results:

Researcher:	A lot of people are having kind of open houses at home and not funerals.
Sharon:	Well, we've already had one of those. We didn't really mean it to be that.
Researcher:	Who was it for?
Sharon:	Well, it was for me. [Laughs] We were sitting around planning something, and Bob said they had got everything over with, and Lyle said, "everything but the funeral." And Bob said, "Oh we had that this morning." And I said, "Instead of a funeral, you could have my last three days be a funeral."

Connie:	Well, Sharon, how do you know when your last three days are?
Sharon:	Because we'll make 'em that.

As we were making our farewells on this visit, Sharon said the following:

Sharon:	If I get a chance to *kick off*, you won't care if I do, will you?
Researcher:	Should I rejoice?
Sharon:	Yeah.
Researcher:	Then I'll rejoice with you.

Semi-Open Awareness: Avoiding Terms for Death While Accepting the Fact of It

"Getting it over with": Walt

Like many people, Walt and Dorothy avoiding using the words *die* and *death* before Walt died. They used these words to describe people who had died long ago—such as Walt's father, who had been "dead for 17 years"—but apparently had difficulty using them in the current context. Walt was very aware that his condition was terminal and that his days were numbered, but—in our presence, at least—avoided saying that he was dying. His references were euphemistic, but in no sense did they dodge the fact of his impending death:

I look forward to getting *this* over with. I'd just as soon *be asleep* tomorrow.

Even more oblique references to death appeared in references to Walt's condition and how his doctor informed him of this condition:

The doctor said, "There is a bed and you'd be more comfortable. The more you use it, the more comfortable you'll be."

In referring to her husband's terminal condition in his presence, Dorothy adopted medical terminology but avoided saying *terminal, dead,* or *died.*

He's got congestive heart failure and hardening of the arteries, and lungs are bad. They put him on Comfort One at that time. We got a letter from the doctor to the estate of Walt.

Dorothy used the words *die* and *death* sparingly—and not until after her husband had actually died:

Since last spring I knew that he was *dying*.

He knew he was *dying*.

When Dorothy recalled discussions with Walt prior to his death, however, she avoided saying "die" words, preferring instead the words *go* and *leave*:

He'd say, "Why do I have to go on? Isn't there some way I can leave?" I'd say, "Walt, when your time comes and your body and your spirit says it's time for you to go, you will go." He was ready to go. It was a relief when he was finally gone.

"I read a book on death": Sarah

Nobody could be clearer about her terminal condition than Sarah. She told us that she had bone cancer that had spread from earlier breast cancer and was now affecting her back. It was clear to her that there was no cure for this illness. At the same time, just how imminent her death might be was muddied by the fact that she did not die in Hospice House, as everyone expected, and eventually moved to another care facility during our study. We visited her over a period of six months, during which time Sarah accepted the fact that she was dying but carefully avoided using the words *death* and *die*.

Sarah described her admission to Hospice House in terms of her doctor's kind explanation: "You'd be good for the people there." Despite her avoidance of the words *death* and *dying* in relationship to herself, Sarah had no qualms about using these words in reference to others:

I read that book . . . it's on *death*.

There was lots of *deaths* at the nursing home where I was before.

The blind lady [her good friend], she *died*.

My doctor almost *died* himself.

My brother . . . *died* on the motorcycle.

Closed Awareness: Using Terms of Death Impersonally and Avoiding the Fact

Fantasizing about Her Condition: Kitty

Kitty maintained, throughout our visits with her, that she was doing just fine. She never acknowledged the seriousness of her illness or the imminence of death. For her, death was still a long way off in the future:

> I think I'm doing pretty good.

> I'm doing just fine. I think I am.

> I'm in very good condition . . . just the fact that I black out, you know.

> I've really got no complaints, you know. I think I'm getting better all the time.

Although Kitty maintained that her condition was stable—even improving— she seemed comfortable talking abstractly about death and using the words *dying* and *die.*

> I trust I won't be here then [in 5 to 10 years].

> After all, *dying* is a very personal and lonely thing you have to do by yourself.

> I always figured I was gonna *die* in my sleep, you know . . . and then all of a sudden I guess it was the doctor that said, "Well, you know, that isn't the way it happens."

> I told the doctor, I said, "Now I just presumed I'd *die* in my sleep in my bed [laughs], and he said, "Most of us feel that way, but it doesn't always work."

> My mother *died* in a fire, in a chair like that, sitting right there. She either dropped a cigarette or when she went to light the lighter it fell in her lap. And she caught on fire. It was very tragic, you know, very traumatic for me.

Death in the Abstract: Barbara

Barbara often spoke about her terminal condition in an impersonal and abstract way, usually in the passive voice. In our first meeting with her, for example, she discussed terminal illness in the abstract. She began with "I" statements about her lung surgery, then talked in general about terminal illness, then concluded with "I" statements about her doctor's inability to be clear with her:

> I had the lung surgery, and my psychosocial self wouldn't accept that I had major surgery and it had cut down on my physical ability to do certain things, so I was trying to be where I was without surgery and it wasn't working. And I just couldn't understand it. It was depressing. But anyway, looking at connections for *a patient* who has moved into, let's say a Phase IV or a terminal phase of chronic illness, if *they* could be connected by *their* doctor so that *they* feel that the support of *their*, for example, my doctor seems very hesitant to talk with me about terminal issues.

Barbara continued this focus on the need for doctors to connect patients to a support network when there is terminal illness several times throughout our visits:

> Let me tell you my vision. I would like to see doctors connect the patient to a support network in a more aggressive way, especially when the word *terminal* is being used. The doctors should give *you* a name and number when *you're* at Phase IV, so you can find services, connections to others.

Note how Barbara uses the word *you* instead of the first person pronoun. Her "you" in this example is equivalent to "one" or "a person"—impersonal and abstract rather than personal and immediate. Barbara also uses "a person" and "someone" as an abstract representation of self:

> When *a person* is diagnosed as terminal, then the support system out there takes it upon themselves to contact *them*. I really believe that if there is a connection with the doctor's office that's handling chronically, terminally ill people that can notify the agency that *this person* has been moved into this category, they might need some extraordinary support and they're willing to talk to *someone like yourself* to improve the quality of life.

Barbara also uses abstract representations of her illness when she describes the financial burden it places on her family:

> One thing that's important is the financial issue, who's working and who's not, when *there's* a terminal illness.

At times, Barbara abstracts her condition in the context of the lack of counseling available for children of patients—again not citing her own case but instead generalizing to "a parent":

> With children, I would say between the ages of say, 7 and 15, there seems to be a gap in services as far as being able to address their needs when they're dealing with *a parent* that is chronically ill or is possibly terminal. I've found Missoula really lacking.

Even when Barbara appears to deal with her terminal condition, she distances the issue by abstracting it from herself. Note that she does not say "my death" or even "my end-of-life issues."

> I'm dealing with *end-of-life issues* and trying to make some warped sense of it.

Avoiding using the terms *terminal* or *incurable* is another obvious way to abstract the issue. Through her treatment, Barbara learned a great deal about medical terminology and medical uses of language—referring, for example, to "the lungs" and "the surgery," much as doctors do to distance themselves from over-intimacy. In the same vein, Barbara often used the shorthand version when she mentioned her illness, referring to it as "the diagnosis" rather than "terminal cancer."

Accompanying Barbara's abstractions is a frequent glimmer of hope that she is getting better and may have a significantly longer period of time to live:

> I was really on a skyrocket with my blood test since April. It jumped up to 375 something, and then they started the medicine. When I landed in the hospital, it came down 12 percent. And then they had another. This is my second treatment I just finished. They did another blood test, and it showed over 50 percent drop. Really amazing.
>
> I've had remarkable results from the chemo. In just two treatments my tumor marker blood tests CA125 has fallen from 372 down to 144, and I don't know what it is now. My doctor and I both believe that I'm doing very well and will do very well.

Despite Barbara's representations of death in the abstract, at times she indicated clearly that she understood she was dying and spoke rather plainly about her death:

> I was encouraged by my husband to resign my job, enjoy what time I had left, but I don't know how much time I have left.

As a patient in this position of being crunched not only by illness but by emotional issues of, um, dying, of your family's grief and loss, and finances, it would be a novel idea for Missoula [to set up a foundation to assist people caught by financial difficulty when someone is terminal].

This house is actually the last place I am going to live.

Barbara was also able to use the word *die* on a few occasions. One of these occasions was associated with another person who had died, rather than herself:

My friend and colleague got the word that he had lung cancer and that it was just taking off like lightning. He *died* in the spring.

In one instance, Barbara associated death with herself at an earlier time in her illness:

I almost *died* in April.

More indirectly, Barbara gave evidence of her forthcoming death by describing how it might affect her children:

My daughter coming on Saturday is going to be a real gift to me because she is going to help me go through things and give them away or throw them away, donate them. I will feel much better when this is done. Because one thing that was on my mind is when I die so much goes on; I'm Indian, that complicates things.

When I die, I want my children to have these pictures.

Dealing with this whole issue that I *might die* from this creates pain for my children that I can only imagine.

Closed Awareness: Avoiding the Terms and Avoiding the Fact of Death

Two of our patients—Roberta and Mabel—avoided communication about their terminal condition and distanced themselves from it by avoiding the word *die* and any of its derivatives.

"I'm in good health": Roberta

Although Roberta had been on hospice for several months, in none of our conversations did she ever give the slightest indication that she was terminally ill—

or, in fact, that she was ill at all. On the contrary, her stance was that she was quite healthy:

Roberta: I feel good most of the time. Yeah, my health is good. I'm in good health.

Researcher: Sounds like you had a bad spell in the spring.

Roberta: I had a cold, I guess it was. I can fight those things as a rule. I can do pretty well, you know.

Roberta did admit to having a pacemaker, but she did not associate this fact with any serious illness. In fact, she portrayed it more as an aid to her check-ups than as an indication of a continuous problem:

I got a pacemaker. It keeps me going. They can check my heart over the phone, you know.

It's been going on now for a while, so we're kinda used to it and everything's okay. I haven't anything to gripe about.

By the time we met Roberta, her mental abilities were becoming more and more affected by her illness, and her level of cognitive functioning was difficult to determine. Roberta would not talk to us about her imminent death. Her daughter/caregiver, Debbie, tried to help us understand that this was not just a recent change or one caused by her dementia. Roberta had a lifelong aversion to death and dying; she fit the description of someone with high "death anxiety" (Kelly and Corriveau 1985).

Maybe about three years ago she said she wanted to be cremated. And so that was all she said. That was the only time she ever talked about dying. She would not even talk to my dad about death. He had tried various times to talk to her about what would happen if he were to die, just the way he felt about things. After he passed away she found a letter that he had written to her. Instead of talking to her about it, he wrote it down for her. So when the time came later in her life to do things with various things that she had, she wouldn't talk about them. Wouldn't go to funerals, even for her friends. Just would not even talk about people dying. Just totally disliked the idea.

The last part of October [about a month before she died], she'd go to bed at night and she would just be frightened, just scared to lie down, and I realized then that she had a great fear of dying.

The few times Roberta did use the word *die*, it was only as a past tense verb—and describing other people, not herself:

> My husband *died* a long time ago.
> I think my parents *died* very young.

Debbie used the word *die* in her mother's presence, but she also was referring to others who had died in the past, not to Roberta.

Tales of Woe: Mabel

Unlike Roberta, Mabel frequently complained about her ailments; like Roberta, however, Mabel avoided any mention of her own terminal illness. Although Mabel was willing to speak about the deaths of others, she was relatively silent throughout our visits about the possibility or imminence of her own death. Her single, somewhat ambiguous allusion to it came toward the beginning of our first visit as she described how she was told about her bone cancer:

> I couldn't believe it. No way in the world could I believe that I had bone cancer. I didn't never think that I would live to be this old, 86 now. I guess she's [the doctor] did all she can.

In later visits, Mabel insisted that her pains were the result of her hip problems, bursitis, or a bad fall (see chapter 6), rather than her terminal condition. Mabel's conversations about death usually focused on the deaths of others, not her own; her language often took on a more violent tone. She repeated these stories, or tales of woe, every time we visited her:

> My nephew [Rob] killed hisself. How he did it, I don't know.
> My other nephew too shot hisself. I don't know what he did. They thought he shot hisself. At first they thought that he drove the truck down by the river and some way went into the water but it didn't and they don't know what happened. But anyway, they found him dead. Maybe somebody did kill him and drive his car there in back of the hospital. You don't know. You don't know. I don't think he woulda ever killed hisself.
> My nephew, Rob, in the end had cancer. Then at the end he couldn't stand the pain any more and he went out in the back yard and shot hisself. It hasn't been too long that we were up there to see him, then he shot hisself.

In our last visit, Mabel asked her daughter to describe a newspaper story they had just read about "a disease that will make you do things that you wouldn't do." Bernice then described how the government was trying to get a medication off the market because "people were commitin' suicide." Bernice then embellished the story by describing a television program they had seen in which a man was put on Prozac:

> And he was real nice. He never had a mean bone in his body. Two children. And he would have these real bad pains. And then the doctor showed her how she can massage and she would. . . . And she said that one night she was settin' on the couch, and he set down beside her. Put his head on her, and then she felt his head comin' up like that, popped her on the chest. Well, it took her a few seconds to realize that he had just stabbed her. So she got up and went upstairs. Called the kids to lock their doors. She had a 15-year-old and a 16-year-old. . . . Well, by the time she got help there he had shot hisself.

Mabel used the word *died* very infrequently, never in reference to herself and always in association with deceased family members:

> My dad *died* three days after I was born. He had spotted fever. Two ticks bit him.
> My mother had a tough time all her life, and she *died* when she was 47, I was 16.

Mabel's only oblique reference to her own mortality was expressed in a jocular cliché. Note that she uses the general pronoun *you* rather than the first-person pronoun:

Researcher: It's hard for you to get out now?

Mabel: Oh gosh, yes. When you got one foot in the grave and the other sliding in. [Laughs]

Participants' Talk about Suicide

The topic of euthanasia was not an easy one to bring up in our research. Sometimes the participant or caregiver introduced it, but more commonly we inserted it into a conversation, once both parties seemed comfortable enough to handle it. On the whole, our participants did not have much interest in suicide—assisted or otherwise. There is some indication that Dennis and Ralph made some remarks about ending their own lives, shortly after their terminal diagnosis was given (the time at which they were most vulnerable). They seemed to have gotten over this feeling quickly, however, if it was a serious thought at all. The rest of our participants gave no indication that such an act was ever a serious possibility.

Maybe Had Some Thoughts Early in His Illness: Dennis

Talking with us three months before his death, Dennis denied any interest in assisted suicide:

> No. I'd rather it be this way. Because it gives you a chance to tie up any loose ends that you may have. And believe me, we all have them. And there's a lot that has to be done. There's a lot that has to be thought of. . . . This way I have a say in everything.

Carrie, Dennis's mother, confirmed her son's statement in one of our after-death meetings with her:

Researcher: Did he ever talk about euthanasia, that he would like to?

Carrie: Huh-uh. No. I've been through this three times now: with my dad, my mother-in-law, and Dennis. And it's uncanny how precious life is. My mother-in-law used to say that if things got that bad for her we should just put her on an iceberg and push her out. But when her time came, no, no. She hung onto life. It's very precious, and it doesn't seem to matter if you're young or old.

Although Dennis's mother may not have recognized any inclination on his part to commit suicide, his brother told us the following, in a separate after-death interview:

> Everybody was always concerned about him. I think he dropped hints to many people that he wanted to call it quits at various times after he was first diagnosed. I think he could see in the crystal ball a little bit and see what was coming. I knew of him talking about those kind of thoughts when he was still physically strong. I think he saw that it was going to be quite miserable.

Just how much of Dennis's hints about suicide can be attributed to male bravado and how much was real, we can't know. If we take the statements by Dennis and his family members literally, however, we would suspect that he apparently had some thoughts of suicide at the point of his greatest vulnerability—just after he was diagnosed as incurable. These thoughts, if they did occur at all, clearly passed quickly; as his condition got worse, Dennis tried harder and harder to hang on to life as long as he could.

"I should have shot myself when I first found out": Ralph

Like Dennis, Ralph made no mention and gave no hint to us that he had ever considered suicide. A week before he died, however, Sandy told us a different story:

> You know, he threatened that in the beginning. When he first started getting to the point where he couldn't do the things that he liked to do, he'd say, "You know, I should've just taken that gun and shot myself when I first found out I was sick." And I says, "No, that wouldn't have accomplished anything." And more and more I think he sees that now, and I don't think he'd do it now because he understands all this so much better now, about dying and going to be with God and everything. I don't think he'd do anything to jeopardize that now.

Ralph had insisted that they bring his little .38 revolver when they moved to Missoula a few months earlier, explaining that he needed the gun to protect them from "strange people in the city." Sandy described what happened after that as follows:

> But for a while when we first moved to the apartment he was so depressed, poor thing. I hid the gun from him for a long time because he was talking funny to me once in a while. Well, he finally got past that point.

"Might have said it as a young man, but not now": Walt

Our visits with Walt occurred during the last two months before he died. He was clearly in the last stages of life, and he had "mellowed from his earlier frustration and anger," as Dorothy put it. He gave us no indication that he had ever even considered suicide. Our after-death visit with his daughter confirmed our suspicion that it was not a viable option for him:

> He never talked about it. As a young, healthy person he might have said, "Well, I'm not gonna die in a nursing home. I'd just as soon go out and kill myself as lay in a nursing home." Those things might have been said.

Dorothy also mentioned to us that they had previous first-hand experience with a kind of suicidal act in their family, through the refusal of further medical treatment:

> Walt's dad pulled all the tubes out of himself. They had him wrapped with a straight jacket when he broke his hip. And he said, "I'm not living any longer." He got out of the straight jacket, pulled all the tubes out and that was it. But that was much different from euthanasia, because the whole family has to be contented with that [euthanasia]. The whole family has to be willing to let go.

From what we learned about how this family struggled to give Walt permission to "go," Dorothy's definition of euthanasia simply did not appear to fit Walt's case. His daughter's speculation that her dad may have felt differently about suicide during his early years fits with Dennis's and Ralph's situations. Early in the diagnosis, thoughts of suicide apparently crossed the minds of some of our patients. Consideration of suicide was apparently less likely as their condition worsened.

"It's against my cultural values": Barbara

After high school, Barbara at first decided on a career in nursing. While in training, she faced the reality of euthanasia up close:

> I first started in nursing and decided that all this about euthanasia was so demanding. It was really a big issue. And I couldn't agree with it. It was against my cultural philosophy. And I really struggled with that because they placed us in a nursing home connected to a hospital where one day your patient would be there and the next day he would be gone. If we asked someone what happened, they'd tell us, "Well, they died last night." Nobody

would talk to you about that. It's like that meant nothing. And so I went into a form of a depression about what I was doing.

Barbara gave absolutely no clues that she might consider suicide for herself. It would seem that this issue was decided by her strong and enduring cultural values against it.

Talks About Suicide by Others But Not Herself: Mabel

Mabel seemed to enjoy telling tales of woe. Several times she recycled the recent unrelated suicides of two nephews. One had occurred four years earlier, and the other occurred a month or two before our first visit with Mabel. She was concerned about why these good and handsome young men had killed themselves. However much these suicides were on her mind, there appeared to be no interest on her part in ending her own life. Mabel's world had always been her family, sisters, children, nieces, and nephews. Any bad things that occurred in her family seemed to shake her understanding of the world itself. These two recent deaths in her family bothered her and found their way into her conversations with apparent ease. Confronted with the possibility of her own suicide, however, she was absolutely clear:

Mabel:	They found his truck back there of the hospital in Hamilton. And he was dead.
Researcher:	That was your nephew, right?
Mabel:	Nephew. Same age of Bernice. Good lookin' and good. He was such a good person. Such a good person.
Researcher:	That really bothers you, doesn't it, Mabel?
Mabel:	Yeah, but Bernice said she bet that this medicine that he was takin' forced him to do that. So, I don't know. 'Cause I don't think he would because he had cancer of the stomach and surgery. Just put an end to it. But I don't know.
Researcher:	Have you ever felt that way? Like you just get so tired and—?
Mabel:	No. Hunh-uh.
Researcher:	It sounds like you're not about to do that.
Mabel:	No.

"Never gave any thought about how I'd go": Kitty

A person who says she never gave any thought about how she might die is not likely to have given any thought to suicide:

> I always figured I was gonna die in my sleep, you know. That was it. I never gave any thought about how I'd go.

Unlike the other participants in our study who were asked the "truck" question, Kitty said that she would rather die quickly than have a lingering illness:

Researcher: One of the big issues now is, would you rather be hit by a truck, or would it be better to have some kind of illness to cope with?

Kitty: You're asking me? I'd rather go suddenly. That stuff is a drain, you know. It's a drain on me and it's a drain on my friends. So I'd just rather it got over quickly if I had my choice. Most of us don't have much to say about it.

On the surface, one might interpret Kitty's answer as a willingness to get it over with by her own hand. But there were no other clues in our visits with her that this would be the case. She clearly recognized the "drain" that her illness was putting on everyone who cared about her, but this acknowledgment did not mean that she would take her own life to remedy the problem. In all other respects, Kitty was the one participant who seemed to take no particular interest in exactly how she would die.

In an after-death visit with one of Kitty's church friends, however, we were told that when Kitty's hospice nurse found her on the floor at home, the day they finally insisted she be moved to Hospice House, she had taken out her IV line:

> She had pulled out the tube that went to the aorta of her heart, to the artery that they were putting the antibiotics in. She pulled it out the day before. I think she thought she could hasten her death because she was losing complete control.

Whether Kitty pulled the tube out intentionally, as her friend suspected, or it was just an accident, we will never know. Control was, indeed, an important quality-of-life issue for Kitty. Perhaps realizing that she no longer had much control led her to make this last effort. If so, however, such an act runs counter to everything she had told us earlier.

"That wasn't her wish": Sharon

Sharon's sister and caregiver, Connie, told us tearfully about how her own husband had stopped his dialysis and chose to die. She had no fears about Sharon taking her own life, though. And Sharon gave no indication to us that she had ever even considered it. Connie's own wishes for assisted suicide if she ever developed Alzheimer's were well known to Sharon. Connie told us, however, that Sharon did not want this for herself:

Researcher:	Did Sharon ever talk about . . . getting help in dying if she really needed it or assisted suicide? Did that ever come up?
Connie:	I don't think she ever talked about that. We kidded about it one day. She was lying in bed and she said that she had just been trying to think how to die. And I said, "Well, you know, we could call Kevorkian." But that's the only time. There was never any talk about it. And she knew about my own directives. But that wasn't hers, though.

Talking about Death with Each Other

Simply because two parties love each other is no guarantee that they can communicate effectively on all topics. Even if they are able to communicate well on most topics, they may not be articulate or willing to talk about difficult topics such as the imminent death of one of the parties. In this section we focus on how the caregivers and their loved ones succeeded or failed to talk to each other about important aspects of death and dying. Our study participants revealed a range of ability to discuss death with each other in our presence, from totally open to guarded avoidance of the topic (Table 2-2). (Kitty and Sarah are

Table 2-2   Communication: Open vs. Avoidance

Open	Avoidance
Dennis and Carrie	Roberta and family
Sharon and Connie	Mabel and Bernice
Walt and Dorothy	Barbara and Dan
Ralph and Sandy	

not discussed in this section. Kitty had no family and Sarah was not living with family during the research period.)

Barbara poses a special problem in categorization because she had two different caregivers during the period of her terminal illness. With her first caregiver, she was as unable to talk openly about her death as he was. During the last month of her life, when her primary caregiver changed, so did the openness of talk about her coming death. We do not discuss this situation further, however, because it impinges too much on the private wishes of the family and because we were unable to maintain contact with her during this time.

Open Awareness

There appeared to be very little that Dennis and his mother could not talk about, including his terminal illness and forthcoming death. In our presence they spoke about his lingering illness as a "dress rehearsal for death," the fact that "we're all going to die," and the recognition that "awareness of death is an opportunity that not everyone gets." Perhaps Dennis put it best:

> I can talk to my family about just about anything. Mom can almost read my mind as to what's going on. We always say we're joined at the hip, and we are.

This caregiver and patient did, indeed, talk about almost anything, including Dennis's imminent death. Interestingly, however, Carrie did not plan Dennis's memorial service with him; his sister did instead. Carrie told us this:

> She [Dennis's sister] was the one that just would sit there and talk about funeral arrangements with Dennis. He told her the pallbearers he wanted and the music he wanted. She wrote everything down. Now I wasn't up to that. But we all have gifts.

Sharon talked openly about her forthcoming death with virtually anyone. She joked about it, in fact. Her caregiver, Connie, was a bit more careful discussing death with her sister, having just gone through her own husband's death four years earlier.

Walt and Dorothy did not talk about death much in front of us. Walt's dying process was very prolonged, however, and they may well have gotten all the necessary things discussed before we even began our research. Over and over again, however, Dorothy spoke about how this family told each other everything and discussed all important matters in the open. Our conversations with other family members supported Dorothy's assertion.

Sandy's candor on all subjects was a delight to behold. She feared nothing, including talking with Ralph about how and when he would die. All of these families—Ralph and Sandy, Walt and Dorothy, Sharon and Connie, Dennis and Carrie—shared an openness of communication that signaled their acceptance of the finality of death and of dying.

Closed Awareness: Avoiding the Topic

In two other families, the topic of death was clearly avoided. These were two of the oldest participants (both eighty-seven). At Mabel's house, her daughter would follow us out to the car to talk and sometimes obliquely refer to "later" or "when this is over." The very indeterminacy of Mabel's condition, bone cancer, did not give them a clear, predictable trajectory to death and further reinforced their difficulty in talking about death.

Roberta's family demonstrated the difficulty many people have in discussing the imminence of death with the person who is dying. As described earlier in this chapter, Roberta was highly anxious about dying, insisting on her good health even at the end of her life, and was characteristically reluctant to discuss death and dying. She would not attend the funerals of friends. Her husband had died suddenly at the breakfast table from a blood clot. His sudden death certainly would have increased her anxiety and avoidance of thoughts and discussions about death.

Thus, at the end of life, Roberta's family had to struggle with honoring her "wishes," while being honest to their own feelings and experience. When Roberta's daughters brought her home from the hospital knowing that she had only days to live, they decided to call in the Chalice of Repose to play at her bedside—something that they had not planned beforehand or even talked about. The two sons-in-law were very upset with this decision because it would signal to her that she was dying:

They felt it would upset Mom. It would not be fair to her to be frightened by it.

Despite the sons-in-laws' objections, Roberta's daughters "went ahead and decided yes." They found the music calming to Roberta even in her comatose state—after an initial startled reaction—and it clearly provided her daughters a significant ritual that signaled their mother's "transition."

Every family solves the problem of meeting their own needs and the needs of the one dying in its own way. Some do so by maintaining the family tradition that "we never talk about death"; others, such as Roberta's, do so by responding directly to how the current experience of actually being present at their loved one's death strikes them and creating new rituals or changing old ones. Although Roberta's daughters were not able to talk with her directly while she was conscious, they found it healing and helpful to be open with each other. After Roberta became comatose, her daughters also talked to her directly about her dying, and said goodbye.

Roberta's family was the most open with those outside the family about the fact of her death. They called everyone they knew after they brought her home from the hospital. The night Roberta died, everyone who could was called to come say goodbye and they called relatives who were out of town to say goodbye to her over the telephone.

Roberta's family provides an illustration of how a large family that had not experienced a death at home before found ways of making this death an open rather than secretive experience. Not only were family members welcomed, but Debbie and her sisters also invited us, as researchers, to come "anytime you want to" while she was dying. So we did, visiting Roberta and her family the day of her death. Other caregivers, who knew us equally well if not better, were not as comfortable with our presence, nor did we consider suggesting it.

Communication in the Subculture of Dying People and Their Families

Sixty years ago, linguist Louise Pound (1936) observed, "One of mankind's gravest problems is to avoid a straightforward mention of dying or burial." For some of the participants in this study, talking about death was a longstanding verbal taboo. Our Victorian ancestors, whose delicate natures did not permit them to utter words such as "leg" in mixed company, created a euphemism that survives to this day: drumstick.

Historians generally recognize that nineteenth-century prudishness grew out of a desire to deny, or at least publicly ignore, the existence of sex and sexual body parts, as well as death and dying. Lest we think lightly of such linguistic practice, consider the fact that the field of medicine often creates similar language changes, as in "mental illness" for "insanity" and "Hansen's disease" for "leprosy." The older patients in our study might well be excused for their discomfort in using the "die" words in relation to themselves. Mabel, Roberta, and Walt—all octogenarians—may simply have inherited their generation's discomfort with saying "die" or "death." What, then, enabled Kitty, Ralph, Sharon, and Sarah—who were almost the same age—to use these words in conversation? Kitty appeared to be fantasizing: Even though she could use the words freely, she strongly avoided the fact that death related to her personally. Sharon, Ralph, and Sarah had clearly made their peace on this earth and forged ahead to whatever might be, making their use of these words natural and easy. They were not afraid to say that they were dying.

This absence of fear of death may be a form of power in itself. One cannot control death, but one can have a degree of power over it by acknowledging its existence. Ralph, Sharon, and Dennis gave particularly clear evidence of having some degree of power over their deaths. This power not only enabled them to say where they would die, who would be with them, and what their memorial services would be like; it also enabled them to choose how they would talk about their condition and ultimate death. They appeared to feel empowered to use the words.

Those who seek the power of ending their own lives have open to them the avenue of suicide. Our participants did not appear to want such power, even though there were reports that Dennis and Ralph had made such remarks about the possibility years earlier. Control is an elusive concept, and what appears to be a powerful action (such as killing oneself) actually may be a less powerful characteristic than sustaining the powerful will to live.

Chapter 3

Planning and Choices

People often plan for vacations, schooling, retirement, family, weddings, and many other things, but they seldom plan carefully for their own deaths. A plan, quite simply, is a method for achieving an end. Planning consists of conceptualizing, setting goals, and considering alternatives—including forecasting the advantages and disadvantages of different possible actions.

Purchasing life insurance engages one in at least one kind of planning for death. But there are other plans to be made as well. Within the subculture of the terminally ill patient, planning—for care, for medical treatment, or for death itself—offers at least the appearance of exercising some control over an event for which little sense of control seems possible. One may not be able to control the fact of dying, but one can at least control where and how it will happen. Seven of the eight participants who died during this study maintained at least some sense of control by choosing to live out their lives at home. These terminally ill patients had no realistic hope of remaining alive for a long time, but their final plans about where they would die appeared to give them at least a short-term sense of control and dignity. As Seale (1998) points out, planning to ameliorate the consequences of one's own death is a positive act of control.

Some aspects of existence are once-in-a-lifetime events for which most people have no experience whatsoever. For example, most people are novices at buying engagement rings, homes, or other tangible things that usually are purchased rarely in a lifetime, if at all. As a result, they sometimes do such things badly. Being diagnosed with a terminal illness is another once-in-a-lifetime event. A diagnosed terminal illness is not one for which many people are prepared emotionally, rationally, financially, or spiritually. For this reason, we paid attention to how participants and caregivers managed to make plans for care, how they dealt with unanticipated events when things didn't go "as planned," and how they planned for decisions about possible medical treatment, including heroic measures.

Some people are natural planners. Others seem only to react to whatever comes along in life. Not surprisingly, some of the families in this study planned what would happen to them very carefully, whereas others did not. Our observations suggest that people who are predisposed to plan carefully tend to make good use of this ability. Nonplanners may not manage as well—at least, not without some help. The participants and families in this study illustrate the spectrum of planning, or lack thereof, in this matter. This chapter describes several aspects of planning and decision making at the end of life: participants' planning or lack of planning for care, their unanticipated choices and decisions, their planning for medical treatment, and the influences of finances on their planning and choices.

Planning for Care

Perhaps the most thorough plan for care in our study was the one devised by Walt and his caregiver, Dorothy. Dorothy is one of those people who sees long range, considers and weighs various alternatives, then chooses the one that best suits the needs of everyone involved. Deciding to relocate to a place that is more suitable for home care at the end of life is not easy for most people, but Walt and Dorothy pulled it off with dignity, grace, and economic sense. Another good example of planfulness is the case of Ralph and his caregiver, Sandy, who gave up their dreams of staying on their beloved rural homestead and moved into the city of Missoula during Ralph's last months of life. In this chapter, we contrast these two examples of good care planning with the situations of Barbara and Kitty, whose planning for their own care was somewhat less than satisfactory for themselves and for those around them.

"We had it all planned": Walt

On our first visit to Walt, we noticed a lift-up bed, a lift-up chair, and other items. We asked if Medicare helped with these things. Dorothy replied, "No, I bought these before we went on hospice; we've had 'em for a long time." Walt had suffered with his heart condition for 11 years to that point; Dorothy obviously was thinking ahead. But evidence of this foresight is more dramatic in her description of how they came to live in their current home—a new, one-story duplex with wide doorways and a bathroom right next to Walt's bed:

> The kids built this house. We knew he was going to get to the point he couldn't take care of himself. Our house was big, plus yard—too big. I couldn't take care of him and the house and yard. I had it all

planned. I'd been trying to do it for several years 'cause I knew what he was going down to. And I think you should make yourself as comfortable as you can.

At our second visit, Walt elaborated a bit on how they managed a new house for his care:

When we sold that house there was some money. And it would have been some money left over to build this. But the youngest daughter here, she didn't have a home and didn't have any real prospects of getting a home of her own. So Dorothy and I decided that we can't take this money with us and do us any good. So why not just whack it up amongst the kids now, right now. We can build this for us and we'll have it completely clear and then my daughter, she'll have a good start living in the other half of the house.

Neither Walt nor Dorothy was totally clear to us about the details of what appeared to us to be a rather unique housing arrangement, orchestrated by the entire family. So we spoke with Walt's middle daughter a few weeks after his death. She verified that Dorothy was "the planner" but added that she, herself, was the financial manager of the family:

Mom's always been a planner for the future, okay. You know, "If your dad dies while I'm tryin' to raise you kids, I can't afford the house payments so I'm gonna go out and buy mortgage insurance." So the house payments would be made.

                        ∼ ∼ ∼

Mom had been running down the Bitterroot a lot taking care of Dad's folks. And so she has always claimed that when it got to be her time that she wanted things as convenient for us as possible, not like it was for her. So she's kind of always made these plans. She hadn't done anything much to their house. She'd taken care of it but there wasn't time for some major updating. There was a lot of contemplating about what she was gonna do because she knew Dad was getting to the point that he couldn't do the hedges and she couldn't keep up the yard work and the house work, and they were getting overwhelmed with their bigger place. A simpler, smaller house. Downsizing so she could maintain what she had.

                        ∼ ∼ ∼

And she always talked to us kids about what to do. And one of her first things, my sister who now lives next door and her husband have always had financial problems. They lived in a little rat hole for quite a few years, and Mom decided, well, maybe she'd build onto her house where my sister and her husband could live next door and take care of things. But the city planning and development and all that would not go along with it. So adding onto the house was not an option. And we could not find any duplexes that gave us any handicapped features. So Mom finally decided, "Well, let's just sell it. We'll take all the money we've got and build a duplex and my daughter can live on one side and take care of us." My sister and her husband do a lot for 'em. If nothin' else, they are always there as company. Made her feel a little more secure and safe.

Once it was decided that a new duplex would be built, the family took stock of available resources and planned how to make what they had stretch to fulfill their plans. The middle daughter elaborated:

Mom and Dad only had like $———. We worked on that budget, I'll tell you. Left and right. And see, they took and gave their money to us kids. And we put it all in a partnership. So the estate's basically already divided up. None of that can be fought over. And so our goal now is for the five of us to take care of 'em. We'll wait and see how Mom does. And if Mom gets to the point that she needs to go into a care facility of some type, we have the duplex to sell and maintain her on that. Or, if there's money providing, rent her side out, leave my sister and her husband on their side. Mom was afraid that the financial strain on Dad's situation would wipe her out. She really worried about that. That's why she set up the partnership. I manage the finances.

With the partnership in place, the family went about trying to find a suitable place to build. Here they met unexpected opposition from Missoula's zoning regulations. They also had to marshal their limited resources carefully. The middle sister explained how they did this:

There isn't much land where you can build duplexes in this town. And so we had to take the lot that we had, design the duplex for Mom and Dad all on the one level. My sister ended up with basically no living room and no eating area. They ended up with a really small area downstairs, but their half has a pretty nice upstairs bedroom area.

~ ~ ~

My two brothers did the plumbing. My brother and I did all the waste underneath in the crawl space during that cold snap. We were down there and almost froze to death at 7:00 one night. We did all the plumbing. My other brother did the electrical. And we got a friend to come in and do the venting on the boilers for the heating system. We hired a contractor for the construction. And then we all went in and did the painting.

Together, Walt's family planned to provide a suitable care facility for their terminally ill father. Although this example may not be common, it is instructive and inspirational. It was a particularly wise plan in that it also offered provisions for the mother if and when she needed it in the future. In addition, it solved both the financial problem and the housing problem of one of the children. Equally important, it resolved any inheritance issues well in advance of the deaths of both parents.

"If we ever did anything right": Ralph

Ralph, an older emphysema patient, tells another story of how he and his caregiver, Sandy, prepared for his care. In March 1996, he began treatments for pneumonia and a massive lung infection at the Veterans Hospital in Helena for several months. When his condition improved enough for him to leave the care of the VA hospital, he needed rehabilitation to help get him back on his feet. He described these events as follows:

You see, I was over at Fort Harrison, and they sent me over here (to Missoula), originally to a physical therapist. I couldn't walk, and they said that if anybody could make me walk, these people in Missoula could. So they sent me over here for a month—six weeks, I guess—before I got to where I could walk again. They kept me there as long as they could. You see, they had some kind of a deal worked out between Medicare and the Vets over there. I don't know how they had it doped out, you see, but I was getting my room and board, you might say, over there. Then the Vets sent me over here for the physical therapy. When my physical therapy benefits ran out, then hospice came along. And they took me and got me on Medicare, but we had to come and pick up a place to live and all that stuff.

In later visits, Sandy elaborated a bit on their move into Missoula. When they came to Missoula for physical therapy, Ralph had to have a local doctor. So he went to his brother's physician—who, as it turns out, was the one who suggested hospice. Because there was no hospice service in their area, they decided that the only thing they could do was to move to town. Sandy also described Ralph's misgivings about finding housing in the city:

> All this time that we were talking about living in town, Ralph had all the reasons of never getting an apartment, looking at the back of some brick building all the time. So I told him, I said, "Now, I've found an apartment on the ground floor that's all set up for wheelchairs and handicapped people." When we were moving in, I took him out there on the porch, and here was, you know, grass and trees and a river and birds and he was just flabbergasted. . . . Even a long time after we moved all our stuff in here, he couldn't feature in his mind where these apartment buildings were, and we were in this apartment a month before I finally got it through his head where he was. So after I got him home and he was on his feet better and we were walking around and doin' stuff, I took him for a ride out there and showed him where it was so that he could get the idea. If I had taken him back to the ranch instead of this apartment, he couldn't go for walks like he can here. Back home the only place for him to go that's level enough to walk for that wheelchair is out there on the gravel road. People would go by in their cars and, whew, the dust. So I told him, I said, "That isn't going to work."

Two weeks before Ralph died, the topic of their good luck in finding this apartment came up again:

Researcher: I'm really impressed that you found a place that's handicapped-accessible and where you can get out so well.

Sandy: Right. And this is what Ralph says all the time. He's so grateful for having this place. He said, "Boy. if you ever did anything right in your life, you found this place."

In this instance, Ralph and Sandy assessed the alternatives and planned for Ralph's last months in the wisest way possible, even though it separated them from the most motivating and central part of their lives—the beautiful Swan valley. Planning is easy when the alternatives are all good ones. Moving into the city was a frightening prospect to Ralph, and he exhibited the courage to follow that plan cheerfully and, in the long run, to make the best of it.

Difficulty in Planning for Care

In contrast to Ralph and Walt, the normal human instinct to survive, to think about "getting well," made acceptance of dying and the need to plan for end-of-life care very difficult for two other participants: Barbara and Kitty.

"I keep telling myself I'm doing fine": Kitty

Kitty, a single woman in her eighties, said, "I always figured I was going to die in my sleep. That was it. I never gave any thought about it." Kitty had worked in the medical field as a technician for 40 years, but this experience did not lead to a greater willingness to plan for a terminal illness, which was not clearly defined. It also was never clear from our conversations with Kitty how well she understood her illness or declining condition.

In fact, Kitty did have a very clear plan for the end of her life: She would go on living in her own home, with her beloved animals that she had rescued from the Humane Society. Kitty assumed that she would be able to stay by herself and simply die one night—even though she was an "orphan," with no relatives in Missoula to help her accomplish this goal. Kitty reported that her physician talked very directly with her in spring 1997, after she had a car accident when she blacked out while she was driving:

> I said I assumed I'd die in my sleep. He said that isn't the way it happens.

Apparently, Kitty's doctor spent some time with her in spring 1997 trying to develop a plan for her care. She was characteristically cryptic about this discussion, even when asked:

> They wanted me to go to Hospice House, and then I didn't want to right now, you know, so I didn't. [Laugh] They wanted to put me out at Hospice House, and I wouldn't go. I figured I could do better at home, by myself, having somebody look in on me, of course.

Only after Kitty's death, when we met and talked at length with friends from her church, did we discover the opportunities she was given to plan for and make choices about her care—and her refusal to do so. A friend explained:

At that point, Stu [Kitty's physician] talked her into going to Hospice [House]. She was in the hospital ready to go to Hospice. . . . She was ready to go because I think she was afraid she couldn't take care of herself anymore, and she got a burst of energy that morning and said, "I'm not going." And so Stu and I said to her, "You may die in some pretty miserable circumstances." Kitty said, "What difference will that make to me?" And so we said, "Somebody's got to see you every day." And she agreed to let home health do it.

Kitty did accept the provision of hospice services in her own home, at the insistence of her doctor and church family:

When I got out of the hospital the first time, the doctor arranged, he wanted to send me out to Hospice. I said no, I'm not going to. So I think he thought maybe getting a hospice nurse in would. . . . [Laugh] I didn't object because I want to make sure that I get my medicines all taken at the proper time.

During our first visit, however, Kitty seemed reluctant to acknowledge that hospice was providing her care at home. From her perspective, hospice was still in the future—in the form of Hospice House—but not now, even though she had a hospice nurse visiting weekly.

Researcher: Do you have hospice?

Kitty: Yeah, I think it's hospice. It might be . . . well, there's hospice and Partners, and to tell you the truth, I don't ask who they are when they come in.

Some of Kitty's confusion about who was actually providing her care probably is attributable to her increasing dementia, which also made her more suspicious and unwilling to talk about her own personal needs or care. As researchers, we were confused about her care and her understanding about her care because she was so unclear about her own care needs or who provided assistance for her. During her life, she explicitly requested that we not talk to any of her friends about her situation.

When we first visited, Kitty said that she would go to Hospice House "when the time comes." She was increasingly conditional or vague in her responses, however, about when that time would be, perhaps because of the effects of her illness on cognition. We asked how she would know "when the time came": "What would be a sign to you that you probably should go?" Her response:

> Well, if I get so tired that just trying to do anything around the house . . . that will be a sign that the medication is not keeping my blood pressure up. It will be time for me to get some help, or to, to go to Hospice House. I know that if I continue to have these blackout spells that eventually I probably will end up there.

The "if I get tired" conditional clause and the continued ambivalence about "getting some help or going to Hospice House" reflect Kitty's denial not of death itself but of dying. This attitude persisted in the face of decreasing mobility, incontinence, and obvious fatigue that everyone else noticed. In subsequent visits during the next three months, Kitty continued to assert that she was doing fine:

> I keep telling myself I'm doing fine . . . I think I am. Others don't think so, but I'm getting better.

Up to and including our last visit in Kitty's home, two days before she had to move to Hospice House, she never felt "tired enough" to think that she was ready to go. Even in our brief visits, her increasing impairment in judgment, difficulty in processing ordinary conversation, and difficulty in evaluating her own situation and functioning were evident.

Earlier, we were amazed at how well she was doing—staying at home with no one else living there—given the seriousness of her illness. We asked her how she did it. She described to us the kinds of help she received:

> I tell you, the health care people are just keeping excellent track of me. There's a girl that comes about 9:30 in the morning, every day. And then I get Meals on Wheels. Then there's another girl that came in, I had her run some errands for me. I had to have some calcium supplement picked up at Osco. And so I asked her if she'd do it, and she said she would. . . . There's people that call, bring flowers from the altar, and bring communion. The clergy and the lay leaders call on me, the clergy try to, and then they have a group called the lay ministers. They bring communion to us shut-ins.

Because other participants in our study had one or more full-time family caregivers to manage complicated medications, visits, and so forth, Kitty's apparent single-handed mastery of her care planning, with no caregiver, was even more astounding to us. When we expressed our amazement at all this, she said she didn't really know how she did it.

Researcher: I wonder how you do it. How is that you organize your life so well? How do you think about it? What do you plan? Do you write yourself notes? [Both laugh]

Kitty: No. . . . I don't know. Maybe just think about it once in a while. No definite sitting down and saying to myself, "Now, you're going to do this and this and this at such and such a time." Nothing like that. In that respect, I'm very disorganized. I don't have any definite plan of organizing my life, no.

In our after-death conversation with Kitty's church friends, the missing link in her care was revealed: Her priest had spent the last nine months of Kitty's life planning *for* her, without much cooperation on her part for most of that time. His stress was evident as he spoke about what orchestrating her care required:

That's a tough one. . . . How much time do I have to put it together? We knew we were Kitty's family. We just got on the phone and started putting a system together. The hardest part was getting her to accept it. When the daily visits [from a home health care nurse] stopped, I called four parishioners, two of them nurses. And they would try to visit her, each once a week. And then [the assistant priest] would call five days out of the week to make sure.

When Kitty developed a foot infection, her church friends took turns taking her into the doctor's office for two weeks of daily IV antibiotic treatments. Even with all their efforts, Kitty obviously needed much more daily help by the time she was a month from death. Only when the hospice nurse found her confused and incontinent early one Monday morning, having pulled out the IV line herself, was she able to convince Kitty that the time had come to go to Hospice House.

Kitty certainly had the outlines of a plan for the end of her life, but her planning was marked by unwillingness or increasing cognitive inability (or both) to recognize the level of care she needed. She had no family to become her partners in planning, nor did she have friends she trusted enough to take on this role. Nor did she trust even her parish priest or her long-time physician to make those decisions for her. She maintained that she would know and that she could decide rationally. This belief in her own rationality proved to be an illusion. Confronting and challenging this belief with someone who has always been independent and able to make sound decisions concerning her own life is particularly difficult.

"I don't know what to do next": *Barbara*

Barbara—a woman in the prime of life at forty-six, with many successes and prestige in her profession—had confronted cancer in various guises since 1991. At each serious encounter, with surgery or other treatment, she had another remission. Her experience of girding for battle over and over—using all the resources of both the medical world and her own Native American traditions—helps explain why she deferred planning for her end-of-life care while she prepared for the next battle.

Planning may be facilitated by having a consistent, unambiguous message about one's prognosis and nearness to death. Walt, who had congestive heart failure, and Ralph, who had emphysema, saw themselves as receiving such information from multiple sources—from their disease, from their physicians, from their own bodies, and from their stage in life as senior citizens. Barbara had none of these messages. Her disease was sometimes in retreat; her physician didn't seem to want to talk with her about being terminal, even when she said she wanted to; she had periods when her body gave her many signs of getting better; and she was relatively young, with children still at home.

So Barbara planned well for her continuous fight with her illness but not for her end-of-life care. Until two months before her death, she remained hopeful that her advanced cancer had once more gone into remission. Even when she discussed her terminal condition with us, she noted that

> It was very dim in April and May, but with the response to the medicine and the help of Divine healing, my doctor and I both believe that I'm doing very well and will do very well.

In Barbara's case, hope for a remission could not coexist with planning for end-of-life care. In such cases, a family member may be the best one to take on the task of planning for care. Barbara's husband shared her hopes, however, and—despite his acknowledgment that the doctors "say that it's terminal"— found it equally difficult to talk about or help her plan for her death as drawing closer during the time we visited them:

> The hospice guy, he said if we needed him, give him a call. We haven't needed him. We might . . . in the future sometime, I guess. When she's ready. These tests are showing that [the cancer] is going down. And that doesn't make sense to me. When the test is coming

down, that means better. . . . She could be around for half a year, or a year, or five years, you know. It's hard telling.

Barbara's husband seemed ill-prepared or unwilling to assume responsibility for planning her care; nor is there any evidence from our data that Barbara would have wanted him to. At one point Barbara seemed to be particularly confused by not "knowing" with certainty what lay ahead for her. Barbara was an intelligent person who had learned to use information well and to rely on objective, factual information in her work. Her education and advanced degrees, her intelligence and administrative skills, were of little help to her when she confronted the ambiguities, the state of "not-knowing," the unpredictability of illness and death. These ambiguities were not part of her advanced university education or work life. Four months before her death, she described her difficulty with not knowing:

I have no idea what the end of my life will be like. I could very well be in a hospital somewhere with an infection, and I have no control over that. So we just don't know. That's one of those difficult aspects of illness, that I don't know . . . what to do next.

In this statement, there is a sense that if Barbara had been given definite information—as happens with some illnesses and some kinds of cancer (though not ovarian cancer)—that "you will die within three months," she would have acted quickly to make plans. She had lived for six years, however, because of aggressive cancer treatment, because of hope, and because of her own "resilience" (her word).

We were not able to maintain contact with Barbara in the last three months before her death; thus, we have no first-hand information from her perspective about this end-time. We learned from family members after her death that her family felt shut out and not involved in the decision making during much of this time—and that the consequences were serious: Lack of adequate home nursing care resulted in two extended hospital admissions. There were conflicts within the family over where she should be during her last days and how aggressive her care should be. Until family members intervened, there had been no planning for her children's future after her death.

Both Kitty and Barbara held onto hopes for a longer life until just weeks before they died and made little apparent preparation or plans on their own for their actual end-of-life care. As a consequence of their basic stance of not giving in or acknowledging death's coming, neither of them discussed with others or planned for the care they would need as they neared death.

Unanticipated Choices and Decisions

Each terminal illness has an expected trajectory. Although physicians cannot say with certainty when death will come, the inexorable progression of symptoms as the body's organs are affected and "shut down" is well understood. Study participants who wanted to know what lay ahead for them found out and planned accordingly. Yet there may be twists and turns on the path of a terminal illness that nobody can predict. Two participants in our study provided examples of unanticipated events, resulting in the need to make choices for which they could not have planned.

Importance of "Full Knowledge" in Making Unexpected Decisions

Roberta's family confronted the sudden need to absorb a large amount of new technical medical information, understand it, and make decisions that were right for them—within hours and days. This information was more difficult because it was not what they had expected, based on their understanding of their mother's heart condition.

Once Roberta was "declared hospice" and palliative care had begun, her daughter Debbie planned to keep her at home until she died and was assured by Roberta's physician and by hospice that this was possible—that Roberta shouldn't have to be hospitalized again. Avoiding the hospital was the paramount goal of Debbie's planning for her mother's end-of-life care.

Yet Roberta *was* hospitalized again, despite her daughter's plans. The first time, in September (two months before death), Roberta became dehydrated suddenly and was admitted overnight to correct it. In October, she had a sudden blood pressure drop, and the hospice nurse "wanted to know if the doctor could look at her at the hospital." Roberta said she didn't want to go, and Debbie decided that they would see what they could do at home, with the assistance of hospice, to correct it. Debbie considered the anxiety and distress Roberta might experience in the hospital a threat to the quality of her life, even though trying to treat her at home might risk shortening her life.

Because of the nurse's concern, Roberta's physician insisted that she come into the office for an X-ray. The strain of leaving the house to go to the physician's office was such that Roberta's daughter, a week later, was adamant in telling us,

> I decided that we would never do this again to her . . . to go through the routine of seeing a doctor, or the hospital, unless it's really, really important.

Despite Debbie's clear decision not to hospitalize Roberta for tests or treatment for her heart after the October incident, another choice of whether or not

to hospitalize—and to treat—was presented to the family for an entirely different reason. Again, the family had to consider choosing between quantity and
quality of life.

In November, Roberta got up at night and fell when her hip fractured. In
great pain, she was taken immediately to the hospital. The family initially
chose surgery for a modified hip replacement, even though they regarded this
decision as a "hard choice": Without surgery, Roberta could not sit up and
would remain in constant pain—a truly diminished quality of life. The surgery
would be a major stress to a weak heart and system, however, and might result
in shortening her life. In making decisions to respond to this unanticipated
event, Debbie stressed that her choices were made easier because she received
what she felt was "full knowledge" about the choices available:

> At the hospital, when the nurse was talking with the orthopedic
> surgeon about Mom's condition, I saw this, that other options were
> being presented to us and to Mom. I was just . . . I was just
> overwhelmed. I could see what was happening and I thought,
> "Wow, I've got to be open-minded about this stuff, as far as
> listening to what really is available and knowing what the choices
> were. . . . I had no idea.

≈ ≈ ≈

> She [the hospice nurse] gave me a picture of the whole thing,
> instead of saying, like the doctors, "This is what we're going to do."
> It was more detailed and in depth, and I felt comfortable with full
> knowledge. I felt much more comfortable after I heard all this.

Roberta's own physician, as well as the surgeon, also was part of the family's decision process. He counseled waiting a day to conduct more tests and to
be sure her vital signs were stable. Debbie spoke of being "taken aback" by the
marked differences in medical opinions being presented: "go ahead with
surgery immediately" and "better wait to see how she is doing." Debbie said,
"I was really weighing things carefully again." In this period between the early
Monday morning admission after Roberta's hip fractured and Wednesday
morning [the day scheduled for the surgery], her kidneys failed. Her daughters
took this as "a clear message": "I think the choice was made for us." They were
no longer faced with the unsatisfactory choice between "quality" of life or
"quantity."

When kidney failure was confirmed, the family was asked whether they
wanted to choose Hospice House, home care with hospice, or a nursing home
for her final days. Roberta's physician did not suggest leaving her in the hos-

pital. The family chose home care. "There were no other choices," as Debbie put it. Roberta was brought home in traction to allow her to rest more comfortably with the broken hip. She died the next evening, in peace and comfort for herself and her family.

During Roberta's last week, Debbie's conversations with us revolved around the "hard choices" facing her family. Before her mother's death as well as afterwards, Debbie voiced her concern about whether "doing surgery right away" would have helped. But she felt satisfied with her mother's care despite the crisis, and she felt a sense of peace with her mother's death. Debbie stressed the importance to her of having information from trusted sources whom she already knew: the hospice nurse and her mother's long-time physician, who were very open and willing to listen to her, to hear her concerns, and to answer her questions.

As exacerbations of symptoms occur, patients and families are confronted with new choices about further treatment, even when they have made the general choice of palliative care. Palliative treatment, which is designed to comfort and improve the quality of life, encompasses a very wide range of care—and still involves choices and decisions.

Unanticipated Outcomes and New Choices

Sarah also faced a decision for which she and her caregiver were totally unprepared. After Sarah had been living for about four years in a senior residence center, her doctor determined that she could no longer manage her own medication schedule and other daily activities and suggested that she "would be good for the other patients at Hospice House." Sarah willingly moved there in June 1997 and told us, on our initial visit with her, "This is my home now." But this was not to be. By November 1997, Sarah's condition appeared to improve, and hospice finally asked that she move somewhere else. Sarah's daughter Karen told us that the doctor gave her the news gently: "Your mom can be moved."

When Sarah entered Hospice House, her condition was considered to be clearly terminal. Karen reports that the doctor told her that Sarah's cancer cells then went into her blood and spread from there. She had a series of tumors on her spine, about which Karen told us:

> This last time, when they found the last tumors, the doctor said three big ones were wrapped around the spine. And I asked him, "Whoa, where it's near the spine, what's the prognosis?" And he looked at me and he just shook his head and said, "Karen, the average person, once the cancer is in the bone, takes maybe four months."

Sarah's physician, Karen, and possibly Sarah herself believed that Sarah would die at Hospice House, but she didn't. With hospice's attention to her medications for pain, she actually seemed to get better. Hospice House was not able to keep patients for long periods of time, so Karen had to find somewhere else for her mother to live. There was no room for her mother in her own home, and the search began again—five months after they thought everything was settled for good.

It was a bittersweet choice to make. Glad that Sarah was still alive but pained by the need to move her once again, Karen sought out several afford-able nursing homes. High-quality nursing homes cost two to three times the amount of Sarah's benefits. The first two places they tried were unsatisfactory. Karen reports that these places tried to keep her mother in bed all day, whereas her doctor wanted her up and walking as much as possible.

> We found out they really were trying to push the dope on Mom. You know, "Let's give her a pill for this. Let's give her a pill for that."

Other places had different problems. Sarah's normal optimism and cheer-fulness dissolved. She cried a lot. Karen couldn't stand it. She finally located a home that was licensed for personal care that took in eight women (most with dementia) who did not require twenty-four-hour nursing care. The atmosphere was friendly. The home was clean and nicely appointed. We visited Sarah there and found that she was much like her old self again.

But Karen's problems were not over. This home charged more than her mother's social security benefits. Without hospice service, Karen also had to find a way to pay for her mother's expensive medications. Meanwhile, Sarah's cancer benefits had run out, and she could not get any more reimbursements for another five months. Karen reported, "I'm getting a little panicky."

Unanticipated choices often are a central part of the care of patients with incurable illnesses. In Sarah's case, the major unanticipated event was that Sarah kept on living much longer than anyone anticipated—the result of her strong determination to live and possibly the good care and nurturing envi-ronment she enjoyed at Hospice House.

Planning for Medical Treatment

We have distinguished in this study between planning for care at the end of life and specific planning for end-of-life medical treatment, most popularly con-veyed in the form of advance directives. Advance directives include legal documents such as "living wills" and DPOAs for health care, DNR orders on hospital charts, and the Comfort One designation used in Montana to alert emergency medical technicians not to resuscitate terminally ill patients who have suffered cardiovascular arrest at home or in public. There is increasing interest in having every adult engage in such planning for the medical treatment at the end of life. The rationale is that such planning will help to ensure quality of life for persons with terminal or sudden life-threatening illness or injury who are subsequently unable to make their wishes known.

Understanding how participants viewed their choices requires exploring what they actually knew. In contrast to their planning for their care, their choice of medical treatment or nontreatment was less a matter of deliberate planning than of making decisions when a choice was offered to them. This group of study participants is somewhat unusual, in that seven of them had chosen or been recommended for hospice care early in their trajectory of terminal illness, rather than in their last month of life. Their choice of hospice was their primary means of advance planning, from their perspective.

Several different conversations with Connie—whose sister Sharon, a woman in her seventies, was dying of emphysema—reflect a typical attitude about end-of-life care for those who saw hospice care as a form of advance planning:

Connie: Sharon was just having a really hard time breathing, and I called her doctor, and she shocked me with a question, "Is it time for hospice?" And I said, "Oh no. We're not ready for that." But as I thought about that, I decided, if she's eligible for hospice, that's her decision, not mine, to make. So that's how that came about.

Researcher: How did Sharon react to that?

Connie: I think [clears throat] she's given death a lot of thought before that and didn't expect to live this long. But her reaction was greater than I expected. I thought she believed she was near the end of her life anyway. But to be told that is a little different. She began to do some things right away, she began to act as though the end was imminent, any day now. And so she began to do some things that she wanted to take care of before she died.

Researcher: This whole process of advance directives, about what kind of care she would want when she's dying . . . being taken to the hospital if she has a cardiac

	arrest. . . . all these things that can happen. Does hospice have somebody talk to you?
Connie:	Yes. They go over that.
Researcher:	Sharon had a living will, and she'd made some plans?
Connie:	Right.
Researcher:	Did she give anyone a durable power of attorney?
Connie:	Yes. We were supposed to take care of that, and we didn't. We had the papers and never did get them signed. It's just something we put off. But she had communicated everything to her doctor and to the hospice people.
Researcher:	It doesn't sound like there were any problems with that.
Connie:	No, no, not at all.
Researcher:	So there weren't any differences within her family, her children, about what kind of care?
Connie:	No. I think everybody was prepared. When she first went into hospice, from then on I think there was an acceptance of it and awareness that it was coming. . . .

∾ ∾ ∾

Connie:	[An infection] is what they're expecting. That's what they're counting on.
Researcher:	So that would be something Sharon wouldn't expect them to try to fight aggressively, or you wouldn't?
Connie:	At this point she says no.

All of the participants had DNRs and/or living wills—including the two who had not chosen hospice care (Dennis and Barbara) but had experienced several serious hospitalizations. They had these DNRs and living wills largely because the hospitals, hospice, nursing homes, physicians, had brought up the need for such instruments and encouraged patients to sign them. But the participants differed widely in their knowledge and attitudes about what they had done and their willingness and ability to make choices about end-of-life care. This variation highlights the crucial distinction between simply signing a piece of

Table 3-1   Patient Choices

	Hospice	DNR/Comfort One	Living Will	DPOA-Health
Barbara	No	Yes	Yes	No
Dennis	No	Yes	Yes	No
Kitty	Yes	Yes	Yes	No
Mabel	Yes	Yes	Yes	Yes
Ralph	Yes	Yes	Yes	Yes
Roberta	Yes	Yes	Yes	Yes
Sarah	Yes	No	Yes	No
Sharon	Yes	Yes	Yes	No
Walt	Yes	Yes	Yes	Unknown

paper about a hypothetical event and having thoughtfully considered and shared one's preferences with family, physicians, and other caregivers.

In terms of specific planning for end-of-life medical treatment, most of our participants had made a choice for hospice care; thus, they and their families had been through some kind of discussion about the meaning of palliative care and had agreed with the consequences for their medical treatment. Table 3-1 displays such planning.

What is most instructive in all of the conversations we analyzed was the lack of interest or concern about living wills and DNR orders, relative to other concerns. Among younger or healthier people, there is often an interest in "making sure I don't live on as a vegetable," but our participants did not seem particularly worried about this possibility. Patients and families appeared to feel that choosing hospice took care of any advance directives about medical treatment. They did not bring up the topic until specifically asked—one indication that it wasn't of much concern to them.

Our participants were not always clear about the meaning of specific terms such as "Comfort One" or "advanced directive." They didn't engage in much conversation about these instruments because they did not seem to know much about what they were. Kitty said:

> I've got a Comfort One pamphlet taped to the refrigerator, but I don't know what it is. I don't know. It's just up there, and I don't know whether one of the hospice gals put it up there for me or what.

Others knew what specific terms such as "living will" meant, but not the more generic term:

Researcher:	Does the term "advance directive" mean anything to you?
Sarah:	Advance directive?
Researcher:	Things like, well, some people sign things that say "If I'm a vegetable, do not resuscitate me."
Sarah:	Oh, we've got a living will..

∾ ∾ ∾

Researcher:	Have you gone through advanced care planning, advance directives with your doctor?
Kitty:	No. I think he asked me, and I said, "I just presumed I'd die in my sleep in my bed." And he said, "Most of us do feel that way, but it doesn't always work."
Researcher:	Related to this advance directives thing, since you live alone right now, is there anyone that you designate to speak for you? If you had another blackout, ended up in the hospital, couldn't manage for yourself, do you choose someone as a kind of care planner?
Kitty:	Kind of a living will sort of thing you mean? Oh, the doctor has one, my lawyer has one, the church office has one. I've got them scattered all over the place.

Some caregivers were equally unsure about palliative care:

Researcher:	Did your doctor ever talk with you about what palliative care means, or explain the kind of—
Sandy:	No.
Researcher:	—care that goes on in the medical field?
Sandy:	Yeah, Yeah. You know, I know I've read the word palliative, but I don't really know what it means.

∾ ∾ ∾

Researcher:	Can you explain what you think palliative care is?

Connie: I understand that to mean, care for the dying in the last period of life. I think of as just making the dying a better quality.

Other caregivers, such as Barbara's husband, Dan, clearly recognized that they had discussed and agreed to no heroic measures to keep someone alive:

Researcher: Have you gone through any discussions about advanced . . . what advance directives mean? Agreed upon plans for the last days? Like "do not resuscitate"?

Dan: Oh yeah. We've got that all written down there. We got that, um, is that a living will?

Researcher: Do you remember how you define that?

Dan: Yeah, No resuscitation please. Nothing where she could have a bunch of . . . you know, she just doesn't want to be a vegetable. No way.

An Example of the Effect of Advanced Care Planning for Medical Treatment on Last-Minute Decision Making

Our data appear to suggest that some people began planning for the eventuality of their dying long before death—usually because of a serious health event or emergency in which they thought they might, or actually did, come close to death. Having experienced the psychological reality of this event aided them in making clear plans, involving their families and probable caregivers, in decisions concerning living wills, DNRs, and DPOAs for health care.

Roberta's experience is a good example of how earlier serious episodes provided her and her family with opportunities to discuss medical treatment well before she was diagnosed as terminally ill. These opportunities helped her family—her daughter Debbie, in particular—become comfortable with the decisions they would have to make at the end. Closer to Roberta's death, when Roberta grew frightened and very anxious about dying, their earlier planning and decisions held firm. Because they had discussed their concerns much earlier, Roberta's daughters did not feel guilty or pressured to try to extend her life.

Debbie explained that her mother's had been asked to sign DNR orders several years earlier. Roberta had been very anxious about death all of her life; she was unwilling to go to funerals and unwilling to talk about death with her husband before he died. According to Debbie, however, an encounter with an emergency room physician early on in her illness had helped Roberta to make an initial decision regarding medical treatment:

One time we had her in the hospital when her heart was fibrillating. The emergency room doctor said to me during her examination, "Does she have a Do Not Resuscitate?" And it shocked Mom terribly. She didn't feel like she was any where near this state, to be considered terminal. And she said, "Of course you resuscitate me. Of course you do." And Mom was totally upset with that suggestion. Well, that was the first time she talked about it. [But] after that she didn't really argue about it. She wanted [it], and yet it kind of shocked her.

∼ ∼ ∼

Before she had gotten to the point where she wasn't able to take care of herself, we had talked about this. In fact, this is the third "Do Not Resuscitate" order she has signed in the last eight or nine years. In the hospital the first time, about eight years ago, her heart started doing funny things, and at that point she decided that "Do Not Resuscitate" would be the thing to do because she didn't want to ever linger.

These early conversations before Roberta became seriously ill clearly helped her daughter deal with her mother's increased anxiety at the very end of her life, when her dementia was interfering more with her reasoning. During her last few months, her daughter reports:

One side of her was saying, "I don't want to do this." So as time went by, the fact that she would have to accept her death, by saying "Do Not Resuscitate," was bothering her a lot.

The doctor pursued this with her at the hospital last time. And Mom was frightened about this "Do Not Resuscitate," frightened of not being saved. I was kind of sorry that this was broached, because Mom just doesn't feel this way right now. I just tell her we want to do whatever she needs.

Age clearly is a factor in encouraging planning for medical treatment at the end of life because advanced age usually provides more opportunities for near-death events. After such events, patients and physicians alike may be more willing or find it easier to bring up the subject the next time. Dying is not just the enemy—which may still be vanquished for the next 30 years by the doctor's science and art—but more like a neighbor, waiting quietly around the corner for another opportunity to come over and stay.

Roberta's family also had a DPOA for health care that they executed when they were unable to find her living will after she was admitted to the hospital, six months before her death. Debbie reported:

We have the durable power of attorney. She had a living will, a long time ago. The durable power of attorney we had decided on last spring. She was comfortable with that. The reason we did have one for Mom is because we couldn't find her living will . . . and the living will was later found, at a doctor's office!

The final decision that Roberta's daughter had to make—in the twenty-four hours before her mother's death—was whether to ask for an IV line to provide fluids. Again, her reasoning about this choice was affected by her knowledge of her mother's preferences when she was still mentally alert:

That night I got this harebrained idea. I thought, "Why do we think that her kidneys are failing? How do we know this for sure? Why don't we give her an IV? Why can't we give her some kind of something to make sure that she's, you know, not shutting down?" I really wanted to do everything I could to help sustain some more life in her. And I was having a real difficult time adjusting to this possibility that she wasn't functioning, that I'm not doing anything to help her. It was hard.

Debbie's last-minute internal struggle and doubt may be common for caregivers, as families confront unanticipated choices during the last moments of life. In this case, Debbie's earlier opportunities to talk with her mother—and the knowledge that her mother did trust her to make decisions she couldn't make for herself—helped Debbie resolve her doubts without lingering guilt. In an after-death interview, Debbie expressed her comfort with her mother's death and with the family's decisions concerning her care.

Implications

Among our study participants, having living wills or DNR orders was not consistently correlated with their preferred end-of-life care. In fact, there may be no easy connection at all for a patient between engaging in hypothetical decisions about specific medical treatments and being willing or able to talk with family and physician about what one *does* want. As described above, Walt and Ralph had spent much time and effort with their families talking and deciding how they would live out their lives: finding good care, help for caregivers, a beautiful setting in which to live, settling financial concerns. They had DNR orders and had completed advance directives such as living wills. Others in our study, such as Barbara and Kitty, also had living wills and DNRs but apparently had not engaged in planning or decision making concerning actual end-of-life care—or made decisions that avoided stress for those closest to them.

Influence of Finances on Planning and Choices

Worries

Although Ralph and his caregiver Sandy had engaged in helpful financial planning, they were not immune to worries. Ralph told us, "When you're only making Social Security, you don't live very fast." Sandy reported that when she was about to start receiving her own pension, Ralph still worried about expenses:

> I told him, "I can bear some of this cost myself and we'll be all right." But he still frets about the cost. He was a little put out, though, when I got my Social Security because it was more than his.

Sarah also had strong worries about the cost of her illness. When she had to leave Hospice House, she said:

> I don't know how much—I can't stay here much longer 'cause the money's going down so fast. I had insurance when my husband died and that's what I'm on now. I think it runs out this spring. So I'll have to do something. I don't know what yet.

If Sarah was concerned about finances, her daughter was even more concerned. According to Karen, Sarah was not totally aware of how her care was being financed:

> Us girls are just gonna make up the difference of what she's short in her checks. We decided we wouldn't get Christmas presents for each other, and we'll just put it on mom's care.

Four months later, after Sarah had moved from Hospice House to the private home, her expenses escalated, and Karen said:

> I don't know what I'm gonna do. We haven't told Mom. She gets less than it costs to stay in there. And we're paying for her medicines plus what she's short on the rent. Her cancer benefits just ran out, and she isn't able to get any more till August. I'm getting a little panicky. Every day I sit and I try to figure out what I'm gonna do but I'm out of my money. There's places that might be okay but, gosh, two-three thousand a month. Very few can do that.

Barbara, who was younger and did not have retirement benefits or Medicare, had even more worries about finances; she and her husband were close to bankruptcy after six years of her illness:

We were really at a point in May of having a very difficult discussion about whether to file bankruptcy or not. We do not receive any type of assistance outside of my job and insurance other than Missoula County Cancer [the local American Cancer Society chapter]. They pay medication. They pay 20 percent of medication, up to a certain dollar amount. They have bought me a couple of wigs in the last six years. That's the type of assistance we received. So it doesn't matter if there's two weeks left before my next paycheck and we might need food. We don't qualify for nothing. That's a real stress issue. If you have what looks like a legitimate full paycheck coming in, society believes that everything is okay even though you can't see in the door. I mean it's an illusion. When you look at the number of bills that you're paying, it's extraordinary—with the hospital, the clinic, the radiologist, the pathologist, the home health care, the solutions, the psychiatry. And then you look at what your family needs, if they have a problem. My daughter is in need of dental work. And you know that's like my priority. And she's not covered by any insurance. And I don't want her teeth to crumble in her mouth. And so I've got to look into that and see if I can come up with something, even a payment plan or something. But dental work is very expensive.

$\sim \ \sim \ \sim$

Everybody has a different financial picture, and we were at a point of should we just give up? Dump it legally? I really felt very strongly that I didn't want to file bankruptcy because I had come and worked so hard to get to a certain point and now give that all up. I realize that sometimes it's a pride thing; you reach a point where you may have to let go of that for your family's sake.

Selling Off Property

One common way that our study participants managed to survive financially was to sell off their property. Ralph's caregiver Sandy told us that early in Ralph's illness they began to sell things:

He used to have a little J3 Piper Cub. . . . And then of course he had to sell it because that was one of the first things to go. And he hated that. If he'da had his way, he'da hung onto it till he was gone, you know.

Sarah also told us that she had to sell things to keep afloat financially. One of the first things she had to do after her husband died was to sell their house:

> I just couldn't keep it up. By then it was an older house, and everything was going wrong. We had to put in a new toilet and all that stuff. And I was pretty broke by then. Didn't have much money. Then I started selling stuff. We had to hook into the sewer then. You had to. There was no choice. So I started selling stuff to get money, enough to live on. But it all worked out all right with what's comin' in each month. I never had much left over, but it reaches if you stretch hard enough.

Loss of Income

Financial needs also caused some caregivers and family members to quit their jobs to care for their loved ones. Roberta's son-in-law stopped working for this purpose. Barbara's husband did the same. In one of our early visits, Barbara brought the subject up in the context of their recent purchase of a bungalow where Barbara would be more comfortable on one floor:

> Let me throw one out at you that I think is important: the financial issue of who's working and who's not when there's a terminal illness. My husband left a very good truck driving job to be home now as my caregiver. He was almost penalized by the real estate agent because he wasn't working. Society demands that the man be the wage earner, not the woman. And here I am, still working. I've got a sick leave pool, etc. That's a real issue.

As their financial condition grew worse, Barbara's husband tried to go back to work but found it difficult to do. In a separate visit, he told us about the problem:

> Twice I got called home because of Barbara's illness, and now they won't hire me back because of her condition. Won't let me go out on the road because they don't want to have to send me home every week. And now I can't get a job with another company because of my job history with the first company. I have to put that down because I need to show experience. You know they call and they say, "Well, his wife has this and this," and it just doesn't work. I don't know what to do.

Unpaid Debts

Our study participants also described the debts they had piled up because of the illness. Barbara hypothesized what she would say if she ever met a potential benefactor:

> "We have this family and they've got $5,000 in clear debt. They'll lose their car." [In fact we already have lost ours; it was a '93.] "And they can't pay their rent. What is the possibility of a donation? This is a clear hardship case. They don't qualify for public assistance or anything."

Barbara's frustration was clear in her own reaction to the above hypothetical conversation:

> I would be very interested to find out if their benefactor-heart goes that direction, as opposed to getting their name on a plaque at an institution. If we didn't have someone give to us a couple thousand dollars the first of June, we would've gone under.

Barbara described one other financial scrape that she and her husband had recently faced:

> I almost feel that it's very ironic that I can spend 25 days in the hospital—and I really like that hospital; I appreciate it—and my insurance company pays 100 percent because I'm at that point of stop-loss benefits and they'll pay 100 percent of my care there. And I see the printouts that they send me of what they've paid. And it goes over $103,000 for that amount of care. And they turn me in to the collection agency for $142. And they write me letters, they're nagging me. My husband told them, when he started managing, that instead of paying $50 a month or $100 a month, it's gonna have to go down to $25. I was just looking at the notice from the Missoula Credit Bureau. It impacts me immensely because they tell you that it doesn't go on your credit report, but yet it does. To the hospital, and I think you know, it doesn't matter. It's all about money. And you need their care, and it's a legitimate bill, legally, and it's got to be paid, but not instead of feeding your child.

Seemingly little things, such as household repairs, can become large stumbling blocks to patients with very limited resources. Mabel's refrigerator broke down at about the time her caregiver/daughter, Bernice, was to get medical treatment for herself. Then the car needed a new oil pan. As a result, Bernice never got the treatment she needed. Her mother's care came first.

Kitty explained to us more than once that she had no financial stresses. In one of our visits she said:

> No, I don't have any problems. Eventually, I suppose, I might run into some difficulty as far as money goes. Eventually. Eventually. But right now my finances are fine because I haven't had to put out very much.

Yet in our after-death visit with a friend, we were told a quite different story:

> When Kitty got in the wreck, we found out that she had no driver's license, no insurance. She and I have always been friends. So I was the one she called. And it looked like she was gonna be fined in the thousands, so we got that taken care of. Then I looked at her checkbook. And had a fellow parishioner who is an accountant examine it. But she was in trouble way before that. But we didn't know it.

What Helped

The seven participants who were on hospice all, in one way or another, gave hospice the credit for saving them from financial ruin. Connie reported to us that her sister, Sharon, saw hospice as the only way she could afford her medications:

> I guess what we saw as the primary advantage to start with was the fact that it would take over her medication. She doesn't have insurance for medication, so that was a real expense, just a terrible expense for her. So, we thought, that just from that standpoint it would be useful to have hospice.

Roberta's caregiver, Debbie, said essentially the same thing:

> The doctor declared mother hospice so that (expense) is taken care of, thank goodness.

Ralph gave the credit to hospice and Social Security. Walt credited his Pipes, Trades, and Trust insurance, in addition to hospice, with saving his family from financial doom. Dennis, who was not receiving hospice care, credited Indian

Health and Medicare with protecting him financially. His mother confirmed this assessment in an after-death visit:

> What Medicare doesn't pick up, then Indian Health would. So we did have that luxury of not having to worry about financial things. His Fentanyl and antibiotics and that ran, oh gosh, somewhere around thousands and thousands.

Barbara, like Dennis, was not on hospice, nor did she have any clear understanding about how hospice worked:

> I have a concern about hospice. I know what I've read. I have concerns because it is expensive and it shouldn't be. Why have it if one can't afford it?

By the end of the study, Sarah and Mabel could no longer qualify for hospice services under the Medicare Hospice benefit, and they and their children faced considerable future financial burdens.

Planning and Choices in the Subculture of Terminally Ill Participants

Although planning is essential, the end of life often contains surprises. There are always unexpected events, and even the best plans cannot anticipate every eventuality. Most of the study participants—those who planned carefully and those who did not—encountered surprises at the end and found that there are limits to the decisions they could make in advance. Some of the surprises were only minimal, others were shattering.

- Dennis talked frequently about consciousness, about being aware, and he and his mother apparently expected that Dennis would be conscious and able to say "goodbye" to her at the moment of death. His final comatose state led to a quiet, early morning death, with his mother in the other room.

- Ralph had always planned to live out his life on his ranch, not in the "big city" of Missoula. After Ralph and Sandy moved to Missoula, they expected, from all they were told, that Ralph would slip into a coma at the end. Instead, he had a "bleed-out" [gastrointestinal hemorrhage] and became delusional and paranoid, suspicious of everyone, and had to be sedated and moved to Hospice House for his last days.

- Roberta's daughters expected their mother to die peacefully at home of congestive heart failure. Neither they nor their hospice nurse could have predicted that her hip would fracture and that she would be hospitalized for hip replacement surgery the week she died.

- Sarah planned to live out her days at Hospice House. She didn't plan on getting better, becoming more stable, and having to leave Hospice House and the hospice program for more than a year. (She lived long enough to reenter hospice care for the last few months of her life, and she died at Hospice House.)

- Kitty planned to die at home, alone, "like an animal." She may even have tried to hasten her death by pulling out the PIK IV line the day she was moved to Hospice House. She died at Hospice House, rather than in her own home.

- Barbara admitted that she didn't know what to plan for. But she apparently believed that she would be able to maintain control and make her own decisions until her last day of life. Her eventual decline and incapacity led to family conflicts and removed decision making from her own hands.

Death, like birth, seems to be an experience that is full of surprises and sometimes unexpected twists in the road. Only Walt and Sharon had the deaths they might have envisioned and had been led to expect.

At some point control becomes impossible for the dying person because death, by definition, entails loss of control. Thus, our observations suggest that everyone who is facing death needs a trusted family member or friend who can make good decisions when increasing dementia, immobility, or medications limit one's judgment. Unlike Walt and Ralph, neither Barbara nor Kitty had trusted family caregivers who could or would make plans for their care as they were dying.

There is another reason for having a surrogate decision maker appointed early in the course of a terminal illness. There is an inherent cognitive difficulty in making plans for two opposing possibilities at the same time—that one may live another two years and that one may not last three months. For many patients, retaining hope that life will continue is essential. Consciously asking someone else to take charge of planning for if, or when, life doesn't continue may be the only way to avoid the conflict. Patients with cancer and their physicians emphasize the role of hope as a prime source of lengthening life or even bringing about a complete remission, particularly in younger patients. In such circumstances, a family member may be better able than the patient to take on the task of planning and guiding decision making if treatments fail.

Intensified medical treatment, medication, therapy, and other services can be expected to bring additional financial stress to most people. Walt's and Ralph's experiences offer evidence that careful financial planning can at least reduce some of the financial burden of dying. In Ralph's case, the solution was simply finding an affordable, handicapped-accessible apartment. In Walt's case, it was a matter of improving the physical location for his final care and at the same time solving the issues of inheritance and making life easier for his caregiver and his children.

The fragile social networks of terminally ill patients can be solidified—as attested by Sharon, Kitty, Walt, and other patients who chose to stay at home during their last months. Ralph's decision to move into Missoula for accessibility to medical treatment and hospice help was a decision to cut himself off from his friends back home in the Swan. Sarah had the outgoing, pleasant personality that enabled her to extend her social network wherever she happened to be. Dennis chose to have a very tight social network, with his mother as the center of his last months of life and very few others around him. Dennis appeared to work more on his inward development than on social connections at the end.

Comfort is a relative term. One could hardly say that our participants had any conventional sense of physical comfort; but under the circumstances some seemed to achieve more comfort than others. Physical discomfort is to be expected, but emotional and spiritual comfort are still available to those who work at getting it. For example, Walt was confined to bed 99 percent of the time. But at least it was his own bed in his own home. As he himself pointed out, his worst problem was boredom, not physical discomfort.

Ralph's constant struggle for breath and the loss of his beloved surroundings certainly were not socially comfortable for him, but he would have had physical discomfort in any other context, so he opted for a place that could offer the most help for it. This choice was the best he could do. Transplanted, he achieved the physical comfort of having hospice care and a doctor nearby. Even then, Sandy and Ralph were comfortable enough in their handicapped-accessible apartment overlooking the Clark Fork River. In fact, they often celebrated their good fortune in having that home.

The inevitable conclusion is that most dying patients will have to surrender their former mobility. Only two of our participants could walk more than a few steps. Most were in wheelchairs or needed walkers. Caregivers for those in wheelchairs found transporting their loved ones, even for doctor visits, very difficult.

Sandy finally decided that trucking Ralph for two-hour trips to and from Missoula was more than either of them could take. Carrie managed to drive her son, Dennis, on the one-hour trip to see his doctor in Missoula on a weekly basis for many months. Karen, Sarah's daughter, lived far enough outside town that she had to take a half-day of her busy schedule to see that her mother got to scheduled appointments with her doctor. Loss of mobility in the patient led to multiple increased demands on their caregivers to replace this diminished quality of life.

Chapter 4

Professional Care and Doctor-Patient Communication

Participants Talk about Professional Care

We do not attempt here to evaluate or even discuss the quality of care provided by doctors, nurses, and other medical professionals. When the patients and caregivers brought up the subject of their professional care, however, we listened and recorded what they told us, in the spirit of ethnographic research. We make no claim about the accuracy of what they reported to us, but, like so many other things, subjective reactions turn out to be guideposts for potential changes. We also paid attention to the participants' reports of and reactions to what their professional caregivers said to them about their illness, as well as the choices that they were given. We report on some aspects of communication in chapter 3. In this chapter we report on conversations concerning participants' professional care because these conversations also were important to those involved in the process.

To provide a framework for understanding the perspectives of the participants, we first provide a summary of their professional care settings and caregivers during the last year of their life—or from the time they received a terminal diagnosis (see Table 4-1). This table includes the type of physician(s) who treated them; the home health care services they had, including hospice care; and the length of time individual health professionals were involved. This summary is based on their conversations with us; it does not reflect their medical records or include specialists and other medical personnel they may have seen but did not mention to us. It is meant to provide only a general context for understanding the patient and family perspective and their comments concerning professional care.

Table 4-1   Profile of Professional Care

Patient	Care Settings	Health Care Personnel	Contact/Length
Dennis	Home:	Oncologist and staff	Outpatient, weekly for 6 years
		Home health nurses	Various, weekly for 12 months
Barbara	Home:	Oncologist [moved away]	Outpatient and hospital, 6 years
	Hospital—several weeks:	New oncologist	Outpatient and hospital, 6 months
		Home health nurses	Weekly IV, same nurses 2 years
	Hospice/Hospice House:	Hospice nurse/staff	Last 4 days of life
Ralph	Missoula apartment:	Brother's physician	Outpatient, referred hospice
		Hospice nurse	Weekly, 16 months
		Hospice physician	Periodic home visits, 16 months
Sharon	Sister's home:	Physician 2+ years	Outpatient, home visit
		Hospice nurse	Weekly, 5 months
Walt	Home:	Physician	Outpatient, hospital, 10 years
		Hospice nurse	Weekly, 12 months
		Hospice physician	Occasional visits
Sarah	Physician's office:	Physician/oncologist	Outpatient, many years
	Hospice House:	Hospice House staff	Daily, 4 months' residence
	Board and care home:	Home health aides	Weekly personal care

Table continues on facing page.

Table 4-1 (*continued*)   Profile of Professional Care

Patient	Care Settings	Health Care Personnel	Contact/Length
Kitty	Physician's office:	Oncologist	Outpatient, every 3 weeks
	Home:	Hospice nurse	Weekly, last 7 months
		Home health nurses	Daily, various staff, 2–3 months
	Hospice House:	Hospice House staff	Last 3 weeks of life
Mabel	Home/Physician's office:	Oncologist	Outpatient, home visits
		Hospice nurse	14 months
		Home health service	Monthly nurse visits after hospice ended
Roberta	Physician's office:	Physician	Outpatient
	Daughter's home:	Health aide (private)	Daily, last 6 months
	Hospital:	Physician/surgeon	3 days
		Hospice nurse	Weekly, last 6 months

"He's as gentle as can be": Dennis and Carrie

Patients and caregivers alike had nothing but praise for their doctors, nurses, social workers, hospice staff, and others who helped them at this difficult time. For example, Dennis related:

> Everybody who's been involved in my care and with my treatments has been wonderful. I've met some really wonderful people through the health care process. My doctor has really been very close with me in being able to tell me things. The other day he even went so far as to say, "If you lived in Missoula, I would come to your house rather than have you come in here because I know what a difficulty it is for you to travel."

Carrie echoed Dennis' sentiments:

> He's trying very hard. And he's so good. Gosh, he's wonderful.
> And he will tell it as it is. And you can tell that it's hard sometimes,
> but he's as gentle as he can be.

Because Dennis lived sixty miles away on traditional reservation lands and
could claim Native American ancestry, his care was included under the Indian
Health Care Plan:

> I have visitations from a nurse at least twice a week, and they take
> my vitals, change out my pain medication. And I'm also visited by a
> social worker. And I see them, if not every week, once a week, and
> they also have provided a housekeeper that comes in, spells my
> mother, because Mom puts in a lot of time. We've really had an
> ordeal with that. It's been terrible because we haven't been able to
> have any consistency with the housekeeping part.

Finding good housekeeping help for Dennis was not Carrie's only problem.
Even when he was hospitalized at various times, Carrie, using her everyday
experience taking care of her son, had to help the trained medical people with
Dennis's care:

> They had to experiment in the hospital in Seattle because he was in
> a terrible, terrible way. He was on a special flotation bed for burn
> victims. And it took a team of eight the first day. Then I was able to
> be with them for the next days. They had to lift a mattress cover and
> it had been allowed to stick to him, on his lesions. He had lesions so
> terrible on his back. Well, I figured how to use a rolled pillow so
> that nothing would touch them. But that was the only way he could
> be tended to. His lesions were so bad he couldn't even lather
> himself in the shower. So I'd mix a solution in a spray bottle of soap
> and spray it all over him, hair included. And then he could get in
> the shower and tolerate the pain. Like when he was taken to the
> hospital by ambulance in February. I drove there separately. When I
> walked in, two nurses were standing in his room asking me, "How
> do you handle him? What do you do? Show us." So it's like we've
> done a lot of pioneer work. The pharmacist at the hospital said to
> me, "You are very perceptive." It's a gift maybe that I have. The
> simplest thing that's used for one thing, I can see the possibilities of
> using it in another.

At one point, Dennis was admitted briefly to a hospital nearer to his home, "just to keep him on Fentanyl":

> When I got there, he was laying straight on regular sheets, no blue one underneath him. And I said to the male nurses there, "Oh God, give him one of those blue sheets." And they had to raise him up and put it down, 'cause otherwise the sheets would adhere to him like glue and they'd be ripping the hide off his skin.

The one thing that Dennis feared most was that at some point he might have to go to the hospital to die:

> If something happens, then they're just going to have to deal with my pain medication, and if I have to get 24-hour nursing, or constant nursing, then that's what I'll get. But the hospital atmosphere just [sighs] depresses me to no end. And I don't want to be there if that's going to be my dying place.

In July we asked Dennis if he really thought that he could get the kind of help he would need if he remained at home. He said:

> Yeah. I think I can. I haven't really investigated it. I suppose I should. But from what I understand, there is that type of, uh, help out there where they can stay most of the day and then they go to their homes at night and they're on call, so to speak. But it would put me more at ease to be in my own digs rather than in the hospital where, for one thing, you can't rest. And it's just not an atmosphere that's conducive to how I might want to pass away. You know, with sterile atmosphere and very cold.

In August, as Dennis's condition grew worse, outside of his presence Carrie reported that taking Dennis to Missoula twice a week for treatment was becoming more and more difficult:

> Last night his legs bothered him so bad that he couldn't even step over the tub to stand in the tub for me to give him a saline wash. He's been sleeping sitting up so his legs won't touch the recliner as it went backwards. The pain travels, and it gets unbelievable wherever it decides to be. So last night he said, "I don't even think I can get in the car to come to the doctor's," and so I said to him, "Why don't we go into the hospital now, and you can get your

blood transfusion in the hospital and you can at least get there?"
And he said, "I'm NOT going to the hospital!"

When we asked Carrie to describe some of her other inventions in the care
of Dennis, she told us:

> He had lesions on his rear end. And because of the muscle tissue
> would hurt if he would sit or stand. So I had a bed sheet that I
> would put over his clothing and have him flex the buttocks real
> hard, and then I would tie it, I'd roll it in a certain way, then tie it
> real tight, and it was like a girdle. I knew that he couldn't get into a
> girdle of any kind to give him support, so I just made one.

Dennis also was getting help from a psychiatrist in July, when we first began to
visit him:

> I do see a psychiatrist once a week now. I saw him last week, and
> I'll be seeing him again tomorrow. And he kind of gets me through
> those stumbling blocks about how this illness can be allowed and
> whether I deserve this. That type of thinking is more the child that
> is within me, not the person I am.

Dennis did not have hospice care, even at the very end of life. After Dennis
died, Carrie told us:

> Hospice was brought up all the time, and there was some reason
> why it wouldn't work out. It was because of the changeability of the
> schedule. Night and day meant nothing to us.

Carrie did not say more, but Dennis's insistence on pursuing any treatment
that might bring some remission of his disease clearly oriented him away from
seeking palliative care.

"She's a jewel": Barbara

Barbara had been seeing the same doctor since her cancer was diagnosed in
1991. She was very attached to him. He decided to make a career change and
moved away, however, just as she was released from the hospital and began a
new course of chemotherapy, six months before her death. Barbara was devas-
tated by this loss:

His last day was Friday. So I am now with a different doctor. I know him and I like him and I trust him. But I felt very sad. I got to say goodbye to him and write him a note, and I told him, "I'll really miss you." And he said, "I'll miss you too." Just a wonderful, dedicated man. I've seen him every single week since 1991. He seemed to want to be encouraging as opposed to discouraging. Because I did make it through a very difficult period. He continued to monitor me, even though I was under the surgeon's care. He made a decision that morphine wasn't good for me. He's a good person and he had a personal way about him, and I think that he gets to know people so much that it's a struggle. Oncology's hard.

Barbara also had very good things to say about the home health service that had provided home nursing care during her several acute crises over the years:

I've had two main nurses that have worked with me for two years now. One just left and moved to Spokane, because she could get, I guess, a better wage and more work there with IV therapy. And I was sad to see her go. She just became a friend of ours. The other nurse I like equally as well. She's a jewel.

We hear in Barbara's account the strong value of continuity of professional caregivers: "I've seen him every single week since 1991"; "for two years now"; "she became a friend"; "he continued to monitor me."

"We can't say enough about hospice": Ralph and Sandy

At the very beginning of our first visit with Ralph, he sang the praise of hospice:

I got people around me who would, you know, help some. That has worked out real good here for us with the people that's come in. They're people from the hospice society here. It was the doctors that mainly done it.

That's the reason we're here is on account of hospice. It's been just a wonderful thing. To start with, neither of us had ever experienced anything like this. We didn't know what to do, you know. This hospice, I think it's the greatest thing going. It's the help they give a person, showing you how and talking to you, telling you the ways to do some of this stuff and talking to these bigger outfits, you know. Yeah, I've sure learned a lot from this hospice outfit here. I mean I just can't say nothing bad about it. There's no way I can say anything bad about it. I can't say enough good.

Nor could Ralph "say enough good" about his hospice doctor. In late October, Ralph told us that the doctor had stopped in to see him on his way back from the airport:

He come in here, and he hadn't even been home yet. This guy come walkin' in, just knocked on the door and come walkin' in. I've thought of it on occasion. Stoppin' by when he came from the airport. Thought of me before his own family.

∿ ∿ ∿

The doctors tell me I'm about six years overdue now. They look at me and they figure, they don't know why I'm here, but I am. I was fortunate enough by lastin' so long, through this hospice thing, to have a lot more time to talk about, think about takin' care of things, the trees and animals and birds and fish and all that stuff.

The fact that Ralph managed to outlive the predictions of his terminal illness caused him some concern on behalf of his doctor, as reported by Sandy:

It's like the other day when the doctor was here, Ralph says to him because Medicare's been raising such a fit, investigating all these frauds and everything. He says, "Are they on to you because I've lasted this whole year when I should have been dead a year ago?" The doctor said, "I wish they would. I've wanted nothing more than one of them come out here and examine you and tell me you aren't dying."

From what Sandy reported to us, the hospice nurses apparently kept Ralph well informed about what to expect:

She's been tellin' Ralph for months that this was what was gonna happen to him. That eventually he would just get sleepier and sleepier and sleepier until one of these days he'll quit. She says, "Well, that's his disease. And the less air goes into your brain, the sleepier you get."

When we visited Sandy after Ralph's death, she also sang the praises of hospice:

Well, I'll tell you, I've been telling everybody who will listen about hospice and how wonderful it is and how it just makes everything so much easier.

Ralph also got physical therapy during his last months of life, as Sandy reported:

The therapy gal, he canceled her for a while 'cause he didn't feel like settin' up there, you know, lettin' her do that ultrasound. Well, now she's come back, so we're back to Thursday nights. Wednesday the Reiki guy comes back. The hospice nurse has been doin' Reiki while he's been gone. She took a class on it one weekend. So she's been doin' it while he was away, but when he comes back, he'll be comin' Wednesday morning at 10:00.

After Ralph's death, Sandy told us about how he appreciated Reiki and the harp music a hospice volunteer would play for him:

He tried the Chalice of Repose once, but he don't like that. He loved the harp music, but he hated the chanting. And the Reiki, he really looked forward to that.

"We're so lucky": Walt and Dorothy

Like the other participants on hospice care, Walt and Dorothy had nothing but deep appreciation and admiration for hospice, as they told us in our first visit with them:

Walt:	A volunteer comes once a week.
Dorothy:	Sometimes he comes three or four times a week.
Walt:	He stops in when he's got time.
Dorothy:	We don't have any regular hours either. Whenever he wants to come, he shows up. Doesn't make any difference. We're always here. Things don't change. They're absolutely wonderful. One came today—gave him a bath while I changed his bed. Our nurse is one in a million. I just can't ask for any better help in this world. They're all wonderful. And it's so nice not to have to worry about pain medications through them.

That really helps a lot when you have limited income. That helps an awfully lot. I just can't think of what we would do without them. I don't have to take him in to the doctor since he's been on hospice. The nurse takes care of that and talks to the doctor when we were having troubles. It's free, with your Medicare. The oxygen is furnished by them. His potty chair is furnished, and things like that.

A few days before Walt died, Dorothy was still singing the praises of hospice, this time referring to the hospice nurse:

Walt's comfortable. The hospice nurse made sure of that. She's sure wonderful. Gosh, we're so lucky to have someone like that to come in. She's a jewel.

In our after-death visit with Dorothy, she told us a bit more about how the hospice nurse helped Walt at the end:

The day he died, he talked to all the children, and then the hospice nurse came in. His temperature was high, his blood pressure was low, and we knew he was about gone. So she cleaned him up, and before she left she said, "Now Walt, it's time for you to think. If you want to go, you just go ahead and go." And he sighed a couple times and that was it. It was very nice. And then the hospice nurse came for me and took care of the situation and saw that the body was removed, and so it was very nice.

And Dorothy had still more to say about the advantages of hospice care:

We no longer had to take him to the doctor. I couldn't take him in much longer. Sometimes he would pass out in the doctor's office, you know. So it was a real blessing to us. And I can't say that a single one of the hospice workers that ever came out wasn't caring. The hospice nurse was a pure joy, and the bath girl was pure delight. He always looked forward to the two male volunteers that were his same age. Having people around that were his age was really supportive.

Walt no longer saw his personal physician during his last year, but he remembered him as helpful:

I really think a lot of our doctors, too. They've been wonderful. I really appreciate our doctor over the years. He's been a good doctor.

"My doctor's like my friend": Sarah

Our initial visits to Sarah were at Hospice House, shortly after she had moved in there. She had nothing but praise for this facility and the care that she got there:

I heard all the good things. And then we came out to look, you know, and see what it was all about, and we liked everything about it. Well, it's just actually an awful lot like home. Can't say enough about it.

After Sarah had left Hospice House, she moved to a licensed personal care home. She loved it as well:

It's a private home, and she takes just what she can handle, and there's two girls and they drop in and help out and it's real nice. . . . The people here kid with me all the time. [Laughs] You know, "Don't give Sarah that; that's too good for Sarah." [Laughs} Stuff like that. I can kid back too, but sometimes it's better not to.

Sarah's daughter, Karen, reflected her mother's satisfaction when she told us:

I can't say anything against it. I haven't seen anything that I can complain about. If I was young again, I'd start a place like this myself.

Sarah never had much to say about the specific people who helped her daily, but from the interactions that we observed between Sarah and her professional caregivers, we can only believe that she was very content. She did have a few words about her doctor, however, who had treated her for many years, from the beginning of her breast cancer: "Well, my doctor's just like a friend."

In the brief period after Sarah left Hospice House but before she moved into a private board and care facility, Karen placed her mother in two different nursing homes, both of which turned out to be very bad experiences. Sarah, always tactful and friendly, was guarded about describing her discontent:

Well, I don't know how much I can say; uh, somebody said be careful because they can sue ya. In one of them, dinner was supposed to be at 5. So I was downstairs with the rest at the dining room. And I waited and waited and I waited, and everybody else got up and left. So I called the girl over, and I said, "I didn't have any supper." She said, "Well, your name wasn't on the list." And away she went. And I went until morning. I didn't get any dinner, and, oh, it was just one thing after another like that. They had a bunch of high school kids and nobody over 'em. And their pillows were like rocks. I could go on and on. That's enough.

The theme of continuity of caregiving personnel shows up again and again in Sarah's situation: Hospice House, with eight beds, and the personal care home, with eleven residents, were very small compared to larger nursing homes. The staff was correspondingly small and had fewer changes of personnel than larger facilities.

Karen was more vocal than Sarah about their experience of nursing homes:

Those old people do not deserve that. I don't care how cranky they are. I saw too many things. Bad, bad, bad. Those people just sat there. They were numb. They never spoke to each other. They never laughed. We found out they were trying to push dope on Mom. You know, "Oh, let's give her a pill for this. Let's give her a pill for that."

~ ~ ~

The woman in the room with her, they just walked in Sunday and said, "Your Medicare is up. It won't pay any more after Tuesday. You have to move out." And well, the woman started crying, and she said, "Where am I gonna go?"

Keeping Her Distance from Care: Kitty

Kitty's professional care was complicated by the fact that she was determined to go it alone. She gave the impression that she wanted little to do with doctors. Some months earlier, she had blacked out while driving and, in her words, "took out a dumpster, and now they won't let me drive." This statement led to the following exchange:

Researcher: Was that when you started having to spend more of your time at the doctor's?

Kitty: No, not necessarily. They didn't want to see me any more than I wanted to see them. . . . When I got out of the hospital the doctor wanted to send me out to Hospice [House]. I said, "No, I'm not going, and so I think he thought maybe getting a hospice nurse would. . . . [Laughs]

After describing another such blackout, Kitty noted:

> The doctors don't place any limits on me 'cause, very frankly, they know that I wouldn't obey them. If they wanted to put me out in Hospice House, I wouldn't go.

The nurses who came to Kitty's home got a somewhat better report card from her, although she seemed confused about, or unwilling to identify, exactly what service they represented:

Researcher: Does somebody come every day?

Kitty: To tell you the truth, I've got so many people looking in on me I can't keep them straight.

Researcher: Does hospice or a nurse come by regularly, as well as your friends?

Kitty: Yeah. Yeah. To tell you the truth, I don't ask who they are when they come in. . . . I don't object because I want to make sure that I get my medicines all taken in proper time. I don't want to seem inhospitable. I'm glad to see anybody.

During our second visit with Kitty, she elaborated a bit on her daily care:

> I tell you, the [home health service] is just keeping such excellent track of me. There's a girl comes about 9:30 in the morning. It isn't the same girl, you know.

In a later visit, Kitty told us only slightly more about her professional care. She reported that she didn't learn much from her doctor but that the home health service (or hospice—she still wasn't sure which it was) watched out for her:

> They're keeping a pretty good eye on me. They're always checking my blood pressure, and then they just check to see how I'm doing.

Kitty's sketchy account of her professional care did not match the description of it given by hospice staff after Kitty had died. Not only had she had weekly visits but her increasing dementia and inability to care for herself were very evident to hospice. In mid-November, when the hospice nurse found Kitty's home strewn with stool and the IV PIC line pulled out and coiled up, Kitty was told she had to go to Hospice House.

In our various visits to Kitty, we were never able to get her to describe what her exact medical problem was. She always said she had blackouts of some unknown origin. After her death, we asked her friend and priest if he or Kitty ever discovered what it was. His response was as follows:

> Kitty never knew. I asked her doctor straight out. He said, "She's older. She's having these spells." I said, "What are they?" He replied, "We're not sure." Kitty once took a friend in with her and said to the doctor, "Whatever you want to tell me, tell her, so somebody knows." And they got no more than that.

"She's did about all she can for me": Mabel

Like Kitty, Mabel's daughter Bernice had kind words for her mother's hospice nurse—although Bernice had considerably less regard for some of Mabel's doctors. Because Mabel was less communicative in most matters, we relied on Bernice for an understanding of her mother's attitude toward her professional care. (For confidentiality, we have coded the doctors as A through E in this account.):

> In '94 we moved in here. And it was at this point, when she had bursitis in her hip, she went to [Dr. A]. And she thought that the only way that she could sleep after she got the artificial hip was on her left side. When she got the artificial hip put in, he injected the cortisone in it for the arthritis. That was why he did it. But apparently mom believes in her heart that he accidentally hit a nerve. That's the point when they ran her through all the tests, did the bone scans and everything. And they did find bone cancer in there. But mom didn't believe it because she couldn't focus beyond the point that she knew he hit a nerve. . . .
>
> But I think the doctors could've handled everything different right from the beginning. [Dr. A] didn't want [Dr. B] to do a biopsy. They kind of got into it on the day of surgery. [Dr. A] was telling [Dr. B], "Let her fully recover from this and then start with a mammogram and go from to here." Well, [Dr. B] got his way. She had the mastectomy right away. They told her, well, apparently there is enough time in between those surgeries to where that got

into the bone. Well, this is what they said. [Dr. C] was her cancer doctor. They called in [Dr. D]. And of course [Dr. A] was the one that had the ambulance come out to get mom. Well, after she got discharged from the hospital and we had to go to the first week visit, that was when [Dr. C] told us that he was going to be her cancer doctor. And you know, they started her on Tamoxifen when she was in the hospital. Well, mom went off it in three months. She said, "I don't believe it. I know he hit a nerve, and that's all there is to it." And she wouldn't let him treat her for it because she didn't believe she had it. And last year he says, "Mabel, you've got to take your Tamoxifen or you're gonna be bedridden." Well there's several times I told [Dr. C] , "She's white as a ghost."

∿ ∿ ∿

Well, I took her up to [Dr. E] for that second opinion. I said, "Mom, we're gonna to go the drug store and get this Tamoxifen filled, and you're gonna take it, and you're gonna get a second opinion." I took her up to [Dr. E], who talked to us, and she looked at mom and took a little blood. [Dr. E] has been her doctor ever since.

Out of this complicated history, we conclude that Dr. A—the one who did the hip replacement—gets a favorable evaluation from Mabel and Bernice, despite his allegedly hitting a nerve with the cortisone shot. Of him, Bernice said, "[Dr. A] is a good hip replacer." Dr. B gets their blame for doing the mastectomy right away. Dr. C, Mabel's original oncologist, seems to be treated neutrally, perhaps having been no more than the victim of bearing the bad news of her cancer.

In this account, there is no mention of a trusted family physician treating Mabel over time—someone who would have known her and might have played a stronger role in coordinating her care once she needed to see specialists. On the other hand, Mabel and Bernice revered Dr. E, Mabel's oncologist. They called her by her first name. Mabel seldom gave high praise to anyone, but she managed, during our visits, to say of her doctor, "She's real nice; I guess she's did about all she can for me."

Mabel also had great respect for hospice and the nurses sent to help her, noting: "If I didn't have help from them I don't know where I'd be." Of Mabel's hospice nurse, Bernice observed, "She's just a wonderful person." Shortly after our last visit, however, Mabel's hospice service ran out. She continued to receive a monthly visit from a home health service to check her medications; her daughter did the remainder of her home care, including struggling to take Mabel to the doctor's office for outpatient care for another eighteen months.

"Just loved the hospice people": Sharon

Sharon's daughter reported to us a conversation she had with her mother about hospice care:

> She just loved the hospice people. I remember when hospice first came to see her a couple times, she said, "I just may not die. I'm having too much fun." She was totally happy. Totally blown away that everything could be so perfect. She hadn't expected it at all.

Connie, Sharon's sister and caregiver, supported this opinion fully. At one point Connie described how she considered putting Sharon in a nursing home:

> I'm going to meet with the social worker and see what options we might have. I don't know if there are any. Could she be in a nursing home with the kind of level of care she requires? I had thought all along that they couldn't provide this kind of care. They couldn't give her every five minutes the medicine she needs every day. In a way it's almost easier to do it here than to run out there three times a day or whatever it is.

Sharon reported to us that she also appreciated her doctor, even though she had never thought much of doctors on the whole. As she said (with characteristic bluntness):

> I was just really lucky. Ordinarily I've never been very cozy with doctors. You know, I used them only in emergencies. Well, I had to get a test for something. And so I didn't have a doctor, so I just asked the closest person around. And she suggested [my doctor]. She'd never been to her. I guess she'd heard she was good. So I went to her for a shot, and she's wonderful. Yeah, I was really lucky in having her. She makes house calls.

Three months and several visits later, Sharon was still singing the praises of her doctor and hospice team:

> Well, that's one thing I always wanted was to not be depending on anybody for anything, and here I am, almost totally [dependent]. And I'm fortunate to have such kindly people doing it.

"I could never do it without their help": Roberta

When we first visited Roberta, she was already on hospice service. A nurse visited her at Debbie's home once a week, and the bath lady came twice a week. Everyone was quite satisfied with her professional care. Debbie described the hospice nurse as "simply great," adding, "I could never do it without their help; it just couldn't be done. I just can't begin to say enough about her and what she went through for us."

Only the last few days of Roberta's life occasioned any concern about her medical treatment. About a week before her death, Roberta suffered a fractured hip. She was taken to the hospital, where an orthopedist examined her and advised surgery right away. Roberta's regular physician had doubts about this recommendation—as did her hospice caregiver, who came with them to the hospital. But Roberta told them, "Fix it." Debbie's own narrative of this event was as follows:

It hurt her to move. And so she wanted to have it fixed. She wanted to get things back to normal and get home, you know. And this was great. But then as the evening wore on I realized that I needed my other sister here, and she was on her way over. Of course, this postponed the surgery for another day. The doctor said, "Sure, no problem."

≈ ≈ ≈

In the meantime, the orthopedic doctor—I can't remember his name now—did not know mom's history of congestive heart problems and didn't learn about it until Mom's hospice nurse intervened and told him about it. And he didn't know that. And he said, "Oh." So there were things—I mean I could see this interaction going on, and I was just really taken aback by the whole thing. And I was weighing things carefully again. And then she started having a lot of fluid buildup. . . .

In the meantime, [Mom's doctor] was really, really dubious about surgery at that point, and he was advising us, too. He said, "We have to drain this fluid." So they gave her a diuretic to start draining the fluid, and I saw Mom changing about that time. I saw her more lethargic and doing a lot of hand movements. She was doing a lot of gesturing while she was kind of not quite asleep. Things were really startling me. And so they went ahead and set up schedule for the next day for surgery. Mom was very willing to do this and ready to go with it. But I saw her less cognizant and less aware of what was happening. . . .

That night, Tuesday night, her doctor came in. He said, "I'm having second thoughts about this surgery." He was dragging his heels. He didn't know how this was going to work out. He was having a lot of second thoughts. Third and fourth thoughts: We were really gung ho. "Let's do the surgery. We'll do what we need to do, let's get her fixed."

So the next morning he called and said, "I think we're not going to be able to do the surgery because she has kidney failure. She doesn't have much time left." He said, "You have some choices to make here. You can take her to Hospice House or you can take her to a nursing home." I said, "No, she'll come back home with us." There was just no choice. She started with us, and she'll finish with us. So we prepared her for the ambulance ride, and this part was hard because I didn't realize that the only pain medicine they gave her was a mild pain pill. But anyhow, we made the ambulance ride home here. It was hard for her to do this. It was for me too. At that point I thought, "Oh gosh, what have we done to Mom? Why have we moved her? Why have we put her in this situation?" In the long run I'm glad we brought her home because we had everything set up, thanks to Ellie. Thanks to the maneuvering of the nurses and everybody that was concerned. They had everything in place. And the hospice nurse, Ellie, was here waiting for her and had her kind of traction system set up for her hip. Ready to go, and she had made special arrangements for that. And she had gotten some morphine, a new pump for her.

Debbie describes herself as "gung ho" for medicine, and a believer in the omniscience of doctors. When she was faced with very difficult choices about her mother's care, however, she discovered that medical science has limits and valid differences of medical opinions and that in the end, families must make choices about what's best for them.

What Works in Doctor-Patient Communication: A Critical Incident

The descriptions of the professional health care given by the participants and their caregivers is a litany of positives in most cases: "wonderful," "trying hard," "dedicated," "personally interested," "like a friend," "selfless," "one in a million," "a jewel," "a pure joy," "supportive," "real nice," "kindly," "a delight," and "simply great." Even Kitty, who never cared much for doctors, and Mabel, who reported a bad experience, were kindly toward at least some of their professional caregivers. Roberta's case, however, provides a critical incident that illustrates what actually works when doctor-patient—or, in this case, doctor-family—communication is at a crucial, life-determining point.

Debbie elaborated on the three factors in the communication with her mother's physicians and nurses that led to satisfaction with her mother's care during the last week of Roberta's life: She and her sisters were given what she termed "full knowledge" about their choices; they were included in open and frank discussions between the hospice nurse and the physicians about the best treatment plan; and two of the health care professionals already knew her mother and could offer decisions that were based on continuous knowledge of her needs, wishes, and care. Because of these factors, an unexpected, painful, and tragic event that could have led to many recriminations instead was resolved to the satisfaction of the participants involved—including Roberta, who was able to go home for her last day of life.

The Importance of "Full Knowledge" in Planning

We note above that Debbie described herself as physician-oriented: fix, repair, help. She describes her wonderment as the hospice nurse came to the hospital after Roberta was admitted, to join the family as they talked with the orthopedic surgeon and to ask about options other than immediate surgery:

> At the hospital when nurse was talking with the orthopedic surgeon about Mom's condition. When I saw this, that other options were being presented to us and to Mom, I was just. . . . I was just overwhelmed. I could see what was happening, and I thought, "Wow, I've got to be open-minded about this stuff," as far as listening to what really is available and knowing what the choices were. . . . I had no idea.

Debbie said she was still in doubt at this point because "without the surgery mom was still in pain." The hospice nurse explained the other option of taking her to Hospice House, in traction, so that she would be comfortable and not in pain. Debbie said:

> She gave me a picture of the whole thing. It was more detailed and in depth, and I felt comfortable with full knowledge. I felt much more comfortable after I heard all this.

Debbie acknowledges that this "full knowledge" may not be for everyone:

> Maybe this is not good for everybody, who don't want to know this. I think for me it's nice to have a choice.

The family, after hearing all the options, still had agreed to the surgery on Monday. What Debbie remembered best about this stressful period was that at this crucial time, she was given enough knowledge to make an informed choice.

Openness of Communication about Choices

Debbie pointed to the openness of communication among the professionals treating her mother—and their openness with her—as the second major factor that led her to be satisfied with her mother's care:

Debbie: The way the doctors and hospice nurse communicated with us in the room, and Mom's doctor was so up front about his conversation with hospice that night. I was just really pleased with that.

Researcher: You said the nurse was asking if he'd explored some of these options, which you wouldn't have known about?

Debbie: Absolutely not. And she was not backing down. This young person—I was just overwhelmed by her. I didn't have any idea of the choices at first. I started feeling much more relaxed, after she said, "You don't have to have surgery, you can do this." She was kind of giving me a picture of the whole thing, instead of saying, you know, like the doctors, this is what we're going to do, we're going to cut this open and sew her up.

Debbie felt that her mother's primary physician also had been open and given the family information about the choices they had:

He said, "You have some choices to make here. You can take her to Hospice House or you can take her to a nursing home." He was totally understanding, when I told him we were taking Mom home. That was our decision. And he said, "I need to tell you, I have enjoyed working with you. I admire your decision making." And that was a compliment, you know, that doctors don't usually have time or take time for.

The Importance of Continuity of Professional Caregivers

Faced with new and unanticipated choices, Roberta and her family also were fortunate that two long-term caregivers, both of whom had extensive knowledge of Roberta and her medical condition—the hospice nurse and Roberta's own personal physician—were part of the hospital assessment and decision making. The hospice nurse went with the family to the hospital and participated in the first meeting with the orthopedic surgeon. The family was doubly appreciative of her presence:

> Actually with the surgeon that we're seeing, he doesn't know her. He came in and was ready to do surgery and stuff, and the hospice mentioned—the hospice nurse said to the doctor, "You know, she has quite advanced CHF." And he hadn't looked at her chart! And so the nurse kind of filled him in on her condition.

Later the same day, Roberta's own physician assumed her care in preparation for surgery. He became more dubious about her condition and insisted on waiting another day to be sure she could undergo surgery at all, saying, "I'm having second, third, and fourth thoughts." His counsel to wait, despite the daughter's eagerness to help her mom at that point, turned out to be the best decision, as Roberta's body responded to the trauma by shutting down.

Debbie found that the hospice nurse was willing to keep explaining what was happening and discussing her choices, right up to the end of her mother's life. After they brought Roberta home, Debbie fretted all night about whether they were doing the right thing by not treating her mother, who was no longer conscious and no longer able to eat or drink. The hospice nurse checked with them regularly, and the following night Debbie had a long conversation with her:

> She came over about 6:30 in the evening. She came in the living room, sat down, and I shared with her my thoughts. "Can we have an IV? Can we try and make sure that her kidneys haven't shut down? What can we do for her?" And this dear person said, "Yes, we can do that." Not telling me, "No, we couldn't do that." You know, I knew that this was the answer, but she said, "Yes, we can do that. Let me tell you a little more about what's happening to her." So I listened to her, and she carefully explained things to me that made me understand what was happening to Mom and why it was so important for me to let go of her. And she was very kind, and I felt a lot of compassion from her and her explanation of what was happening to Mom's system and everything. Medically, why it would be harmful for them to start giving her fluids and how her system wouldn't absorb it, and she would get this fluid back into her again and cause some more problems. And I could understand that. I looked over to my sister, and I says, "Okay, I can let go of her now." I asked, "Is that okay with you?" And she said, "Yes."

Professional Care and the Subculture of Terminally Ill People

The idea of professional care is one in which patients and their caregivers, by definition, give up elements of power and control. By accepting hospice care they are saying, in essence, "I no longer have control of things, and I have little or no power to make individual decisions." They expect such decisions to be made for them by doctors, nurses, or hospice workers.

For example, Walt, Sharon, Roberta, Sarah, and Ralph were perfectly willing to give such power and control to their caregivers and medical professionals. In contrast, Dennis, who was much younger, held tenaciously onto whatever control he could still manage; Kitty, who was much older, held on to power by distancing herself from her caregivers. Under no circumstances would Dennis permit anyone to take him to the hospital to die. Nor would he even let his mother make this decision for him. She, in turn, held onto certain power and control in her relationship with nurses concerning her son's care. One of the recurring topics throughout our visits was that she had to instruct the professionals, who had never experienced a case like her son's, in how to bathe him, change his linens, and many other things. Although she did not have power and control over Dennis, she was able to maintain such power and control where she could.

Continuity was particularly relevant in the area of professional care. Connection over time with the same persons, who know the patient and whom patient and family trust because of that knowledge, was a crucial element in patient attitudes and satisfaction. Dennis and Carrie were deeply troubled by the lack of continuity they felt in an ever-changing set of home health care workers. On the other hand, they offered only praise for the physician who had treated Dennis over the course of his long illness. Dennis, Walt, and Kitty also strongly demanded the continuity of staying in their own homes until they would die. Barbara was troubled by having to switch doctors when her long-time physician moved away from Missoula. The continuity in her home health service nurses, on the other hand, contributed to her satisfaction with their services.

For others, the early choice of hospice provided an unexpected benefit: continuity of the same hospice nurse throughout their illness and death. In Roberta's case, the hospice nurse also was present to help the family understand the consequences of choices they had to make about their mother's care.

Chapter 5

Knowledge of Illness and Attitudes toward Pain and Death

Introduction: Open versus Closed Awareness

One psychological cost of closed awareness is that patients cannot help their caregivers and families with their grief or deal with their own feelings about dying (Glaser and Strauss 1964). Medical personnel are placed in a particularly difficult position as well. In chapter 2 we discuss the issue of closed awareness of the terminal diagnosis and what it implies for the remaining time allotted. There can also be closed awareness—if not ignorance—of the contributing disease itself. The participants' knowledge of their illness and attitudes toward pain and death varied greatly, probably reflecting the variation that one might expect in the larger population. Some patients learned everything they could about their disease. Others tended to sit back and leave all decision making to the medical profession. Our findings do not explicitly reveal the cause of such differences, although they do correlate with age in this group.

How much knowledge participants had may be related to how useful the knowledge was to them. The two youngest, both of whom had cancer, appeared to have a good grasp of their specific illnesses and the course of their disease. Their cancers, which occurred in their early thirties and forties, were unexpected and untimely invasions, and they both actively sought medical knowledge to better fight their battles. Two participants in their early seventies, both dying of emphysema, also had a better understanding of the changes in their body and their terminal decline than did the more elderly participants (those age eighty or over).

Likewise, attitudes toward the terminal illness, pain, and death seemed to vary according to age. The two younger participants fought their illness in every way they could. They mentioned pain more than the older patients. The older participants more commonly discussed illnesses or discomfort that were unrelated or marginal to the cause of their terminal condition. The two younger people continued to do some of the things they had loved to do when healthy, such as play golf or go on camping trips. The older participants, especially the males, seemed to have resigned themselves, as much as they loved the things they did before their illness, to the fact that such activity was no longer possible.

Knowledge of Illness

Characteristic comments from participants reveal the variation in knowledge of and attitude toward illness, in relation to age:

"I knew that it was coming back again." (Barbara, age forty-six)
"I am quite a rarity." (Dennis, age thirty-nine)
"So here comes this emphysema." (Ralph, age seventy)
"Breathing has been hard for me for a long time." (Sharon, age seventy-four)
"I'm in good condition, it's just that I black out." (Kitty, age eighty)
"It's my heart, isn't it dear?" (Walt, age eighty)
"I just take what comes." (Sarah, age eighty)
"I'm in good health." (Roberta, age eighty-five)
"I couldn't believe I had cancer." (Mabel, age eighty-seven)

People in Their Forties: Illness as Enemy to Be Studied and Fought

The two participants in their forties, Dennis and Barbara, worked very hard to learn all they could about their illness. They learned the names of drugs, treatments, and specialists. They used the language of the medical profession, including procedures, abbreviations (i.e., "meds," "chemo"), and even the distancing terms common in medical talk—such as "the leg" rather than "my leg."

"I knew that it was coming back again": Barbara

Barbara talked about her inner awareness of the disease—about how she knew it had returned—rather than her clinical symptoms:

What happened in '94 was that I started developing some shortness of breath around October, and feeling tired. And it didn't trigger to me at the time that the cancer might be returning, until December. I decided to go out to Now Care in the mall and have them tell me if I had pneumonia or not. And so when I had an X-ray there, the doctor came in and said that I needed to go right down to the emergency room, that there was a lot of fluid in my right lung, and so I knew immediately then that it was cancer. He didn't have to tell me. So we started in on chemotherapy again, and that worked well, and I had basically from March until August where it wasn't active again.

∼ ∼ ∼

In '95 [August] I took a trip with my folks to Denver, and in the morning that we left, I knew it was back, the way I felt. My vision was not clear, I felt heavy, felt a little tired, and I knew, I knew exactly, the way I was feeling, that it was coming back again.

"I am quite a rarity": Dennis

Dennis and his caregiver-mother, Carrie, not only became experts in his rare form of cancer; they also were very proud of their expertise. Without doubt, Dennis was the participant who best knew many of the details of his illness—perhaps because it was so rare. In a sense, he and his mother were learning about it along with the medical profession. He described himself as a "pioneer" in this sense:

Medically, my disease is, uh, nontreatable actually. They can only put it into short-term remissions. And by that I mean a matter of weeks, a month, maybe. And then I am not expected to live past the summer. But actually I've kept a real good attitude towards things, and everybody who's been involved with my care and with my treatments have been wonderful.

A recurring topic throughout our visits was how rare Dennis's disease was:

This disease is something else. I'll give you one statistic. This is so rare. It's called mycosis fungoides, or they have a new name for it called peripheral T-cell lymphoma. And the latest statistic is 500 people per year in the United States will contract this disease. Usually older than me. And they usually die of something else, because of their age. I am quite a rarity. They're quite interested when they hear my age. I've visited quite a few specialists, and anything from environmental physicians to a doctor that flew over from Sweden.

According to Dennis, the medical profession was learning a great deal from him, and he spoke from their perspective—using the pronoun "we," not "they":

We don't know what the disease's full symptoms and characteristics are. Because it seems to change every day. And the doctors, neither do they know. They kind of learn from me as I tell them what symptoms are going on.

In our second visit, Dennis told us how he took the opportunity of his illness to learn a great deal about it. He was not a mere passive recipient of medical treatment. Instead, he gave evidence of learning a great deal more about the practice of medicine than do most:

I had everything from giving myself injections of Interferon to full body radiation to topical nitrogen mustard applications to UVA exposures enhanced by Methoxoralin pills. In 1990 I had full body radiation. I had the maximum that the body can receive. And head to toe, all the folds in the body, everything that would avail me about 5 to 10 years remission. But it was back in 8 months. So then they recategorized me as an aggressive type of mycosis fungoides, which lowered my prognosis considerably. Only 500 people contract this disease per year in the United States. I'd have a better chance of winning the lottery.

Near the end of this visit, we had a tape-recording malfunction, and we were unable to record Dennis's description of his then-current chemotherapy treatment. Our field notes, however, recorded these comments:

Chemotherapy takes six and a half hours every time I go down to the doctor's suite. [He then named several of the medications he was on, using their technical names in a very precise manner]. . . .

This is aggressive treatment, but it's about to stop. That's very scary because of all *that* means. . . .

I'm willing to do it because it buys me time and even a little quality of life. But now the chemo is going to have worse side effects than benefits. The doctor says we're about to stop.

The sophistication that Dennis and his mother exhibited regarding the treatment of his disease is evident in their dialogue during a visit to their physician's oncology suite:

Dennis: I have to wait and see the other doctor. Because I have a bug in my blood. I have a thing called pseudomonas, which is, according to the oncologist, a bad-ass bug. He said, "You're on about the best medication that you could be, but we gotta watch you like a hawk." He said it's a bad one. You treat it with antibiotics and hope that the antibiotic doesn't trigger something else to go.

Carrie: Well, are they talking isolation again because of it?

Dennis: No, he didn't say anything about that. . . . And he said how fast the things come on.

Carrie: Yeah, that's the nature of it.

Dennis: He said it's what they're doing. But there's nothing new. I just go to my 10 milligrams of Prednisone tomorrow. It sounds like I'm gonna get a lot more Zolson again, after the other doctor sees me.

Carrie: Well, I don't see miracles happening with that, do you? With that Zolson?

Dennis: No, I don't. But it's supposed to be pretty good.

Carrie: Yeah, maybe it has held it from going. I mean can this particular bug cause pneumonia?

Dennis: He didn't go into it. All I got to hear is it's a bad-ass bug and that's it. I pretty much know what that means.

Soon, Dennis had to return to the doctor's office to see a second specialist about his new infection. After he left us, Carrie talked about the bug and her own understanding of "what that means":

It's just a matter of time before something like that will invade. It will be resistant to any kind of medicine. That's why I asked if this one could cause pneumonia. And I imagine it can. There's all kinds of pneumonia. To me pneumonia's a blessing. It'll probably take him in a matter of days. It's just a matter of the last stage of life.

People in their Seventies: Acceptance

"So here comes this emphysema": Ralph

In contrast with Dennis's clarity and knowledge about his illness, Ralph had only a general understanding. He knew that he had emphysema, but things got a bit fuzzy from there. On our first visit with him, he gave the following account of his medical history:

> I guess it was probably between six and seven years ago. They told me I got a real bad case of pneumonia. I went into the Vet's hospital over at Helena; never been in the hospital. Well, I got a bad toe one time. So I went into this Vet's hospital over there; boy, was I sick. And they said, "You've got pneumonia." And they put me right in the bed. And they kept me over there, and they got me cleared up. I got to talking to them every day, like you do, and they said, "You got emphysema and you got"—what's that where your bones deteriorate? [Researcher suggests "osteoporosis."] Yeah. "You got that." Within that year I broke my back twice to add to it. And when they were lookin' at that, they find, you know, these bones are all deteriorated. So here comes this emphysema. It's a-comin' along there all the time.

In our next visit, Ralph elaborated a bit on how he came to break his back. He had run his truck into the ditch in a snowstorm and was about to get out of the truck and get a buddy to pull him out:

> I reached over to get my seat belt. I turned around like that and reached to unhook the seat belt and twisted my back off. I believe three vertebras twisted so bad. They called it a compression fracture, 'cause they squashed together when I was jumping up and down or whatever. I passed out from the pain. Man, I told them just as true as I'm tellin' you about what had happened, and the doctor says, "That happens all the time." If you twist your muscles to where they're not holding in a good line, you twist them right out of place. I didn't know that. But they're still all gone. That's from— oh, what's that disease that you get? [Researcher suggests "osteoporosis" again.] Osteoporosis, yeah. You see, I've got that now, too, along with emphysema, bad heart.

"Breathing has been hard for me for a long time": Sharon

Sharon, who had emphysema, simply never brought up the topic of her illness to us. On our first visit, she let her sister explain her symptoms and would refer us to her sister when we asked specifically about them. Only once, in response to a question about whether she felt "comfortable," did she say that "breathing has been hard for me for a long time."

Part of Sharon's lack of concern, or complaint, was the increasing short-term memory loss and gentle confusion that accompanied her late-stage emphysema, which made it difficult for her to remember recent experiences—even uncomfortable ones. Sharon could not remember "struggling to breathe" in the morning—as her sister described it—because, in Sharon's words, "I'm always struggling to breathe." She seemed unwilling to complain about the symptoms of a disease that had occurred because of her cigarette smoking. Sharon continued to smoke even when she was on twenty-four-hour oxygen, unhooking the nose clip to light a cigarette; she never expressed any regrets about smoking, or not stopping.

People in their Eighties: Illness as Old Age

Among the older participants in our study we observed little explicit knowledge of their diseases. Walt and Kitty, in particular, seemed unsure of the specific cause of their terminal conditions. At best, their descriptions were broad and nonspecific. Roberta insisted that she felt fine and was in good health, and Mabel often seemed unsure if she had cancer or just complications from falls and hip surgery. Perhaps the cause of their terminal illness was not so important now that they had entered that most final medical category. Nothing could be done anyway. Curiously enough, when they gave little information about their disease, their caregivers did the same.

"I'm in good condition. It's just that I black out": Kitty

Kitty, who was beginning her eightieth year, only mentioned that she had "blackouts" and low blood pressure. She had told the MDP researcher who first contacted her for the Pilot Clinical Profile that she didn't know why she was part of the study (even though she had just agreed to participate) because she wasn't really sick. After her death, her friend clarified for us that he and Kitty had been told by her physician simply that she was old:

Researcher: Do you know if she ever told anybody what her illness was?

Friend: She doesn't know. She never knew. I asked her doctor straight out. He said, "She's older. She's having these spells." What are they? "We're not sure." She had these little transient things that her doctor never would

explain, and I don't know that he knows, but he never
explained what they were, but she would blank out.

Kitty continued to receive good medical care, visiting her physician regularly and taking whatever medications he and hospice prescribed to control symptoms.

"It's my heart, isn't it, dear?": Walt

Walt and Dorothy had relatively little to say about Walt's medical condition and problems. After a decade of ill health from cardiovascular disease and several serious heart attacks, the topic may no longer have held any interest for them. Walt just knew that he had a "bad heart." Walt's family was most in accord with the view that dying of a chronic illness when one is seventy-five or eighty is a death from "old age," rather than from the ravages of a specific disease (Nuland 1993)—a view we explore in more depth at the end of this chapter. After Walt's death, his daughter responded to the question, "What do you understand to be the cause of his death?":

> Why he died? I truthfully think and feel that it was just old age, and the wearing out of all the different organs. Well, I guess, if maybe he'd taken better care of himself as a child, he wouldn't have had these injuries that would have caused him problems. But you don't change your circulation. You don't change some of those things. So it just happens. It seemed very natural to me that he should pass on.

"I just take what comes": Sarah

Sarah also knew that she had cancer in her bones, but she was not always very clear about the details—often admitting her own confusion in the process. The following quotations, ranging over a six-month period of time, reveal Sarah's knowledge about her illness:

Researcher: What is the nature of your illness? What do you have?

Sarah: Well, I have bone cancer, and then I had surgery on my back—three openings, it was. And I always get this wrong; anyway, it was calcium buildup.

∽ ∽ ∽

Researcher: So when is it you found out you had bone cancer?

Sarah:	Oh, about ten years ago, but it wasn't real bad, you know. It kind of sneaked in. I think it was about ten years ago.

At our next visit, Sarah showed us her swollen arm:

Sarah:	Got an arm that's swelling. When I do that, kneel in that position, it hurts—kinda in the bone, I don't know.
Researcher:	Was it like when your leg was swelling?
Sarah:	Yeah, but it's not the same thing. This was when I had the breast off.
Researcher:	You had your breast off? Did you have breast cancer also?
Sarah:	Yeah.
Researcher:	So it's, uh, sort of spreading around different places?
Sarah:	Yeah. Yeah.
Researcher:	But your swollen leg was from the stroke, you said.
Sarah:	Well, I had surgery on my back and when they done that they hit a nerve. And it got angry. Still gets angry.

At our third visit, Sarah still attributed her physical discomfort to her strokes:

I was allergic to so many pain pills, but then I had a stroke. I had strokes. I think that's what's working on me now.

The two oldest people in the study, Roberta and Mabel, seemed the least cognizant of their particular illness, and showed the most dementia and difficulty in understanding over the course of our visits with them.

"I'm in good health": Roberta

Roberta, who was eighty-five, asserted that she was in good health; she remembered her recent heart problems as only a cold or flu. Her increasing memory loss and confusion made it impossible to be certain what she knew or understood. Her daughter affirmed that her mother continued to assert that she was in "good health" for most of her last few months.

"I couldn't believe I had bone cancer": Mabel

Mabel's understanding of her illness and symptoms was similarly difficult to discern. She described her reaction to being told she had bone cancer:

> I couldn't believe it. No way in the world could I believe that I had bone cancer. I didn't never think that I would live to be this old [eighty-seven].

Mabel's daughter believed that her mother didn't initially understand her illness and continued to believe that her pain was caused by an injection for arthritis. As a result, Mabel refused treatment for cancer at first:

> Mom firmly believes in her heart, and I firmly believe, that he accidentally hit a nerve. They ran her through all the tests, did the bone scans and everything, and they did find the bone cancer in there. Mom didn't believe it because she couldn't focus beyond the point that she knew he hit a nerve.

> $\sim$ $\sim$ $\sim$

> They had started her on the Tamoxifen when she was in the hospital, in '94. Well, Mom went off of it in three months. "I don't believe it. I know he hit a nerve, and that's all there is to it." And then in '96, she fractured [something]. Well, she told him, "I don't have cancer." And she wouldn't let him treat her for it because she didn't believe she had it.

Mabel's understanding of the world was that it was a very malevolent place that caused illness and problems. Thus, her belief that her pain was caused by a misplaced cortisone shot rather than the ravages of cancer made sense. In contrast to Walt and his family, who saw his decline as natural and his illness that of "old age," for Mabel any disease needed a specific, external cause.

Attitudes Toward Pain and Other Symptoms

We found a great deal of variation in participants' experience of and attitude toward their symptoms, including pain; these variations were related to their specific illnesses, their own character, and the context in which they found themselves. The data on which these observations are based come from what we observed and what participants reported during their final months and weeks of life, during the time when they could communicate and were still at home. (During their last day or two of life, the period of "actively dying"—a state of fairly rapid transition between life and death—their experience of pain and other symptoms and of their treatments often differed. We report these experiences chapter 11.) Recall that seven of the nine participants had chosen extended hospice care: Ralph, Sharon, Walt, Roberta, Mabel, Sarah, and Kitty. Dennis did not choose hospice. Barbara's family decided on hospice care only in the last day or two of her life.

> "I'm in constant pain." (Dennis)
>> "I feel awful—I don't know if I'm dead or alive." (Mabel)
>> "I don't talk much about it." (Barbara)
>> "What pain?" (Kitty, Walt, Roberta)
>> "Side effects." (Sarah)
>> "I'll suffer enough." (Ralph)

"I'm in constant pain": Dennis

Dennis was in almost constant pain, for which he bolused whenever he felt it necessary. The pain grew worse while he was sitting, so he frequently would get up and walk around to help relieve it. He described this pain to us on our first visit:

> I sit for a minimal amount of time, and then it gets uncomfortable; then I'll get up and walk around. And this pack here is a pain pack that you'll see me punch once in a while. I don't go anywhere without it. Through all the bolusing I do, I tend to get sleepy. I had a kind of a long night, and with my pain medication, I have to bolus to catch up. All the ones that I've missed during the night. And then when I reach the comfortable state, I'm kind of tired, and my mental facilities are not as crisp as they should be.

Dennis described how difficult it was for him to get to the medical treatment that his illness required:

> Well, the transportation . . . riding in a car is very difficult for me because I have lesions that are ulcerated. They're in different parts of my body. Mostly right now they're on my bottom, which is hard to adjust to, to get comfortable. And cars are very confining, but you do the best you can. But the trip down to Missoula and back makes me very sore, very stiff, and tired. And from when I get into the car to when I come back to the house, there's a whole

readjustment again of bolusing, trying to get the pain under control. Appetite has been fine. But it's the constant pain, the battle with pain, trying to keep it under control. One part of me may hurt one day, another part the next day, and another part the following day. And the lesions are everywhere. I have them from my bottom to my legs, as you can see, to the fold areas. For seven months I've been sleeping on my back. It's the most comfortable. But the other night now I just happened to want to sleep on my right side, which was a revelation. And it was great. I could feel comfortable and I woke up and felt pretty rested. But the whole day is pretty much devoted to getting the pain under control so I can have some quality of life.

Dennis's mother, Carrie, then described an incident a few weeks prior to our visit:

He had a pump failure a few weeks back. And at two in the morning we realized how artificially dependent he is on it for his existence. He's gone from morphine to Fentanyl. The morphine zonked him, the amount. And so he's on this, which gives him a better quality. He can be more lucid. It goes in faster, but it goes out faster too.

Dennis elaborated on how this switch from morphine to Fentanyl came about—in response to his strong preference to remain conscious and coherent:

The switch to Fentanyl was due to the doctor and the pharmacist at the hospital experimenting. They realized that the more they had to raise me on the morphine, the more problems I was having with being coherent and everything. So the Fentanyl seems to let me remain alert and have a pretty stable thinking process. I can remember what's going on and remember the day before. So it's really worked out good in that way, and it's also helped the pain.

By August, Dennis's deteriorating condition made it more and more difficult for us to talk with him. Carrie spoke with us willingly, however, whenever she found the time to see us. One of our visits took place at the physician's suite in Missoula on their regular weekly appointment. As usual, Carrie had driven the sixty miles in the morning; she arranged to meet us at an outside picnic table, adjacent to the doctor's waiting room. While Dennis received treatment, Carrie told us how difficult the past year had been and of her hopes that Dennis could remain conscious until the end, despite the pain:

There were months where comfort was all you strove for—not comfort, but tolerable pain is what we struggled for. And that's what we still struggle for. . . .

It's just a matter of the last stage of life. My dad had cancer and was in a lot of pain. But he died of a heart attack, a lot quicker and easier than suffering with cancer. Dennis will have a lot of pain unless he's out. And that's horrible. I hate that. Out. I don't know where his line is. I know that you can get this what they call CNS, Central Nervous System Syndrome where you're, you know, movement and stuff. But you know I'd rather see him in tolerable pain than out, unconscious. I'd rather see him communicating.

Part of Dennis's (and Carrie's) tolerance for pain until the final days of his life came from the high value they both placed on a "sober mind" and consciousness.

"I feel awful—I don't know if I'm dead or alive": Mabel

Mabel was full of complaints. During the three months we visited Mabel frequently, she complained of pains in various parts of her body, of uncertain cause. Her list of pains was lengthy, and statements such as those quoted below often constituted an entire turn in the conversation:

"My bones hurt . . . ."
　"It hurts a lot, my hip . . . ."
　"It hurts when I walk . . . ."
　"The pain is so bad . . . ."
　"I feel awful anymore—don't know if I'm dead or alive . . . ."
　"Pain in my head, sometimes in my leg . . . ."
　"I got pain in my neck, all the time . . . ."

Mabel believed that her neck pain and the bumps on her head were caused by a fall against a dresser four years earlier. She repeated the story each time she told us how much her neck hurt:

Mabel:　　　　The pain's still the same. Still hurts. All the time.

Researcher:　　What does the hospice nurse say about it?

Mabel:　　　　She don't know. I fell on that book case, every shelf going down. And I don't know if that's what caused it or what.

Mabel's daughter verified the painfulness of her mother's condition:

I know it's really difficult for Mom because she feels so awful all the time.

From our conversations with Mabel and her daughter, we could never be sure we understood what Mabel's pains were, or how severe. Her discomfort was very evident, however. She had a seventy-two-hour pain patch (Fentanyl) for the cancer in her bones, which Bernice changed for her. At the end of the seventy-two-hour period, Mabel was very uncomfortable and would have to lie down until the patch could be changed. Bernice explained:

You have to change them every 72 hours. When the patch is on the low side, that's when more of the pain breaks through. Her legs jerk. On the third day of her patch, she had a little thing she goes through, where she gets real cold, can't get warm. Her legs shake, and I have to give her the Ativan. I have Ativan and the Percocet. The Ativan seems to help the shaking a little bit.

When we first began visiting, Mabel also was complaining about bursitis in her hip. When pain medications failed to help her, Bernice managed to take her to a local orthopedic specialist, who gave her another cortisone shot. This injection provided relief from the pain in her hip. Mabel's other pains persisted, however—worsened, Bernice said, by her sensitivity to medications:

The hospice nurse suggested last Friday that she take Aleve because it kicked in quicker when her neck hurts. She said, "If you take the Aleve, Mabel, it would help you." So only two tablets of Aleve just really puffed her feet right up. I mean, I couldn't keep up with the fluid retention. "Well," the hospice nurse says, "just forget it, and just give her the Percocet when she hurts."

Mabel also was reluctant to take some of the pain medications provided by hospice because they upset her stomach. When the nurse tried a liquid form of Roxanol without Tylenol so that she could take more of it, Mabel didn't like it:

Mom said she didn't want anything cold on her stomach. I said, "Mom, it's at room temperature." I brought it into her in the living room, and she smelled it, and said, "Ugh—you take it." And she tells me the pain pills "don't do any good."

Mabel's hearing and vision were limited; thus, she was more a captive of her body. To her, the loss of vision was as distressing as the continual pain she experienced:

> The worst thing could happen to me is to lose my eyesight. . . . I can't see [TV], just sit here and listen.

Because of these limitations, Mabel had relatively few opportunities to be distracted from pain by social events, TV, reading, or other everyday activities. Mother and daughter rarely had outside visitors, except for the hospice nurse. When Mabel got a phone call from her equally ill and housebound older sister, however, she was more animated as she engaged in that lively fifteen-minute conversation. Mabel's eyes sparkled when she remembered going dancing as a teenager, and she still enjoyed listening to music.

Mabel's continuing complaints provide an argument that medical assistance and good pain medication alone are not sufficient for persons with terminal illness. Pain treatment also requires social support and interactions, interesting activities, and possibly complementary, nonmedical therapies to alleviate discomfort.

"I don't talk much about it": Barbara

For people such as Barbara, a stoic mental attitude toward pain seems to work best. Four months before her death from cancer, during her last remission stage, Barbara called pain "a side issue:"

> I think the pain is kind of a side issue now. It wasn't as great as it was after the surgery. It's gotten a lot better, to where it's not like an important part of my day, because it's not there as much as it was. Even just within the last week's time I've noticed a big difference in the pain level, and that's gratifying. I don't have to have the pain medications as much as I used to. So you know, what does that mean? Am I healing more? That was a concern of mine because pain kind of takes over your mind and helps you feel not comfortable.

Barbara explained her reluctance to dwell on her pain this way:

> One thing about the pain is that I find myself trying not to talk about it much. I think it's the burden. I don't talk about the pain

much with my husband or my kids. One aspect is not having them worry. Or they get in this little panic state, and I don't like to see them do that when all I might have to do is talk with my doctor a little more and adjust it. And that would be better. And a lot of it is my reticence to say, "I don't feel like doing that today." So I go ahead and do it, just so we're together.

Barbara's "reticence" about pain protected her family from having to confront her illness at every moment; if she could manage to "go ahead and do" whatever family activity was planned, they could enjoy it, and she could be with them. Barbara's attitude was that pain was an intruder that she tried to handle by herself, with her doctor's help. She would ignore it if she could; until the last few weeks of her illness, her pain was controlled to her satisfaction with oral medication.

In contrast with Mabel, for whom pain sometimes may have been helpful in getting attention—and who had few distractions from its unceasing presence—Barbara had activities that she loved to provide relief from her pain. She continued to work throughout her illness and was able to take two long trips during her last summer of life to visit friends and to see the ocean one last time.

"What pain?": Kitty, Walt, Roberta, Sharon

For the three participants with congestive heart failure as well as for Sharon, who had emphysema, pain was less of a problem. None of them complained of pain, and they and their caregivers were satisfied with whatever pain medications they needed. Roberta, in fact, had to take only Tylenol for any discomfort related to her heart problems. At the end of her life, she was on a morphine pump because of the fractured hip. Other symptoms were more troublesome for them or their caregivers: fatigue and blackouts for Kitty, immobility and fatigue for Walt, and increasing dementia for Roberta. Kitty several times described her concerns:

Researcher: Do you have much pain?

Kitty: No. Right now I'm having a little bit, just in my lower back. Really, it's because I've been so lazy. I haven't felt quite strong enough to get out and do any gardening.

∾ ∾ ∾

Kitty: They wanted me to go to Hospice House, and I didn't want to go right now, so I didn't. If I continue to have these blackout spells, eventually I probably will end up there. If I get so tired, you know, that just trying to do anything. . . . I don't want to fall, so I move very cautiously, very slowly, and I use my cane, and I'm doing fine. I think I am.

In our conversations, Kitty failed to mention or downplayed some symptoms that were troublesome and of great concern to those who cared for her—specifically, uncontrolled diarrhea (which predated her most recent illness) and the painful infection of her leg and foot that affected her at the end. She mentioned that her foot hurt but insisted that it was "getting better." Kitty's friend described some of her symptoms for us after Kitty's death:

The trip to Oregon wasn't a particularly good trip from her friend's point of view. That's when we finally discovered that Kitty couldn't control the diarrhea. . . . That foot of hers was extremely painful. She was having pretty heavy doses of medication at that point.

For these people, physical discomforts were not the most important part of their day, and they talked about them with reluctance, if at all. For these three, and for Sharon, hospice care appeared to be providing good treatment of their most troublesome symptoms.

"The side-effects": Sarah

Although Sarah did not complain much about pain, she apparently experienced a good deal of it, controlled with medication. In our first visit with her, she reported:

Researcher: Do you have pain now?

Sarah: Oh yeah, I'm on pills all the time.

Six months later, it was the same story:

Researcher: Do you have much pain anymore?

Sarah: Not especially, since this morning.

Researcher: This [radiation treatment] has really helped it?

Sarah: Yeah, boy, it was before, ooh.

Sarah's struggle with pain was not so much with the pain itself as with the medications she was given at various times. She had experienced this problem a year earlier:

> Well, right at first when it [the bone cancer] first started out, I had medicine I was taking. I was allergic to it, but I got to where they were giving it to me for pain, and it was working for pain fine. But it was driving me nuts. I was goofy.

Sarah's daughter Karen reported that had "gone round and round" with Sarah's doctor about this situation:

> You know, I had the worst time getting the doctor to listen to me. I said, "It's those painkillers that are doing this to her." He said, "Oh, no, no, it's gotta be something else." And we went round and round. And I realize that their [the doctor's] main thing is comfort, but there comes a time when just pumping that pain medicine into people isn't the answer. And I'm all for taking care of the pain. [But] I thought, we've got to find something before the end comes because that's gonna be really bad.

Subsequently, Karen told us that Sarah was on a new pain medication:

> Before, she was completely out of it when she was on those painkillers, but now she's very mentally aware. As long as we keep her off the painkillers she's OK. It's a non-narcotic that's brand new. The only problem is the side effect is liver damage. So we have to get her off as fast as we can.

The battle between physical comfort and social/emotional connection and comfort apparently was not over. Sarah, like Dennis, opted for maintaining her mental coherence and functioning over relieving physical pain or possible long-range side effects.

"I'll suffer enough": Ralph

Of all the topics that Ralph brought up in our visits, pain was one of the least common. He clearly had great difficulty getting his breath and in many ways was uncomfortable. Analyzing the pain was not Ralph's way, however. According to Sandy, Ralph complained about his failing vision, about not having any useful work to do, and about the burden his illness placed on her. He did not complain about pain, however. He fully realized his terminal condition but chose to reflect on the positive things in his life rather than dwell on his forthcoming death.

One of Ralph's few conversations relating to pain was the following:

> Before I retired I said to myself, "On Mom's side there were long-lived people. On Dad's side there were short." And I said to myself, "I want to hit the long-lived side. But I didn't. I hit the shorter side. It's gettin' to the point where a very, very little bit more and I'd be a lot better off. I suffer quite a bit. My doctor says I won't suffer too bad. But I won't suffer, probably, too bad, but I am gonna suffer enough. They don't want to give me too much of that stuff [pain medication] because, well, first, they're not supposed to. Second, if I reach the top then I'm in a heck of a shape. If I took too much then I'd get immune to it, and then I'd be in really bad shape.

Two weeks before Ralph died, Sandy described his attitude toward pain in a way that was clearer than anything we had heard Ralph say himself:

> Well, and Ralph says, "It isn't the pain," he says. "I can bear the pain. It isn't the discomfort. It isn't the choking and that. It's this uselessness, this not being able to do anything." He can't hardly wait to die and go to heaven so he can go to work. That's all he talks about. Just to get to heaven and, "Oh, I hope they got somethin' for me to do when I get there."

Frequency of Topic Introduction as an Indication of Salience

Discourse analysts have found that one of the best indicators of people's major concerns can be discerned in the topics they bring up in a conversation. For example, Walt and his caregiver, Dorothy, did not bring up the topic of his medical problems or condition with any degree of frequency. Of the sixty topics that Walt introduced with us, only eight dealt with his health, and only four with his current condition (Table 5-1).

The "uncertainties" are from the following conversation:

Researcher: I don't know what your condition is.

Walt: Heart, isn't it dear?

Dorothy:	Congestive heart failure and hardening of the arteries, and lungs are bad.
Walt:	The damn congestion or whatever it is. I don't know what it is.

≈ ≈ ≈

Researcher:	You have pain with that?
Walt:	The doctor would know more about that than I do.
Dorothy:	Yeah. He's on morphine 45 grams, three times a day. Every eight hours and Roxanol sometimes.

Walt's eight topics relating to his past and current medical condition represent only 13 percent of all the topics he brought up during our visits. Dorothy introduced this topic even less frequently than Walt: Only four of her eighty-seven topics (4.5 percent) related to Walt's physical condition.

Similarly, in our visits with Ralph, he introduced a total of 108 topics—only ten of which had anything to do with his medical condition. In our conversations with his caregiver, Sandy, she brought up a total of 240 topics, only thirteen of which had anything to do with Ralph's medical condition. (See Table 5-2.)

This infrequency of topics related to Ralph's physical complaints (9 percent of Ralph's topics and 5 percent of Sandy's) is startling in light of the seriousness of his condition. Their minds appeared to be on other things.

In contrast to Walt and Ralph, twenty-one of Dennis's seventy-seven topics (27 percent) were related to his physical condition, and twelve of Carrie's sixty topics (20 percent) were on the same subject. Clearly, Dennis and Carrie often brought up the subject of his physical condition. Comparing the combined

Table 5-1   Topics about Medical Problems: Walt

Previous medical problems	
Broken leg in the service	1
Cut off ends of fingers twice	2
Broken pelvis	1
Current medical problems	
Heart attack 18 months earlier	1
"Doctor said I have a bad heart"	1
Uncertainties	2

ratios of pain topics to all topics introduced by these three patients and their caregivers, we see the results in Table 5-3.

The methodological implication of this analysis concerns the use of quantitative research within a more qualitative research framework. Analysis of the quantity of topics introduced by patients and their caregivers can provide a useful numerical picture of their individual agendas and concerns. We believe that a more structured questionnaire or interview approach would not have revealed such quantitative discrimination. More indirect, ethnographic methods of data gathering allow for multiple occurrences of a topic; such data can serve as a basis for comparison with the quantity of that same topic brought up by other participants. In addition, such an approach has the advantage of letting the participants determine their own agendas, self-generating whatever they want to say rather than being led by the researcher's concerns.

Knowledge of Illness and Attitudes about Pain in the Subculture of Terminally Ill People

The major differences among the participants in this study seemed to center on how they managed the loss of power and control; how they dealt with self-recognition and dignity, at a time when there did not seem to be much chance

Table 5-2   Topics about Medical Problems: Ralph and Sandy

	Ralph	Sandy
Medical history background	2	3
Problems with his back	3	0
Problems breathing	1	4
Problems with vision	1	0
Problems with circulation	1	0
Problems with sleeping	0	3
Common colds	0	1
Appetite loss	0	1
Pain	0	1
"I suffer a lot"	1	0
"I'm just plain sick"	1	0
Total	**10**	**13**

Table 5-3   Topics about Medical Problems: Three Families

Topic: Physical condition, pain, etc.	Topic Ratio	%
Dennis and Carrie combined	33 of 137	24
Walt and Dorothy combined	12 of 120	8
Ralph and Sandy combined	23 of 348	6.5

for any; and in what ways they could continue to grow, even in the last days of life.

Control

Dennis gave up power and control very grudgingly. He clearly wanted to control his body, play golf and take walks. He managed to maintain some control over the issue of remaining at home and avoiding hospitalization. He won that issue, although it took a toll on his caregiver and family. Walt, Sarah, Ralph, and Sharon seemed to have no need to control things any longer. They put all their trust in their caregivers and doctors.

Ralph had no particular need to control anything. He had put all his trust in his caregiver and doctors.

Roberta's only evidence of a need to control was focused more on herself rather than on others. She appeared to have a need to maintain her personal dignity and self-respect, even as her body failed her. She was the family matriarch, regal in manner and appearance, and she was always in "good health."

Mabel had a very small universe in which to exercise any possible control: her daughter, her doctor, and the few medical helpers that were admitted. She displayed her control when she refused to accept the doctor's diagnosis of her bone cancer and—for a while, at least—the prescribed medications for it.

Dignity

The older patients—especially Walt, Sarah, Sharon, and Ralph (but not Roberta)—did not evidence a need to have much dignity during their last months. They claimed to have had a "good life." They recognized that their lives were all but over. They were ready to die—and said so. In contrast, Dennis, who was much younger, frequently brought up the topic of how his rare disease placed him in the limelight, telling us rather proudly that he was one of only 500 in the United States with peripheral T-cell lymphoma:

I am quite a rarity. They're quite interested when they hear my age. I've visited quite a few specialists, anything from environmental physicians to a doctor that flew over from Sweden.

Dennis clearly appreciated the self-recognition and dignity that his illness brought. He took whatever positive advantages he could find in a situation that held absolutely no physical benefits. He learned about medicine, especially as it related to his condition. Because his illness was so unusual, he often was learning along with his doctors. He and his mother learned a great deal more about caregiving for this particular illness than his hospital nurses because they had daily, first-hand experience that nurses seldom get. Dennis spoke of growing intellectually and finding some meaning as a pioneer, helping his physicians learn about his disease.

Our other younger participant, Barbara, did not emulate Dennis in this regard. As her illness grew worse, she expressed more concerned about her family and was uninterested in her illness as a source of self-worth.

Growth

Barbara and Dennis, the younger patients, also exhibited signs of personal growth in their last months of life. Elsewhere we describe their continuous spiritual growth. Dennis also showed growth intellectually, as he acquired knowledge of his disease. Such growth does not appear to be common in the subculture of the terminally ill—at least not in the people we studied.

Some Implications of "Knowing" One's Illness

At first, the contrast between the detailed knowledge and open awareness of the younger patients, on one hand, and the vague or even factually incorrect understanding of some of the more elderly patients on the other concerned us. Sherwin Nuland argues convincingly in *How We Die*, however, that "old age" is a respectable and inevitable cause of death and that elderly persons should be allowed the dignity of dying of old age, without aggressive and ultimately useless interventions or the vanity of being given a specific diagnosis for what actually is the general process of aging. Nuland explains that when the body's functioning begins to fail and then shut down, the failure of one or more specific organs can't be blamed for death:

There is plenty of evidence that life does have its natural, inherent limits. . . . When it is possible to identify a disease by giving it a name, its ravages become the subject of treatment, with the potential aim of cure. . . . [But] old age is as insoluble as it is inevitable. By giving scientific names of treatable disease to its manifestations, too many of the specialists from whom the elderly seek care retain their riddle and their fascination with the disease pathology itself. They also believe they give patients some kind of hope, though in the end the hope must always prove to be unjustified. These days, it is not politically correct to admit that some people die of old age (Nuland 1993, 70, 72).

Nuland argues that the general debility that accompanies aging, not the specific organ that fails first, should be considered the cause of death in the elder years, and such assessment should guide the philosophy of treatment. His perspective is reflected in the knowledge and attitudes of some of the more elderly participants in our study. These eighty-year-olds, along with their physicians (as they reported to us), knew that they were dying of old age and were correspondingly less interested in or knowledgeable about the specific organ or system that was failing them.

Mabel's continuing complaints provide an argument that medical assistance and good pain medication alone are not sufficient for persons with terminal illness. Pain treatment also requires social support and interactions, interesting activities, and possibly complementary, nonmedical therapies to alleviate discomfort.

Chapter 6

Daily Life and Meaningful Activities

We commonly think of dying patients as pale, bedridden, passive, and silent. Equally commonly, we describe terminally ill persons only from the perspective of their medical condition. Although the medical perspective is important, observing and understanding a person's everyday activities and routines as a significant part of their existence also is important. Equally important, we should consider the fact that some aspects of life remain enjoyable and meaningful for these persons. We were curious and a little apprehensive about visiting people who were terminally ill because we had only hospital experiences to fall back on. We had much to learn about the last months, weeks, and days of persons with terminal illnesses.

Seale (1998)—a sociologist who studies the meaning of death in modern culture—has argued persuasively that because human life is "embodied," the daily activities involving the body are essential for remaining *human*. People who are dying fear a "falling out of culture"—spiraling down into an isolated, inhuman existence while they are still alive. These fears are well-founded: Chronic illness and dying directly disrupt the life of the body—particularly the customary routines of grooming and personal care, social contacts, and bodily functions such as eating and sleeping that require coordination with others. "To resist such a descent, people engage in two broad strategies to reconstruct their lives, one at the practical level, one at the symbolic level" (Seale 1998, 26). Because our study participants remained at home for most of their last days, they had many practical opportunities to maintain their social bonds through everyday life activities.

In this chapter we document the various practical strategies that these participants used to maintain their social existence and humanness through daily life. Being able to eat with someone; to walk to the bathroom and use it in private, unaided; to talk with a friend; to watch a favorite TV show; to hold a grandchild—these mundane activities of daily living at the end of life can become symbolic acts of the greatest importance. Small routines and rituals—a walk in the sunshine, a dish of favorite ice cream—take on cosmic significance as one approaches death. (Thus, some of the information in this chapter easily could have been included in chapter 9, "Personal Growth, Meaning, and Spirituality.")

As participant-observers, we found that the small details of daily living became salient and meaningful in relation to each individual's life context, age, illness, and stance or attitude toward life and death. Comparisons and generalizations across this small group of participants seemed to trivialize their experience. Hence, in this chapter we focus on the significant aspects of each participant's daily life. We pay attention (and encourage readers to do likewise) to the details involved in maintaining ordinary daily activities as death approaches. A summary at the end of this chapter indicates some of the commonalties among participants, for readers who want a quick overview of what the participants shared in common. The most important finding, however, is the degree to which participants in this study found ways to maintain connections with the people and activities that had always been meaningful to them in their own context—and in so doing to maintain their connection to the culture and social life around them.

Dennis

Daily Routine

Dennis and his mother, Carrie, both described their daily routine as "maintenance." The routine consisted, in their own words, of "stamping out fires" and "keeping him hygienic"—the latter to control spreading fungal and bacterial infections.

Stamping Out Fires and Keeping Him Hygienic

Carrie: It seems we are just chasing fires, stamping out fires. Just eating, pain control, and sponging. That's it. You asked us to keep a record of what our day is like. We decided that we couldn't. Outside of Bob Barker's "The Price is Right," if we didn't have something major at the moment, the rest of the day was maintenance, just pure maintenance. Everything was toward his comfort, his cleanliness.

Dennis: The whole day is pretty much devoted to getting the pain under control so I can have some quality of life.

Since I don't want to be in the hospital, it means a lot of maintenance and a lot of vigilance.

Part of this daily maintenance that Carrie talked about had to do with washing and bathing:

My greatest concern is when and how Dennis is gonna be kept in his last days, hygienically. 'Cause I went through six days of this team effort just to give him a saline wash, which was in place of a shower—bed bath. Where you have to be sedated to turn a person to the side, change the bed and give the saline wash all at the same time, with suction and anesthetic. Suction to catch the water on a floatation bed that you could turn.

Enjoyable Activities

Perhaps because Dennis was younger than the other participants, he appeared to work hard at finding what he called "quality of life." He described his enjoyable activities as golfing, visiting, staying busy, watching television, fishing, playing slot machines, and having "little AA meetings" with his mother.

Golfing

Researcher: If you had a real high spot, a good thing to happen, what would it be?

Dennis: It would be that I would feel good enough to go golfing. That's my love. It's a great release for me. It is some exercise, which I need. And it's so enjoyable for me. And I like to perform for Mom and Dad. Due to my condition, you would think that I would not be able to shoot a good game of golf. But I have actually surprised myself in that it's been real relaxing and fun, and I look forward to each time that I can get out.

Carrie: In May Dennis went out and he golfed eighteen holes. I drove the cart, and he golfed eighteen holes. And I could not believe it. It was a verrrry good day! He had been sick eighteen hours before. He's maybe golfed seven times since then. Sometimes with his dad, sometimes with a buddy, sometimes myself.

Visiting

I enjoy visitors kind of at my leisure, when I want them. I always prefer a phone call prior to somebody dropping over because I may be having a bad day and not want to talk to anybody. But I would say, on the whole, I don't like a whole lot of visitation. Some friends and golf buddies will drop over, but mostly it's been family, though.

∽ ∽ ∽

I have a pastor who likes to drop in. I treat him as I do anybody else that I'm not really familiar with, and that is, "Please call me first." Because he has shown up at the most inopportune times. We've had quite lengthy discussions on dying, etc. And he's offered a lot of comfort in that area. But I can talk to my family about just about anything. Maybe it's the thing that there is death looming over me that loosens my tongue a little bit more, makes me braver, to be more assertive.

Staying Busy

When you're independent, it's really hard to sit back and let people do things for you. I like to cook, fish, and play golf and all kinds of things like that. And when that's kind of taken from you, it's a hard adjustment to say, "Well, how can I entertain myself now?" or "How can I stay busy?" And without involving other people. I have to rely on them for rides or whatever.

Television

TV has become an automatic with me. Whereas before I never watched that much television. But I really have no choice now. I don't read a whole lot. Just never have. I'm not a letter writer. I'm more of an active, outdoorsy person. I do take evening strolls if I can, because I just love this area, the mountains, nor would I want to die in a more beautiful place than this.

Fishing, God, Nature, and Children

What else lifts my spirits? Fishing. The Lord. Uh, I don't find my Lord in the church; I find Him out in the beauty in nature. And fishing—I love to fly fish. I love the different smells and sights and sounds. And I love to travel to different places where I've never been before. And my children, they give me great satisfaction to watch them grow.

Eating

Dennis recalled trying to find something pleasant to do, especially during the long weekly drives for chemotherapy treatment. He spoke of getting a hamburger at a fast food restaurant along the way, starting each day over a good cup of coffee, enjoying a lemon almond-flavored birthday cake from a Missoula bakery, or feasting on Twinkies and chocolate milk. Carrie told us that she would put a donut by his bedside during the last week of his life. She also described a Father's Day dinner for Dennis at the family ranch, a few months earlier, when she cooked Dennis's favorite meal: roast chicken, rice, and good bread.

Playing the Slots

One of the most difficult aspects of daily functioning for Dennis was to travel back and forth to Missoula for treatment. Carrie pointed out that she and Dennis worked hard to find something enjoyable about these trips. One thing was to stop and play the slot machines. As we visited on the patio outside the doctor's office in late July, Carrie elaborated on this activity:

> Dennis had had a serious gambling problem. It caused great hardship in his immediate family. But we come in here and play the machines. I don't care what it takes of my finances. And this might be insane, but the doctor said today, "Have fun," because he didn't think he'd last the summer. And we talked about what you can't do that's fun anymore and that every decision is a "now" decision. How you feel "now." So it lifts our spirits. We chatter a lot the hour we spend driving in. About anything and everything. If we didn't stop at the machines on the way home, what would we do? What would be fun? What would be enjoyable about coming here? There was a time when we spent 47 days in a row for radiation. What would we do? Get a hamburger? There were months when there was nothing to do. There was no golf. Comfort was all you strove for. And not comfort but tolerable pain control is what we struggled for. And that's what we still struggle for. There's a lot to be said when the doctor says, "Have fun." Just that little prize.

The enjoyment Dennis and his mother got from these visits to the slots is evident in their dialogue about such events:

Dennis: And there's a chance of winning money, maybe.

Carrie: And you can take it to the grave, can't you, Dennis?

Dennis: You better believe it [laughing]. I'm gonna.

Carrie:	I mean, people say, "Why do you want to play the machines?" Well, anybody who knows anything about playing machines would know it isn't a matter of money.
Dennis:	It's endorphin release; come on, I mean, you find them any way you can get them. That's what you're looking for.

Having Little AA Meetings

Carrie:	And we love coffee in the morning. We love the morning.
Dennis:	Get all perked up and have our little AA meetings. Solve the troubles of the world [laughs]. We had a good one on the way down today. We just have meetings where we talk back and forth.
Carrie:	Today's topic was the gratefulness of a sober mind. Dennis said, "You have to offer a prayer of thanks when you're given the opportunity to . . . "
Dennis:	. . . to have that second chance.
Carrie:	To have that second chance. And for us, I guess it was a sober mind.
Dennis:	Absolutely. A lot of people don't get that second chance.

Later, when we asked Carrie if she ever managed to attend her AA group during that year, she noted:

There was no time to go. Either you just flopped or you were working on maintenance.

Learning

Dennis also grew cognitively, finding some meaning in this newly acquired knowledge about his disease. He learned about medicine, especially as it related to his condition. Because his illness was so unusual, he often was learning along with his doctors, and this knowledge gave him great satisfaction.

Barbara

Daily Routine and Enjoyable Activities

Barbara's daily routine during the time we visited her was still that of an active woman, working whenever she felt able and taking care of her family. Except for great tiredness and the constant round of tests and doctor's visits, there was little remarkable or unusual about her days until the last month of her life. Although we did not visit with Barbara during her last month—and therefore do not have direct information from her about her daily routine—her sister Irene's account describes a rich and enjoyable time at Irene's home.

Music

She loved classical music. I have a CD player that plays continuous CDs. I played flute music for her.

Friends and Family

Her friends came to my home, and they'd just come in and stand at the foot of her bed. They would stand there . . . just to see her. And when people brought food. Although she wasn't eating, she could see us eating.

I fixed a little couch in the living room, and she was in the living room with all of us. And we sat and visited and talked about her life. This is what we do. And she gets to hear it.

The Baby

We also had a baby there. We had a little four-month-old baby. Barbara couldn't talk any more. But she could see the baby. This little baby did something for her. My other sister would lay the baby right by Barbara. I think that a lot of times at that point, people are afraid to touch 'em. But this little baby would just kind of grab at her and was just laying right on her. And it did something for her. It would calm her.

Food

Her taste was not the best, but I fixed her things that would look good in the beginning. I baked things and I made soups. I would put a little for her, and she'd take two bites.

Smudge

In our culture we like smudge. She was on oxygen, but we'd open up my back door and we'd light the smudge outside and we'd let some of it come in, and then we'd close the door. We didn't know if she was smelling it. But she responded to it.

Stories

I'd say, "Barbara, why don't you just sit back and close your eyes, and I'll tell you a story. Just listen." She loved to hear about our medicine bundle that we belong to. I would tell her stories that had morals in them. I hung my eagle fan above her head because our belief is that's the dream world. When you lay down to rest, that eagle spirit is going to help you to have good dreams.

Ralph

Daily Routine

Ralph seemed to have less problem filling up his days, perhaps because he was much older than Dennis or Barbara. Up to the last week of his life, although he sat in a wheelchair most of the day, he could get to the toilet by himself and could hobble short distances inside his apartment. When we first visited him in mid-August, he spoke of taking "walks" around the apartment area. Even after his walks had to be made with his walker, he was able to get outdoors—a prime requirement for this man of the woods. He began his day by sleeping late, having breakfast, then going back to bed for a while.

Because Ralph was almost blind, Sandy would spend periods of time reading to him. He enjoyed hearing news from the weekly newspaper in the *Swan* as well as the daily *Missoulian*. Sandy also read him the Bible. Often, when we visited the television would be on. Sandy would watch, and Ralph would listen or doze off. Up to his last months, Ralph would go with Sandy on short shopping trips, remaining in the car until she returned. For the most part, however, Ralph's day consisted of medicating, eating, waiting, and sleeping.

Sleeping was one of Ralph's major daily activities at the time we began our visits with him. In September—a month after we met Ralph—Sandy commented about one of Ralph's "bad spells":

I have to do the cleaning around him, but he's asleep most of the time. He's barely been out of bed since last Friday. So we'll just have to see. He'll either come out of it, which he has done before, but now he's getting very discouraged. So I let him sleep all he wants to because when he's asleep, he isn't suffering. The nurse and the doctor have both said that he'll probably just go to sleep into a coma one of these days. 'Cause that's the disease, the progress the disease takes. When he's awake he has to go through all of this gagging and spitting and choking. The choking is the worst. Trying to get the air in. And when he can't get any air, see, he panics. All of us would do that. We gotta just take one day at a time.

Enjoyable Activities

Ralph's enjoyable activities were very limited physically. He whittled (even though he could hardly see what he was doing), watched television (or, more accurately, listened to it), took short walks outside the apartment, accompanied Sandy shopping, was read to, visited with friends and family who drove down to Missoula, and made the long car trip back to his beloved homestead when he could.

Whittling

The last few months, Ralph spent time whittling peach seeds—making tiny baskets out of them. He did this largely by feel because his vision was so weak. This work with a natural material seemed to be a symbolic connection to his lifelong experience working with the land, the environment, and building log homes. When we visited in November, he was talking about the need to protect the environment when we asked:

Researcher:	Are you making something there with that peach pit?
Ralph:	Oh yeah, a little basket. It's to keep my fingers busy.
Researcher:	That's neat. Have you made many of these baskets?
Ralph:	Oh yeah.
Researcher:	I see. You have a little saw and a file. How do you get the hole? Is the center hollow?
Ralph:	Yeah, that's the hollow. You get your pocket knife and dig that out.

Watching Television

The television was usually on when we visited. The extent to which Ralph attended to the programs was unclear, however. Sandy noted that she, at least, watched it some, especially football games. Sandy described a typical Sunday morning in September as follows:

Yesterday morning he got up and we ate breakfast. He has a church service he likes to watch on television. Comes from Jackson, Mississippi—a Baptist minister he likes real well. We listen to that, and then we usually watch "In Touch" with Charles Stanley. He gets a little carried away, but we watch him anyway. This was Sunday morning, you know, and of course now we watch football. Well, I should say, I do. Anyway, we did that yesterday morning, and as soon as breakfast is over he says, "Can I help you with the dishes?" And I said, "No, I think I'll just put 'em in the soap for now." I had my bed made, but I hadn't made his yet. He got up from the table and had all his pills, and he says, "I think I'll go lay down for a little while." And he went in there and he slept for two hours. And then he went back in the afternoon and slept again for a couple hours or so.

Taking Walks along the River

In August and September, Ralph told us that he still tried to get out to take a walk whenever he could and the weather was good:

Researcher: Did you get your walk today?

Ralph: Yep. I walked down there half way, half way down [pointing out the patio door toward the river].

With Ralph's limited air supply, these walks were a struggle, but the river was a beautiful blue mirror, lined with cottonwood trees turning gold in the fall. Even a few steps with a walker and Sandy by his side for support were worth the effort.

Getting Out in the Car

Ralph's daily routine was largely bounded by the apartment, and he had difficulty getting out, even in the car. His one excursion was on Saturday—shopping day for Sandy. Before our first visits with Ralph in August, Sandy used to leave Ralph at the apartment while she bought groceries and made other shopping trips. After August, she was not comfortable leaving him alone:

Ever since the nurse said she would just as soon not have him alone too long, I've been loading him in the car on Saturday morning and going to the grocery store, and he sits in the car and watches the traffic and everything 'cause it was cool early in the mornings and stuff. And there was no traffic or anything, and so that took care of my problem. You know, I can leave him to sit in the car and not have to haul that stupid chair of his in my car. It won't fit in there.

Being Read To

During an October visit Sandy told us that what's "drivin' him nuts right now" was that his vision was growing worse and worse:

> If he could read, then he could read what he wanted to read, you know. But he can't do that, and he's so dependent on me to read to him every day and every night before we go to bed. We read something from the Bible. I have inspirational guides that I've been using, and when the paper comes from home, I read that to him too. But, you know, if I was to sit down and read him a book, it would bore him to death. He's never been one to sit down and read novels and stuff.

Visiting

One of the problems that Ralph had was that in Missoula he was isolated from his many friends back home, in the Swan Valley. Sandy commented to us that in Missoula they didn't really have a network of friends to help out or even visit. Ralph often spoke of his love of simply visiting with people. Most of Ralph's visitors were hospice workers, nurses, volunteers, and, of course, the doctor and chaplain. If Ralph couldn't see his home friends often, he made up for it by claiming these people as his friends as well:

> I really do enjoy visiting with people. That is something that I've talked with the hospice about, and they asked me my opinion. I said there's sure a whole lot to being able to talk to somebody, to get their opinions. Might set you on a little better road to go down too, you know, if you want to listen a little bit, you know. If people come in and talk and tell you about some of their experiences and stuff, like we're doin' here, you know. These people that come in here with me, why, I've gotten a lot of good out of that, a whole bunch of good. Some people say that you don't know how lucky you are about the people you got and that care about you. I didn't know this either until they started comin' out of the woodwork.

Ralph also often spoke to us about his friends back home. A visit from a neighbor was an automatic topic in his conversations with us. In an October visit, for example, he described such a visit:

I had a nice surprise this morning here. It was right after lunchtime, I guess, somewhere right there. I was settin' here and Sandy had stepped out, and there was a knock at the door. And I wondered what in the heck's goin' on. Didn't have no nurses or anything comin' in to look after me, and you people weren't supposed to be here yet. I went over and opened the door, and it was a little girl I know back home. And she had a baby, and she brought the little baby down to show me. I thought that's pretty nice. There's people out there care. It's pretty hard not to cry there. Yeah, I wouldn'ta cared if I'da cried a drop or two. 'Cause that's quite a little bit of effort to drive down, come down here.

Making Visits Back Home

Ralph didn't get to go back to visit his homestead and friends there very often, but the visits he did make certainly were highlights in his life, despite the difficulty he had getting there and back by car. After Ralph's death, Sandy told us:

I brought him up here as many times as he was able to come. The last time I brought him here he said, "I can't ever do this again. It's too hard on me." So I never tried to bring him back again.

When we saw him in October—just after this trip and about a month before he died—Ralph told us:

I made it up there yesterday. It about played me out. But I said, "What difference does it make? I live from morning 'till night anyway. I'm gonna try one more time. I'll be real extra careful." Sandy drove me up there. I had a nice dinner with my sister and her husband and got to look at the old place. Couldn't see it well, but you could feel it all. You could smell it. All that pretty smell of the timber—and from what I could see, I got to look at the clean-up job that the good people had done, and it looked good to me. And the Reliance forester had already looked at it, and he said it was an excellent job that they had done, cleaning it up. So that made me feel good. So I got a day of it. I got a good day. We went up in the morning and stopped several times along it. There's this mountain— looked at things, you know. And went on, on old stops and a few of the places I wanted to see. Especially to see people I was really fond of, the people that have our little store and post office up there. I went especially down to see her 'cause she was a real dear friend of mine. Yeah, it was worth the added. . . .

Ralph stopped his narrative in mid-sentence. Perhaps he realized that he had been doing all the talking, so he said, "Now it's your turn. Tell me a story," noting that he was "out of air." We tried to introduce a new topic, but he quickly interrupted us and recycled his own favorite topic—the Montana Land Reliance and our need to take care of the land. When Ralph had visitors, he seemed to be able to ignore his physical limitations.

Sharon

Daily Routine

As a result of Sharon's advanced emphysema, her daily routine began with several hours of struggling for breath. She would awake early, at five, and then wake and doze fitfully until after 9:00 A.M. or even later. Her sister Connie would get up to help her in her struggle to breathe. Connie would give Sharon her medications, but some mornings Sharon could not get out to the dining room and her recliner until 11:00. She read the paper while she ate breakfast, then stayed in her big chair—eating a little, watching television, and visiting— most of the day. She remained alert and able to be part of conversations during the afternoon. In the evening, she ate in her recliner, watched television, and was in bed by 9:00.

This routine was punctuated by a great number of visitors, including Sharon's three grown children, some grandchildren, friends, and hospice staff and volunteers. "There are enough people coming in," in Sharon's judgment. Connie said that she had to keep track of twenty-three appointments a week.

With chronic emphysema, Sharon had been sedentary for years, so her increasing immobility and limitations did not seem to bother her. Connie remarked, "I thought I'd take her out a lot this summer, but I couldn't get her to go. She really never wants to go."

Enjoyable Activities

Visitors

Visitors—family and friends—were the mainstay and most important part of Sharon's week. The "twenty-three appointments" Connie described included a Senior Companion who turned out to be an old friend of Sharon's, her three adult children, a hospice volunteer, one or two friends from her former church, a second cousin who lived nearby, and eventually, this researcher. Connie's home was open and accessible. We felt comfortable calling in the morning to ask if we could "stop by"; the coffee was always on, and Connie provided a plate of cookies at any hour as a sign of their hospitality. Sharon's ability to talk often was limited, but she enjoyed hearing people talk around her and was an engaged and interested listener, telling us, "I have full days; there's a lot going on."

The pattern of having people come in to share coffee and talk with Sharon while she listened had been part of her life for a long time. Her son describes the "counseling" she used to do at her kitchen table in the rural hamlet they lived in:

> Most of the years I remember her sittin' at the table, the kitchen table. You never knew who'd come and visit. And I mean they had problems, big problems. The wife would come over at times, and then the husband, and she'd spend all day talking to different people, just like a bartender.

Among Sharon's special visitors were some young people she had cared for as a babysitter ten years earlier; these visitors were now in their teens. Sharon reported that one came to visit regularly and played the flute for her during her last months of life:

> When I came to Missoula, I did some babysitting. 'Cause I really enjoyed that. And I didn't have any babies in my family. And they've been a real joy now; I mean, they get to come back and visit me. Some of those babies are grown up.

Parties—Birthday and Other

Sharon's family had two big parties for her during her last months of life; she also planned a third one on her own. The first party was four months before her death, in July, when Sharon's grown children and Connie's children, plus assorted other family, got together to celebrate Sharon's life at Connie's house. A ceremonial four-generation family photograph was taken, stories were told, food shared. Sharon and her family referred to this gathering openly as a kind of memorial service celebrating her life.

Sharon's last birthday was in October, and Connie planned a party for the weekend, with a special cake. She invited different friends and family to visit at different times, so that Sharon wouldn't be overwhelmed. Sharon's daughter came from out of town for the weekend with her teenage son; both of Sharon's sons were there, as was one granddaughter, along with the girlfriend of her other son—also clearly a part of this family. Sharon was in good humor and clearly pleased with her birthday party, despite joking with us a week earlier about hoping she "wouldn't make it." She smoked a cigarette with her son and talked with everyone. There was much joking and teasing and little family strain evident among Sharon's close family one month before her death.

The third party is one that Sharon planned in a conversation with her hospice nurse, during a regular visit. Sharon said that she hoped the nurse "would be here" when she died, and the nurse asked, "Do you want to have a party . . . right at the end?" Sharon's eyes lit up, and she said yes. They began talking about whether to have cocktails, balloons, streamers. Sharon decided on an angel food cake as the most fitting. This planning was done with much laughter and even excitement. Sharon's death was sudden, so there was no time for the actual party, but the planning was as enjoyable for that moment as the party might have been.

Reading Newspapers and Books

Sharon loved to read; she called it her "number one hobby." She often had the local newspaper on her lap, and she seemed to enjoy keeping up with the news. She had assumed that as she became more and more ill, she'd have more time to read. She showed us a pile of books by her chair but said that she found reading more difficult as she grew more ill:

> I'm just real disappointed. I figured that I was gonna have lots of reading time, and I can't. Just can't focus on it.

Talking Books

As Sharon's ability to concentrate lessened, she learned to listen to books on tape. Humorous books by Irma Bombeck were her favorite.

Coffee and Food—"Eat what I want"

Sharon lost much of her taste for food during her last six months, but coffee still tasted good on her seventy-fourth birthday, six weeks before her death: "I can't imagine having too much coffee." As she lost her taste for food, she enjoyed the idea of "eating what I want," rather than having to worry about a balanced diet. Sweets and cakes and other treats still brought her pleasure. Finding a bright side to her loss of appetite and limited intake—and the portents of her system shutting down—was typical of Sharon. She elaborated on this point:

> It really doesn't matter if I eat or not. From now on it's for fun. I can eat what I want!

Cigarettes

Smoking cigarettes had been Sharon's way of declaring her maturity as a teenager in the late 1930s:

> The first thing I did to declare my independence was to start smoking. And I wanted to from the time I was—nobody smoked in

our house, but I always wanted to. Smoking and movies were restricted in our lives. And the only things that I wanted to do was smoke and go to the movies.

Unlike Ralph, Sharon never spoke of regretting that she had smoked. She sometimes would light up a cigarette as she talked with visitors:

I never did stop smoking. Somebody says they remembered me saying I was going to, but I . . . [lights up] I don't remember that.

Sharon may have had only one or two cigarettes a day at the end, but she enjoyed every one. She would carefully unhook the oxygen clip and slip it off while she smoked, then put it back on.

TV—Especially the Gaithers

TV was Sharon's remaining source of entertainment, apart from her visitors, and she watched it whenever nothing else was happening. She had recently discovered the Gaithers' gospel music program on Sunday afternoons. Connie said she never missed their program: "She loved those old hymns."

Walt

Daily Routine

Walt was in bed every time we visited him. He could manage to get to the bathroom, but that was all. He spent his waking hours on his back. More than once Walt complained that his biggest problem was boredom. He claimed that he did not like to watch television very much, but he later admitted that he did like to watch baseball games once in a while. His wife, Dorothy, described Walt's daily activities as follows:

Some days he's practically out for 24 hours. And other days, now like today, he was up for a while and was in the chair a little bit. Sometimes he can't get up at all. I get him awake for the pain medication. And the rest of the day he can sleep until he feels like getting up for a break. Some days he's sick at his stomach and can't eat. Some days he can. It just depends on how he feels. He's in diapers sometimes, and sometimes he isn't. We don't usually have lunch. He usually just has a dish of ice cream. That's usually his afternoon fare.

Enjoyable Activities

By the time we began visiting Walt, he was almost entirely confined to his bed. According to Dorothy, Walt knew that he would die soon and wished that death would come quickly. Under such conditions, finding enjoyable activities is difficult. Walt's family was very closely knit, and it seemed to provide him with most of the joy that he needed. Therefore, visiting—especially with his family—stands out as providing his most enjoyable moments during his last few months. Previously, he had enjoyed getting out, taking rides with his daughter, and seeing the outdoors he loved so much. By the time of our visits, however, he clung to his family most.

Visiting, Especially with Family

It is clear from both Walt and Dorothy that what Walt enjoyed most was having visitors, mostly family members. Dorothy told us, "I wake him up whenever he has 'em coming. I wake him up because that's more important." In our first August visit, Walt's eyes gleamed as he told us about family members coming to see him:

> Well, one of the boys came in this morning and he was here all of a minute. But he was here! Said, "Dad, how you doing?" and "I'm going over to so-and-so, you wanna go with me?" I like to have people come and talk if they don't stay too long. You know what I mean?
>
> Some days all four of 'em is here. One son will come in the middle of the afternoon if he gets the chance. "Well, Dad, I'm not going to bother you." Then he lays down in the bed next to me and takes a nap. Even my daughter in [Eastern city] has been here twice this spring.

Later, also in August, the first topic Walt brought up was about a visit from his nephew and his triplets. Then he recycled this topic three times throughout our visit:

> My wife's nephew was here with his triplet girls. Two girls and one boy they were. Two years old, I think. Boy, they are something! This was a lot of family here.

Dorothy prompted Walt about visits from his granddaughter:

Dorothy: Your kids come to see you all the time. What more do you want in life?

Walt: I'll tell you, they are swell about it. They are really grand.

Dorothy: And when your granddaughter came home from her trip, the first thing she did was to come in and hug you, what more do you want?

Walt: And she didn't even go home to greet her dog first.

After Walt's death, Dorothy reiterated how Walt had loved visitors:

And when he had company, he was good. But when they left, then he was bad. After the kids left, terribly bad.

Getting Outside

Walt had been a plumber who was used to getting out on the job every day. Being cooped up in bed was very difficult for him. Walt and Dorothy's duplex was in a neighborhood with continuous construction going on. Walt could hear the construction, but his bedroom was placed in such a way that he could not get to a window and see it. He lamented this fact to us in an early visit.

One of Walt's daughters, in an after-death visit with us, told us that up to six months before he died, she had taken him out on drives through the town:

I started taking him on a ride once a week, somewhere. And our last ride was down the Bitterroot, to a funeral of one of his relatives. So he got to see a lot of the relatives the day of the funeral. Plus we had gone down to visit some of his uncles that are still alive down in Corvallis. So I was trying to make an effort to take him out to see things. I had to go to Phoenix the middle of March, and I told Dad that when I came back, we'd go up and see some of his friends that he'd been wanting to see up around Arlee. But we never got that far. By the time I got back from Phoenix he couldn't make another trip. There was no taking him out of the house any more.

Sarah

Daily Routine

During the time we visited Sarah, she lived in several different settings, including a senior residence, Hospice House, a regular nursing home, and finally, a private home that takes care of eight elderly women (mostly Alzheimer's patients). Consequently, the information we got about daily routines varied from setting to setting. She mentioned the "entertainments" at her former senior residence several times during our visits with her at more recent settings. She made close friends there, especially with a blind lady who cropped up in her conversation several times. Sarah was pretty much on her own there, except for group meals served in the dining room. We got the impression that she liked this setting, except for the fact that the food was not as good as at Hospice House.

Our first visit with Sarah was after she had left this assisted living facility and moved to Hospice House. She dearly loved her new setting, telling us proudly:

> This is my home now. It's just actually an awful lot like home. Can't say enough for it. The other place [the senior residence] felt more like a restaurant or something like that. You eat there, then you go back to your room and sit for a while. But they did have some entertainments. But they didn't have a kitchen and living room and things like that to go to.

Although Sarah did not specifically describe her daily routine, the field notes of our visits to Hospice House described a setting that suggested things the residents could do there:

> We arrived at 2:00 P.M. and were greeted by a friendly hospice worker who went to Sarah's room to get her. We were ushered into a large and well-appointed, homey living room. Hospice House is just that: a house. It looks like a home in almost every way, except for wheelchairs and walkers in various corners. The living room has a wonderful view of the mountains from the windows. All bedrooms seem to have such views. Residents are not captive to their own rooms here and seem to move around at will. The table in the dining area was set for dinner with four or five placemats for those who could walk (field notes, August 20, 1997).

After Sarah had to leave Hospice House, her daughter, Karen, tried more than one nursing home. She finally settled on a licensed personal care home setting in Missoula, which our field notes describe as follows:

> It is an older, ranch-style home, partly log and added onto, which houses eight ladies. It is very pleasant and clean. There are several large eating tables, lots of sitting room and home decorations. It has NO appearance of being an institution. Each lady has her own private room, with bed, table, chairs, dresser, and television. Sarah's room has a glass patio door leading onto a nice patio and a very

large back yard. There were also two very nice dogs that lived with the host family. Sarah says it's very expensive and that she can't afford to stay there much longer. Sarah likes the family that runs it. A younger couple had to take care of their parents and so they decided to expand and take in other older people as well.

There appears to be no skilled nursing here, and Sarah reports that Medicare "was not available" (perhaps meaning that Medicare did not cover all of the costs). She has just had her last radiation treatment and was a bit fatigued. Her leg has not functioned properly for several months. She hopes that it will improve enough for her to be readmitted to the senior residence where she lived before she went to Hospice House. Residents there are required to be able to get around better than she has been able to lately (field notes, March 24, 1998).

Enjoyable Activities

Sarah's days were sedentary at this phase of her life. She was very easygoing and not at all demanding. She told us that she most enjoyed visiting with people, helping whenever she could, and watching television.

Visiting

Like most of our participants, Sarah often spoke fondly of having visitors come to see her, especially people from her church:

Oh, I've had lots of visitors. The pastor visits all the time. Yeah, well, he's pretty busy. And whenever he can make it. He might come in the evening, or he might come in the afternoon or morning. But whenever he can. But he got out the other day. He was out. Yep.

By early September, Sarah was a bit more precise about the timing of her pastor's visits:

Well, he tries to make it once every two weeks, but he can't always make it. He was so busy.

Other church friends brought the communion elements to Sarah at Hospice House from her church.

It always makes you feel better that somebody cared enough to come. Another thing they do is bring me the flowers from the altar.

Real often they bring them, and then I have 'em for another week. And there's somebody that gets to visit, too, that way.

In March, after Sarah had moved to the board-and-care setting, her church friends continued to visit her:

A lady came here a couple days ago. I still see 'em, and they all tell me, "We're coming," but I'm anxious to see the church now they've done it over. I'm anxious to see the inside. They brought a pink bouquet the other day, a plant.

In this care setting, where the other residents had Alzheimer's disease, Sarah found that she could not engage in the kind of visiting that she did at Hospice House or at her other recent homes. The people who ran the facility provided her with enjoyable conversation, kidding, and chit-chat, however. Sarah also enjoyed visits to her daughter's home. Karen still brought her mother home for dinners whenever possible. Each time we visited, Sarah talked about these dinners at Karen's. After the Christmas holidays, Sarah spoke glowingly about spending Christmas eve at Karen's home along with her other daughter and that daughter's stepchildren.

Helping Other Patients

At our first visit in August, Sarah described how she got to Hospice House—at the same time revealing how much she enjoyed helping other people:

The doctor called them [Hospice House] and asked them if I could come here. He said that he thought I would be real good for the people here. 'Cause I'm not down in bed like, well, most of them are. And if they need the bell or something like that, there's two of us in the room. I was just in a room with this other lady that passed away. I can get around, so there's a lot I can do. That lady wasn't with it, and she'd start to crawl out of bed, you know, and I could always get her to stop. I mean, it was nothing much on my part, but it helped her. . . .

At the other place there was one lady that had a bad foot and leg, and she still calls me. I'd run and get help for her most of the time. It wasn't much different there than it is here, but on a smaller scale.

At the private-care setting, Sarah did not mention helping other residents. The other seven ladies were Alzheimer's patients, all ambulatory. In addition, there were four members of the host family to watch over the eight women, reducing the potential for Sarah to help others.

Watching Television

Only on our last visit to Sarah, in March, did she mention watching television. Her other homes had television in a lobby but not in each room. Now, at the private-care setting, she had her very own television set and not much else to fill her days. So she gave it a try, noting:

> Over the years I couldn't watch a TV program because I was always taking care of the little kids, day care and foster care. So I don't mind settin' and watchin' TV. I like country music and the news. Or just about whatever's on. Oh, there's some that I don't like. And now I can lay down and watch it.

Kitty

Daily Routine

Kitty's day followed a regular and simple pattern. Her dog, Beau, came in to wake her up each morning, and after Kitty got dressed she would unlock the door for her daily visitors. For several months, a home health care aide came in each morning at 9:30 to check on her. The cats and her dog had doors to go in and out of the house by themselves, and she kept fresh water and food for them in the kitchen.

Kitty spent her days in her favorite chair in the living room, with the TV, radio, and her classical music tapes. The Meals on Wheels delivery came about 11:30; the delivery person put the food in the refrigerator for her, so she wouldn't have to get up from her chair. Other visitors from church came on a daily basis. When Kitty was alone, she watched TV and napped in her chair, getting up only to fix lunch and dinner. Kitty described her days this way—an accurate picture:

> Days now are pretty much alike. I get up and have my breakfast, watch a little TV, or listen to the music on KUFM, and sleep. I take naps during the day, anytime I haven't got anything else to do. I'm like an animal, you know. If they haven't got anything else to do, they just curl up and go to sleep. That's the way I am.

Kitty's analogy of being "like an animal," holed up during her last days, was telling. Her small house was cozy and comfortably informal when we first visited, with big overstuffed chairs for visitors and a special chair for her dog. Kitty took a nap in bed in the afternoon and watched the news and other cable channels on TV after dinner. With no one to look after her, she ate "when I get hungry; there's always something in the refrigerator to eat." At night she listened to radio in bed until she fell asleep.

Enjoyable Activities

Visitors: "I like company"

Visitors were the highlight of Kitty's life. With no family as caregivers, she was entirely dependent on people "stopping by" to provide companionship and ensure that her needs were met. On our first visit, Kitty made very clear that we were welcome—and welcome to come back:

> I'm glad to see anybody. I get awful tired of dogs and cats. Conversation with them is a bit limiting. . . . I always welcome visitors because it breaks the monotony. You don't like to just talk to your cats and the dog all day long. [Laugh] Or be alone. I like company. You're my third visitor today.

The visits Kitty wanted were purely social; she had no interest in philosophical introspection or developing new friendships. Unlike some of our other study participants—with whom we developed friendly relations and who talked more openly with us about their fears and their death—Kitty was always guarded and cautious in her conversation. As she grew more ill and confused, she became even more guarded. But her enjoyment of "having a visit" continued, even as she became less able to participate in it. She reiterated this point throughout her last months, even as she became more confused and had more difficulty actually taking part in a conversation or even responding to topics:

> I always enjoy company. People say, "Can we come and visit?" I say, "Of course; you know you always are welcome."

Until Kitty went to Hospice House, her church continued to send in daily visitors or called her during the week, and someone came with communion on Sunday. These daily visits kept Kitty connected to the world she loved and valued most and to the community where she had lived for sixty years, even as she became unable to participate in it actively.

Animals and Birds

Kitty's animals were the center of her emotional life. She spoke of her worry about their fate if anything should happen to her, and much of our conversation centered around the activities of her dog and the two cats:

> I'm very content now, that I can be in my own home and with my animals. This one has a black spot on the nostril. And the other one has practically the same markings except a black chin. They're

littermates, I think. I got them at the Humane Society. I'm a great believer in it. These little waifs at the Humane Society, they're the ones that need the help.

After Kitty's dog died (just six weeks before her own death), she talked of getting another one:

When my foot's all healed up, I'm going to get another one. I've never been without a dog, and I can't imagine living without one. The cats are just angelic, but it's not the same.

One of the barriers to going to Hospice House for Kitty was that she could not take all her animals. Earlier in the summer, she seemed aware that she would have to find other homes for them, but as she lost more mental ability to remember and make judgments, she became convinced that her animals could go with her. Fortunately, in her last weeks at Hospice House, a friend from church began to visit her with her own dog, providing Kitty with an opportunity to have animals in her room even as she was dying. Her priest commented on the importance of this last gift: "That was a wonderful thing for Kitty because animals were her life."

Kitty had a bird feeder outside the large picture window, so that she could see the birds coming to feed. She spoke of a tanager that stopped by in the winter, but as fall drew on, she no longer wanted to open the blinds and kept them closed. In her last months, she enjoyed just looking at the pictures of birds hanging on the wall by her fireplace.

Music

I listen to a lot of music. I listen to KUFM, particularly if they have some good music on that I like—mainly classical. I sometimes go to sleep with it on. They have a lot of nice classical music from time to time that I like to listen to.

Kitty also had hundreds of classical music tapes and a portable tape deck in her home. After she went to Hospice House, she had two weeks of relative comfort and alertness and was able to spend much of her time listening to her tapes on her "boom box."

Dining Out and the Weekly Breakfast Club

For years Kitty had gone to breakfast once a week with a group of women from her church. Amazingly enough, her weekly breakfasts continued throughout her illness, with her friends coming by faithfully to pick her up each week. She had always enjoyed going out to eat, and the breakfast club allowed her to continue until four weeks before she died.

> I like to go out with people, to restaurants or casinos. Any place to get out. I don't care. I'm not proud. I used to like to dine out. . . . I still like that. Now everybody has to take me out.

TV: Animal, Travel, A&E Channels

> If there's anything good on, I'll be watching TV. The animal channel, travel channel, and there's another one . . . A&E [Arts & Entertainment channel on cable].

Radio

> If there isn't anything good on TV, I'll probably be lying in on the bed, listening to KUFM. I listen to Prairie Home Companion every Saturday night. Yeah.

Reading "Whodunits"

> I like whodunits. Light stuff. I used to read a lot of theology and stuff like that, but I'm kind of letting go to that now and just relaxing. I read quite a bit.

Roberta

Daily Routine

At her daughter Debbie's home, Roberta's daily routine remained the same for six months, until the week she died. Each morning she would get up by 9:00 and get dressed. During the first months she wore a pants suit; later in her illness, she wore an elegant dressing robe. Debbie remembers how her mother was about getting dressed:

> She does not want to be in bed. It's a bad thing to be in bed in the daytime, even if you don't feel well. When she's up, that's it, regardless of how bad she feels.

Roberta ate breakfast in the dining room, near her canary's cage, while he sang for her. Sometimes her grandson would fix breakfast for her; more often it was her daughter or son-in-law.

Roberta had a large, comfortable chair in the living room, looking out a large bay window over the street. Watching what was going on, inside and outside the house, was the most important part of her day. When Debbie was at work, a home health aide came in to be with Roberta; the bath aide provided through hospice came once a week to help her with bathing.

Roberta needed assistance with her heart medications but had few other medical needs: no pain medications or oxygen until the end. Her day revolved around waiting for her daughter to come home from her job at 4:00. Evenings were spent in family conversations and watching TV. The house was a social gathering place for Debbie's children and grandchildren, and there was "always something going on."

Enjoyable Activities

Personal Care

Roberta remained an impressive, elegant woman—upright and commanding—until the very last week of her life. She enjoyed personal care. Our field notes record one such instance:

When I came at 4:00, Roberta had just returned from having her hair done. It was cut a bit shorter and not curled, and looked like a young woman's short cut—very youthful. She had enjoyed it thoroughly and spoke of always feeling better after she gets her hair cut (field notes, August 18, 1997).

Roberta's home health aide does her fingernails regularly. Roberta has beautiful hands and long nails (field notes, September 17, 1997).

Waldo the Canary

Waldo was a canary that Roberta brought with her from her home. His cage was in the corner of dining room, so that he could see into the kitchen and the large living room. He sang with good cheer on a regular basis for Roberta and for her visitors. The home health aide remarked:

He'll start when Roberta is at the table in the morning. He'll usually start to whistle for her then. He whistles more when she's there.

Roberta talked about Waldo's importance in her life:

I didn't have other pets. Just a bird. That's all I ever had. I don't like cats. I can't *stand* cats, and I don't like dogs. I like somebody else's dog, but I don't like to own a dog, that gets in the house and all. Birds are easy, heck. Just make sure they've got water, fresh water and food, and they're happy.

TV, Knitting, Reading

Roberta: I watch TV in my room, and if there's nothing on I turn it off and read a book. Let's see, what did I read last that I enjoyed so much? I can't remember. I have to wear glasses when I read, so I don't read too constantly, but I read enough to enjoy it. I like to knit and crochet and things like that.

Debbie: She knits once in a while. She's busy knitting scarves for the little people at school where I work because a lot of them don't have scarves, or they forget them.

Jigsaw Puzzles

Roberta: I like to put jigsaw puzzles together [laughs]. "Oh yippee! I found a piece!" I can be by myself and be pretty happy.

Debbie: We always have a puzzle going for her.

Watching

Being able to sit and look out the large front window, with a view of Mt. Sentinel and the neighborhood street, remained a daily pleasure for Roberta throughout her illness:

I love bay windows. There's nothing like bay windows, believe me. They're so nice, and we got such a pretty view of the mountains. I've always said if I ever had a house or were going to buy a house it would have to have a big bay window in it.

Family Get-Togethers and Social Connections

Debbie's home was the social center of a large family. Most weekends, some of Debbie's children or grandchildren (young adults themselves), nieces and nephews would come over for a lunch or dinner. There was a casual, open quality to this family, and Roberta was always at the center of it for the last six months of her life:

This house is the busiest house on the block—and probably in the city. That's what's fun about it. I've got more to think about than myself. It's fun to have different people coming and going in here. They all just come over here, and we have dinner here. We don't plan ahead at all.

Roberta's daughter Debbie and Roberta's great-grandson, who was living with his grandparents while he attended college, filled in the picture of the family context that surrounded Roberta. Her great-grandson described the family home:

This house gets full on weekends. That's always been true. People from all over will be coming in. My grandmother has a sister that lives in Bozeman, and then one that moved up to the lake. Her sister in Bozeman and her husband stay here fairly frequently. And I have another great uncle, Roberta's brother, who comes up quite a bit. And my dad, my uncles, people from all over, seems like.

Debbie confirmed this picture for us:

We have four sons, and they come in and out; two of them come into town constantly. Earlier this year, our grandson and his dad were both living here because they were both going to school at the same time, so they stayed here. And then we had a lot of company this year. We had Jess from Calcutta, that I had never met before. We housed some people, and it was just fun. I just loved it.

Roberta had never been very comfortable in social settings with people other than her own close family. Debbie described her as reclusive after her move back to Missoula (twenty years earlier, after her husband's death and her retirement). Roberta's family understood and accepted this reclusiveness and lack of social comfort. Debbie spoke of her mom having a "barrier" to close friendships, to letting people outside her family ever get to know her. In Roberta's last illness, she had no friends her age to visit her; her family was enough—and was all she wanted:

I don't have a group of people at all. I mean, I have a few friends, but I don't see them very often. I'm just content with my daughter and her friends, and her husband and kids. They're all very nice.

Birthday Dinners and Other Outings

My birthday was last week. And everybody was so nice. They took me out for dinner, and I was very pleased, and they were just so nice to me. My family are lovely people. Every once in a while we got out to dinner. It's fun. Nice to get out and get something different. And Debbie doesn't have to cook.

Pumpkin Ice Cream and Lollipops

Eating became difficult for Roberta as she grew ill, and during her short stay in a nursing home, she stopped eating much at all. Debbie reported to us:

She was not eating very well the last several years. Well, this summer she *ate*; she couldn't get enough food this summer. It was so fun, I just loved it. She always wanted watermelon, and her lollipops.

For Debbie, Roberta's lack of interest in a favorite ice cream during her last week of life was the most telling symptom during her last week of life that she was dying:

When I tried to give her pumpkin ice cream and she couldn't eat it, I thought that was it. If there was thing that would rouse her, it was the pumpkin ice cream.

Mabel

Daily Routine

With limited sight, hearing, and mobility, Mabel had few pleasures left, and her daily routine did not vary much. She awakened by 9:00 and took care of her bathroom needs herself. She usually wore a brightly colored robe over her nightgown, rather than dressing. Her daughter, Bernice, fixed breakfast for her between 9:30 and 10:00. Mabel usually ate her meals in her large recliner in the front room of the apartment.

Mabel listened to TV and watched the squirrels and birds that crossed the lawn in front of the large patio doors in the living room. Lunch was at 12:30, and Mabel took a nap other afternoons—sometimes going into her bedroom to lie down, often dozing in her chair. The weekly hospice nurse visit was in the afternoon, once a week. There seemed to be no other regular weekly visitors.

Dinner was at 5:30. With increasing difficulty moving and some pain, Mabel no longer sat at the kitchen table but ate on a tray in her chair. After dinner she napped in the chair or watched a favorite TV program until 10:00. Mabel was determined to stay awake until the local news came on. She could not see the TV well, but she could hear it if it was turned up loud. Then she went to bed.

Enjoyable Activities

Mabel had few pleasurable activities left. Her eyesight was rapidly diminishing because of macular degeneration, and her hearing, even with hearing aids, was not good. The bone cancer and consistent pain she experienced made movement difficult. On our visits, Mabel generally complained that she "can't see, can't hear, can't read or write," and had little enjoyment left to her; our field notes recorded some small pleasures that made her days better, however.

Music

Mabel spoke of liking to listen to music. Bernice had a record player, and Mabel had a Sony Walkman that allowed her to listen to tapes without bothering her daughter.

Great-Grandchildren

What gives me joy? The only thing that gives me joy anymore is my grandkids. They come to see me. They haven't been coming lately, though, because they're moving. But they come down a lot.

That little guy there [pointing to pictures on wall behind her], I've only seen him twice. They're coming over some time this month, for a couple of days. He'll be three years old. Ain't he, Bernice?

He's a pretty little thing. He's pretty, all right. And Bernice's son, his wife just had another one. He's got two girls now.

Throughout our months of visiting, Mabel never wavered from her delight and joy in her "grandchildren" (actually great-grandchildren). Only one family lived nearby, in Missoula; other grandchildren and great-grandchildren were scattered from Idaho to Minnesota. Sitting in her chair, Mabel could no longer see the family photographs arranged on the wall, but she had them memorized and could describe each one from memory.

Visitors

Mabel and her daughter had few visitors, outside of occasional family visits from Mabel's other daughter and granddaughter, who lived in Idaho, and from

Bernice's son and daughter-in-law and their children, who lived in Missoula. One former neighbor from Mabel's former home town came a few times during the year. On the other hand, the large sliding glass door opened onto an outside lawn bordered by a small drainage ditch. This area attracted a variety of small animals, pigeons, squirrels, a groundhog, and an occasional duck. Some scampered up to the door looking for food. Despite Mabel's poor vision, she seemed to be able to see these small visitors, and they brightened up her day:

> I was seeing that little pigeon the other day. There's two on the porch. That's the first time I've ever heard them coo. Well, I can see 'em, but it's dim too. Sure had a lot of pigeons out there this morning. Bernice took some food out there and fed them. There sure was a lot. And they fight. We used to have a gopher, and he just disappeared. We think somebody did away with the poor little thing. He was out there every day, looking for somethin' to eat.

On our visits, Mabel usually began her conversations with a litany of her recent complaints, but our notes show that she "remained engaged in our conversation for 45 minutes, seemed bright and alert." Despite her complaints, she enjoyed company. When she felt good, she was able to hear well enough to join in on topics that Bernice was discussing, or to interrupt the conversation to introduce her own topics—usually about news of her family or about local disasters she had heard about.

Christmas Dinner

The happiest time we observed at Mabel's was the day before Christmas. Bernice was planning to cook a full Christmas dinner for her son, daughter-in-law, and their two little girls. Mabel was wheelchair bound and unable to get out without special assistance. Having the family come to their small apartment brought an unusual sense of excitement to their lives.

"Walker, Texas Ranger"

Although Mabel complained that she couldn't see or hear, she unfailingly watched some favorite TV shows, including "Walker, Texas Ranger," and she always watched the 10:00 news at night.

Phone Calls from Her Sister

During one of our visits, the phone next to Mabel's chair rang and she answered it, while we continued to talk with Bernice. The caller was Mabel's older sister, also homebound and ill but still living by herself in another part of

Missoula. When we telephoned their home, Mabel usually answered, but deafness interfered with her ability to understand us, and she would quickly get Bernice on the phone. In contrast, Mabel seemed to have no difficulty hearing and talking at length with her sister. One conversation we observed lasted ten minutes; it consisted of talk about doctors and ailments and about their families and great-grandchildren. They also discussed a recent fire and accidental death in Missoula, which Mabel had heard about on the radio. She also told her sister about our visit and accurately described our ongoing conversation with her daughter. She was very animated and engaged during that telephone conversation and, not surprisingly, showed much more involvement and less confusion than she did in conversations with us, relative strangers.

This phone link with her family appeared to be an important and enjoyable part of Mabel's day. It was one remaining way in which her isolation was lessened.

Local News

Mabel often complained that her poor vision limited her world and was the greatest loss she experienced. Her daughter read the daily newspaper to her, and between listening to Bernice reading the newspaper and listening to the nightly local news, Mabel was able to keep up with local events. She particularly remembered and focused on local disasters, fires, roof cave-ins, and deaths. Local events provided some of the excitement that Mabel seemed to want and found missing in her daily life:

Mabel: I guess they caved that one roof in, right down on the corner.

Researcher: Where is that?

Bernice: Right down there at the Exchange.

Researcher: Oh, I didn't know that.

Mabel: It was in the paper.

On one visit, when Mabel was feeling particularly good, she offered to show the researcher her file of newspaper clippings at our next visit:

Researcher: I'll come back and see you in a couple of weeks. Will that be okay?

Mabel: Probably won't have anything new to tell ya.

Researcher: Well, you never know. If you do—

Mabel:	Might have some pictures to show you, just clippings I've cut out of the paper about different things.
Researcher:	Oh, okay. Things you're interested in.
Mabel:	You probably wouldn't be interested in that.
Researcher:	Oh, I might be.
Mabel:	'Bout old Barney Wilkenson, he fought in the last Big Hole Battle that they had over at Wisdom. I got quite a few pictures. I clip 'em out of the newspaper and save them.

Dancing

Mabel usually complained about her present state or told "tales of woe" about bad things that had happened in the past. On one topic, however, her eyes lit up, and memories of good times returned: dancing:

What do I like about Hamilton? I know me and my sister used to go to the dances all the time at McCormicks'. Everybody I know always went out there on Saturday night. Everybody was friendly up there. . . .

Well, I'll tell you, if I was out and going, I'd go out and get me a boyfriend. We'd go out dancing. Well, that hope's gone forever. With my pain and legs. . . .

I can remember they had a street dance and [laughs] some boys; they had put on wooden shoes, and he wanted to dance with me and I stood up there; heck, I couldn't dance with him with them wooden shoes on, and so I just got off on his feet.

Memories of dancing, and dreams of going dancing again, transformed Mabel's face for a moment. Then the pains and the boredom of her present state returned.

Summary

Our participants' daily routines were similar in matters of medication and sleep or rest. Dennis's day was more taken up with controlling pain and hygiene; Ralph's, Sharon's, and Walt's days were more absorbed in sleep. The others fell somewhere between these extremes, depending on their age, illness, and disease trajectory. One thing to expect in the daily routines of the more elderly population close to death is the increased pattern of sleeping much of the time.

The enjoyable activities mentioned by the participants provide a picture of what they considered to be positive and meaningful in their last days of life. This finding offers implications for the expectations of caregivers and visitors alike. Table 6-1 lists these individual items and offers a measure of comparison.

The foregoing data suggest that watching television, eating, and having visitors—especially young children—appear to be among the broadly enjoyable activities available to persons who are terminally ill. Not surprisingly, male participants in our study hung on to whatever outdoor activities they could, whereas female participants engaged in more indoor activities. Some of the women found ways to bring nature indoors: For example, Roberta had her canary and a view of the mountains from the window, Kitty her pets and the Nature Channel on TV. Books and music were favored by females; eating remained an enjoyable activity for those whose condition permitted it.

Finding enjoyable activities seemed to be more important to Dennis, the patient who seemed most wracked with constant and less controllable pain. All three males in our study found some enjoyment in getting out in nature. Dennis had actual physical activities, such as golfing and fishing. Ralph was satisfied just to get outside the house and visit the homestead or sit in the car while Sandy went shopping. Walt loved being taken for car rides as long as his health permitted.

The females in our study seemed less concerned about getting outside physically. Kitty was quite content in her little nest at home. Even when asked if they would enjoy being taken out—for example, to see the Christmas lights—the female participants were unenthusiastic. All of the participants expressed enjoyment in visiting, but Dennis added the caveat that he preferred that visitors make appointments. Dorothy, Walt's wife, said that anyone could visit Walt any time; she would wake him up if necessary because this activity was so important. Likewise, Kitty's, Ralph's, and Sarah's doors were always open to visitors.

Walt complained of boredom. Dennis seemed to be able to keep busy enough to be satisfied. Ralph complained of his uselessness and prayed that God would find some work for him to do in heaven. In contrast, the females in our study did not openly complain of being bored, although some—such as Mabel and Sarah—clearly had little to occupy them during the day.

Sharing of meals is a particular sign of the social bond and membership in the social community (Seale 1998). Thus, at the end of life, participants and their families focused particularly on eating—how well the dying person could still eat. The daily life of participants was marked by significant food "events," large and small:

Table 6-1 Enjoyable Activities

Enjoyable activities shared by most participants

Dennis	Ralph	Walt	Sarah	Sharon	Barbara	Roberta	Mabel	Kitty
visits, TV	visits, TV	visits, TV	visits, TV	visits, TV	visits	visits, TV	visits, TV	visits, TV

Enjoying food

Dennis	Ralph	Sharon	Barbara	Roberta
junk food	favorite meals	party food	making fry bread	pumpkin ice cream

Outdoor activities/nature

Dennis	Ralph	Walt	Mabel
golf, fishing	walks, going for rides	going for rides	watching animals outside window

Indoor activities

Dennis	Sarah	Sharon	Barbara	Roberta	Walt	Mabel	Kitty
slots	helping others	parties, smoking	working, pet bird, knitting, looking out window	grooming	whittling, radio	telephone, birds	pets

Books, music

Sharon	Barbara	Roberta	Kitty
reading, books on tape	music, hearing stories	reading, jigsaw puzzles	reading, music

birthday parties for Sharon and Roberta; cooking fry bread during Barbara's last two weeks of life at her sister's home; ice cream for Roberta; Ralph making the long drive back to the homestead for a Sunday dinner with his brother; Dennis and his mother sharing a cup of coffee and a hamburger on their painful trips from his home to the doctor's office in Missoula. For others, such as Walt, loss of interest in food and inability to eat at all was a sign of death's nearness.

Daily Life and Meaningful Activities in the Subculture of the Dying

The participants in this study illustrate that members of the subculture of the dying have difficulty achieving former levels of comfort, growth, hope, continuity, control, dignity, mobility, and wide social networks. Their comfort and mobility are, by definition, deeply affected by physical illness. For this group, we observed little remaining energy for active growth, although there was evidence of growth toward meaningful resolution of issues during their past year of life (see chapter 11). Unless there has been careful planning, economic security quickly decays. Hope of living is denied, of course, along with at least some concepts of continuity. Even a person's sense of dignity may come into question. By examining how these participants dealt with their sudden move to the subculture of the dying, we can see different patterns of behavior and thought.

Dennis, the youngest participant in our study, strove valiantly to preserve a sense of hope, continuity, control, mobility, and dignity. He did so by flying in the face of the odds—going out on the golf course and shooting very respectable rounds of golf even in his last months of life. He also ate Twinkies, donuts, and whatever else he wanted. In so doing, he made a statement that he still had control of things, he still had personal value, he was still mobile, he still had some hope. And because he had been an athlete and a golf pro, he also made a statement about his continuity in this field. He was telling the world that it wasn't over quite yet.

Likewise, when Dennis played the slots he expressed his sense of control over the world. He had mastered his gambling problem and could no longer be tempted. In any case, what difference did it make? Just as some dying patients do not worry about becoming addicted to narcotics, Dennis did not worry about a relapse into addictive gambling.

Was this a form of folly on Dennis's part? Didn't he know that he could not stop the onslaught of death even though he acted, temporarily, as though everything was indeed okay? Should he, like Mabel, have just stayed inside and recognized the hopelessness of his plight? Fortunately, this study need not answer these questions.

Most older, terminally ill patients do not fight as hard as Dennis did. Their expressions of control, hope, dignity, and continuity are couched in abstract rather than physical terms. For example, Ralph made a statement about his continuing mobility by talking short walks. He expressed his sense of dignity and continuity by his putting his homestead and ranch into the Montana Land Reliance. He was extremely proud of this action; in his mind, it guaranteed that his land would never come into the hands of real estate developers. This plan also gave Ralph a sense of hope at a time when there was absolutely no hope for the continuation of his own life. This hope, coupled with his belief in life after death, gave Ralph something to look forward to in spite of his impending death.

Walt, Ralph, Sharon, and Sarah had no apparent need for control at this stage of their lives. Walt had surrendered all control to his wife. He was not even humiliated by his need to wear diapers—perhaps the ultimate embarrassment; he cheerfully told us, "It sure does beat the alternative." Ralph was painfully aware that his body was shutting down. In his last weeks, his walks—perhaps the last vestige of a formerly very physical man—were made in a wheelchair. Ralph had no illusions that he could still control his body. Sarah, who had been so active in earlier days, seemed content to let others make decisions for her. Dennis continued to fight, however, for whatever sense of control he might salvage as his body was shutting down. He needed the hope such a fight would bring. He needed the self-dignity that shooting a good round of golf would afford.

The subculture of the dying is characterized by a shrinking social network, especially among the most elderly. Older persons commonly complain that all their friends are gone. This fact in itself obviously reduces the social network. Moreover, some elderly patients seem to prefer isolation. They also can become cranky—as much from not feeling well as from flaws in temperament—leading to further reduction in friends.

These participants reveal a spectrum of positions on the issue of social network. The majority culture often has a wide social network. Minority subcultures often do not. In this sense, the subculture of the dying is like a minority subculture. Loss of mobility alone can reduce social networks. Loss of dignity, control, hope, and economic security also contribute.

In Ralph's case, the need to leave his home area and move 60 miles away to get needed treatment greatly diminished his accessibility to his lifelong social network. In fact, Sandy once told us that they didn't know anybody in Missoula when they first moved there. Ralph's solution to this problem was to make an effort to add locals to his extant network, while maintaining contact with the more distant network back home.

A quite different phenomenon seems to characterize Dennis and Walt, although it is unclear exactly how broad their nonfamily social networks were before they became terminally ill. What we could see during the time we visited them, however, was a narrowing of social networks almost exclusively to their immediate families, especially to their caregivers. Mabel professed to never having many friends, which seems to have contributed to her isolation. Apparently, some terminally ill people and their caregivers expand their social networks at the time of crisis; others contract their friendship circles to focus on their problems.

We have seen how dying persons' everyday, practical strategies for affirming the social bond also become symbolic strategies for transcending its rupture. These participants, by continuing with as many of their daily activities as they could, were able to assert their identity and their continued existence even after being labeled "terminal." Rather than having one "last wish" for a unique experience, they mostly wanted nothing so much as the ordinary, for the ordinary daily activities affirmed their social existence. As chapter 4 shows, these participants were mostly openly "aware" and recognized that they were dying, but they spent very little time dwelling on the presence of that reality in their lives.

Seale (1998) has stressed the centrality of the body to our experience of life itself. Thus, the activities of daily living—which we take for granted when the body is healthy—become of major concern and value when the body is dying. Debbie's observation about her mother's lack of interest in pumpkin ice cream as a signal of her impending death appears to have been accurate. Simple everyday events—such as favorite foods, music, rides in a car, or views of nature—are symbols of life itself to the dying.

Chapter 7

Family Caregiving Experience

We were interested in everything about the family caregiving experience of our participants, particularly because most of them were being cared for at home during their illness by family members or close friends. What, exactly, was involved in caregiving for someone who was terminally ill in Missoula in 1997? What did caregivers find most valuable in the experience—while they were in the middle of it, and looking back? What aspects of this experience did they find most difficult? What kind of support and assistance did they get from others—families, or friends, or the community? What additional help, if any, did they need? What inner resources enabled them to do this, to keep going? How did the particular primary caregiver get "selected" for the job, when several might be available: Why one child of an aging parent, rather than another? Why one sister rather than another?

The picture of the end of life from the patient's perspective that we present in chapters 2 through 6 shows that the most feared aspects of dying—great pain, loneliness, depression, meaninglessness—did not dominate the last days of most of the participants in our study. Pain and other symptoms were controlled; they were able to be with their families and have friends visit; and their preferences—particularly to stay at home—were honored.

The picture from the caregiver's perspective, presented in this chapter, is less rosy. What made the end of life so good for the majority of these participants came from the extra efforts their families made, not just for a few weeks but for many months. The family caregivers had chosen their task, and did it willingly, but the burdens at times seemed overwhelming to them. As a result, this chapter and chapter 8, though accurate and based on direct accounts and observations, may overemphasize or give more space to the family caregivers' day-to-day concerns and the difficulties they were experiencing and underemphasize the deep meaning they found in caregiving for a family member.

In most cases, we may have been the only people who listened to the caregivers; professionals and other family members directed their attention toward the dying person, and to that person's needs. Most of the caregivers were not "complainers," and they seemed unlikely to talk about the difficulties with their own families as openly as they did with us. Because we asked, because we listened, and because they trusted us not to share their concerns with the patient or others in the family, we learned a great deal about how very difficult home caregiving can be, even with good support. This contemporaneous picture of family caregiving, recorded as it was occurring, may not be the picture they would paint now, a few years after the patient's death. Perhaps these data are a bit like what one would find by asking women in the middle of labor how they feel and what their concerns are. Dying can be much like birthing: It can be very difficult and hard work for the dying person, and for their family members who support and get them through it. The value and meaning of both kinds of experiences may be perceived more clearly in retrospect.

This chapter points out that caregiver difficulties from the effects of long-term care of terminally ill loved ones were present even when good communication, open acceptance of death, excellent medical care, family consensus, and physician and family respect for the patient's wishes about care were all present. When any of these factors were *not* present, the level of caregiver stress became extraordinarily high, and undesirable outcomes occurred. Some of these outcomes included unresolved grief, interference with the caregiver's ongoing life after the loved one's death, family conflicts and disruption persisting after death, and even legal difficulties.

This chapter encompasses a wealth of data on caregivers' experiences and perspectives, beginning with a description of caregiver tasks, a "typical day," and the caregiver's acquisition of competence in home care. We describe how particular family caregivers were "selected" and the values and benefits they found in this experience; then we present the most typical difficulties and troublesome symptoms of caregiving for someone who is terminally ill. Chapter 8 discusses the kinds of support caregivers received and the experience of caregivers when some of the support they needed was lacking.

Caregiving Arrangements and Routines

In the families we studied, we observed a diverse range of caregiving responsibilities and roles, as well as a variety of types of individuals who became caregivers. Table 7-1 summarizes the various family arrangements for caregiving as we encountered and observed them.

The care that family caregivers provided ranged from twenty-four-hour home nursing to managing a parent's care while the parent lived at Hospice

Table 7-1 Family Arrangements for Caregiving during Terminal Phase

Arrangement	Number
Living alone, no children, spouse or siblings; church friends provided some assistance	1
Spouse provided care at home	3
Cared for by mother in own home (mother in late sixties)	1
Cared for by adult children (late fifties to sixties), in their homes	2
Cared for by sister in sister's home (sister in seventies)	1
Lived at Hospice House, then in a board and care home, with care management from daughter living near Missoula	1

House and then in a board and care home. Except for one younger family, all of the primary caregivers were themselves in their sixties and seventies.

Tasks and Typical Daily Routines

A typical day for a caregiver begins and ends with caring: seeing that the patient is comfortable, administering medication, monitoring vital signs and systems (appetite, eating, digestion, elimination, breathing, temperature). Patients need help with moving, dressing, bathroom trips, hygiene, and bathing. They need to be fed and kept warm and comfortable, and their human and social needs (attention, conversation, stimulation, affection, and love) have to be met. These tasks are part of any home care for the chronically ill, and these family caregivers did all of this, every day. As the patients became more ill, the number and complexity of the medications typically increased, and the amount of help and attention required for any personal needs increased correspondingly—and often dramatically.

This section brings together the voices of several caregivers, whose experiences represented the typical experiences of most of the participants in this study, and of family caregivers generally:

> I brushed her teeth, I combed her hair. I put makeup on, I painted her fingernails when she wanted them done. I kept her in clean pajamas every day. I put lotion on her. I gave her foot massages. I did everything that you do for a baby. I read to her. I played music for her. (Irene, Barbara's sister)

Much of the daily schedule was determined by the medications, which required precise doses at precise times to keep the patient comfortable:

It just takes a lot of different things to keep her breathing; she has to have them. And she has long ago lost the power to keep track of her own meds. I have to think all the time. (Connie)

Another part of the daily routine was management of the dying person's social life and visitors—including children, grandchildren, and others. For several of the participants, the summer before they died was filled with last visits home from children and grandchildren, nieces and nephews. In addition to nursing and medications, family caregivers found themselves serving as hosts for extended family:

His kids came through on Thursday, but that was a hectic day. We thought it was a day of rest, and it was four people all at once. (Carrie)

Another caregiver also found that much of her energy went into scheduling visitors. As Sharon became less able to use the phone or to remember her own schedule, her sister Connie had to take over and arrange for all visits: Sharon's three children, a few remaining friends, her minister, the Hospice chaplain, a Senior Companion, and an MDP researcher:

But when she has company—and she has a lot of it—then to give her any privacy I have to stay out of the way. And not only that, but I have to be hostess! [Laughs] It's not something I would have thought about at all.

Dorothy's Day

For most caregivers, the most challenging task was learning to keep track of and administer all the medications needed to keep the patients as comfortable and alert as possible. Walt had twelve different medications that Dorothy had to manage for him on a daily basis. On a visit with them before he died, Dorothy was casual in talking about his medications:

Researcher:	Do you have pain with this?
Walt:	Lots of pain pills.
Dorothy:	He's on morphine, 45 grams, three times a day. Every eight hours. Plus Roxanal sometimes.

Walt: When it starts to hurt I take it. I say, "Give me some, what is it, Roxanal?"

Dorothy: Well, that's what I give him when he needs it quick. The morphine I just give him every eight hours, 45 grams.

But after Walt died, Dorothy explained at length what a challenge this routine had been for her. She related that she was able to manage his daily routine only by keeping a written record of his symptoms and vital signs every day, as well as his medication schedule. She explained that this recordkeeping not only helped her with medications, it also allowed her to understand his decline:

I kept records of everything from day to day. I kept a record of his blood pressure. I took, I kept a record of his pulse, I kept a record of everything he'd done. I kept track of all the medications that we changed and why we changed them. And as soon as he started saying, "I can't eat this. I can't swallow it. My taste is leaving," and was having difficulty going to the bathroom . . . and started dropping more weight—he had already gone down from 210 to 165—I knew his body was not doing what it should.

We reproduce Dorothy's handwritten daily records (Fig. 7-1) showing the medications available to Walt and her recording of his pulse, temperature, and oxygen levels at two different times. Taking vital signs and monitoring his medications, appetite, digestion, and elimination became her paramount daily tasks.

Competence

The caregivers we visited demonstrated a high degree of acquired competence in understanding and performing the tasks required for end-of-life care: monitoring and managing medications, hygiene and comfort, vital signs, and troubling symptoms. Two different caregivers' accounts illustrate the competence they had acquired in the preceding months:

Towards the end he was infused at home with . . . right now I'm not thinking of it . . . Vancomycin. We had a Hickman catheter that had a Y, so he could have his Fentanyl, which was necessary, and the other Y for that [antibiotic]. That took about an hour and a half of time. And it entailed a saline flush beforehand, too. It was twice a day, like eight and eight. (Carrie)

∼ ∼ ∼

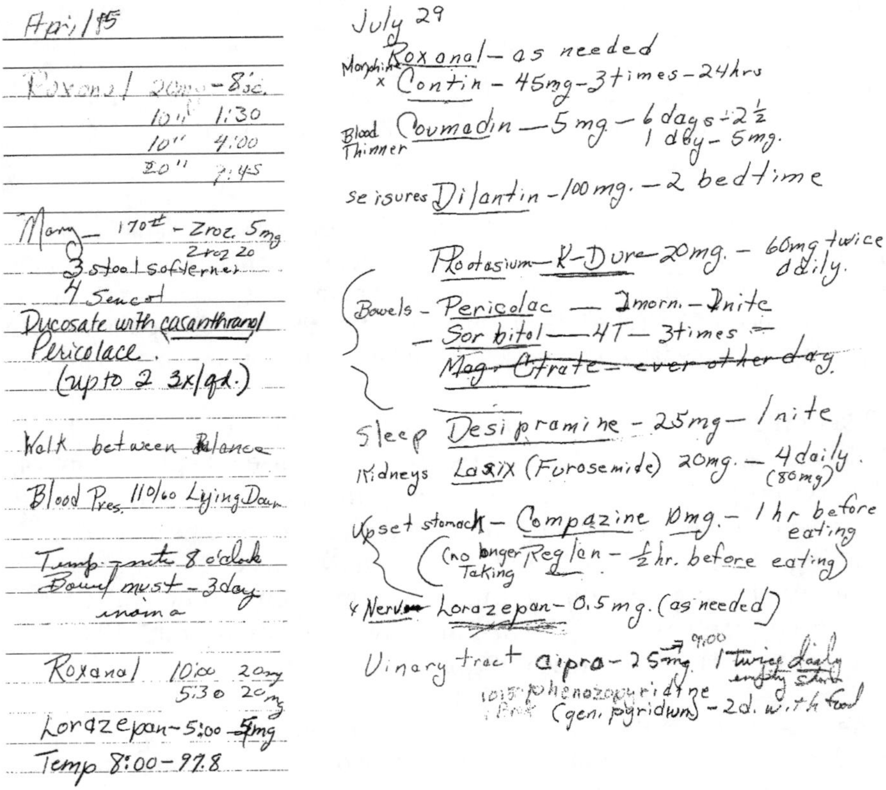

Figure 7-1 Handwritten daily records

Her pain patch is Duragesic. You have to change it every 72 hours. That's when the patch is on the low side, and that's when more of the pain breaks through. Her head didn't feel good this morning. She's pretty tight back there. I took the temperature and blood pressure, the blood sugar. (Bernice)

Organizing for Twenty-four-Hour Care

The high level of medication and monitoring involved in end-of-life palliative care at home means that the family caregiver's life must be as organized as a hospital. Medications have to be given in precise amounts, sometimes at precise times. Someone must always be with the patient, to find the Roxanol or other medication and administer it when there is unexpected pain or nausea. Although the patients in our study varied greatly with regard to their needs for care and assistance, even with the same diagnosis, none of the nine partic-ipants could be left alone for more than a few minutes during the last three to six months of their lives. Even a trip to the grocery store must be carefully planned around finding someone to be in the house—or done with great stress and worry.

One caregiver who was suddenly thrust into three weeks of round-the-clock caregiving when her sister was released from the hospital into her care, was forceful in her assessment of this experience:

> You know, I've never been a nurse. I was a greenhorn. They called me up to the hospital, and they went through all the medicines with me and they told me what time she needed to take them. And you know, I'm a fairly astute learner, but as I started giving her her medicines, I had to make up a chart on my computer and put it on my refrigerator. . . . (Irene)

Another summarized the end of her sister's life:

> It's just all-consuming at the time you're doing it. If it went on for months I don't think I could carry on at that level. (Connie)

This picture of the family caregiving tasks and activities comes from the caregivers' perspectives on what caring for a terminally ill person at home, typ-ically with weekly visits from a Hospice nurse, is like. Our impressions from observing these family caregivers were borne out by their own accounts: Care-giving for someone who is terminally ill is a full-time occupation for more than one person. A single family caregiver for someone who is terminally ill may end up doing the work done by three shifts of nurses at a hospital, nursing home, or Hospice House.

Caregivers: How Chosen?

Caregiving may begin long before the terminal diagnosis, when the ill person is elderly. In these cases, Albert notes:

> Households begin their adaptation to caregiving demands [of an elderly member] long before acute illness forces a relocation of the impaired elder (or relocation of a caregiver to the parent's home). . . . This gradual decline leads future caregivers to alter schedules and begin their socialization into the role of caregiver before caregiving demands precipitate major changes in the household. With increasing parental dependence, we find that caregivers and

impaired parents begin to form *quasi-households* (Albert 1990, 23; emphasis in original).

In our study, four of the caregivers and patients had formed quasi-households years earlier; three were existing households of couples when the person fell seriously ill. Three other situations involved households that formed rather suddenly, following a more unexpected diagnosis of terminal illness (see Table 7-2). Two of these households involved patients in their middle years.

The factors leading to the choice of a caregiver from among available family members have been well-documented in literature on the care of the chronically ill. Caregivers are most likely to be those who are "unmarried, female, not working outside the home" (Albert 1990) or "the only adult child living near, possessing a close relationship with parent in earlier years, strong set of religious/family values" (Silverman and Huelsman 1990). Silverman and Huelsman document that some caregivers assume their role because of a family conflict, which eliminates some other candidates. Albert (1990) also found that caregivers preselect themselves by taking a greater interest in the ill person's care, by staying or moving nearby, and by preparing their own households in advance for the parent's relocation. Data on the individual caregivers in this study validate these findings.

Bernice (Mabel's Caregiver)

Bernice never spoke about how she became her mother's caregiver. Proximity seemed to be the likely answer; although Mabel's other daughter lived in a nearby state, Bernice was living in Missoula when Mabel first had serious health problems:

> We moved in with each other in '92, when she had her mini-stroke. We lived a couple of years together over on North Avenue. And in '94 we moved in here. . . .

Table 7-2 Types of Caregiving Households

Quasi-households	Existing households	Suddenly formed households
Debbie and Roberta	Dorothy and Walt	Barbara and Irene (3 weeks)
Connie and Sharon	Ralph and Sandy	Dennis and Carrie
Mabel and Bernice	Barbara and Dan	Kitty and friends
Sarah and Karen		

With her mini-stroke—that was in November—I kinda figured I would get her home, out of the hospital; well, I took her home with me. Where she was renting the landlord wasn't very nice. And I did get a letter, telling her she had 30 days to get out of there. Okay, so that's it, we're moving in December. And it was so hard on her.

Bernice also appeared to have been "chosen" as the primary caregiver by default. She was less encumbered by other responsibilities or family ties than Mabel's other daughter. Bernice had been divorced for several years when her mother became seriously ill. Bernice's sons were grown and starting families of their own, and she was struggling to support herself financially. Within a year of moving to the new apartment with her mother, Bernice lost her job and was put on disability for three years:

I was in housekeeping, and they called me in once for an interview in distributing. And I turned that down. I still wasn't really over the marriage, and I was like, "Just give me a wall to clean and I'll be happy." If I had it to do over again, I woulda went into distributing because housekeeping was just too much on my legs and my knees. And then, I should not have pushed it the way I did because it really just pushed me over the edge. And between my mind and my legs it was a, um, they had me down as a severe disability. In the meantime, she had her little mini-stroke in '92, and we moved in together at that time. Went through a lot of hell at that time.

Caring for Mabel full-time may have been a welcome responsibility—a task Bernice could take on and do productively at a time when other opportunities seemed closed. Caring for her mother also gave her work she could do well, with a sense of pride. Bernice commented to us at one point that caregiving "is just like a job."

Debbie (Roberta's Caregiver)

Debbie, Roberta's primary caregiver, was the middle of three daughters—all living in Montana, all with their own grown children. Debbie's older sister was recently widowed and might have seemed the obvious choice for primary caregiver. We asked Debbie to tell us how she was the one "selected" in her family. Again, she mentioned proximity, gender influences, and her personal relationship with her mother as factors that helped to determine her appointment. Debbie also described how she began to form a quasi-household with her mother, helping her daily while she lived in her own home:

It started, actually, a long time ago, when Mom was living by herself. For four or five years I've been having to take care of her in one form or another. It seemed like I always kind of was able to tell what she needed. I always knew when she needed something. And it kind of went into the physical things of doing her shopping and taking care of her house, and it got to be more and more. The less she could do, the more we would do. And then my sisters would help, too.

In this family, Debbie's close relationship with her mother did not mean a distant relationship with the other daughters: All three women were close to their mother. Other circumstances in the lives of her sisters, however, militated against their choice:

But my older sister lost her husband several years ago, and it's been hard for her to do this. And she was dealing with an awful lot of those issues, more so than most people. When Mom got sick, I think she was afraid to be involved with it, with Mom's sickness. It was hard for her to do anything like this, really difficult. And Mom knew this.

≈ ≈ ≈

My younger sister hasn't been around in this area too much. And I actually don't think my younger sister's husband would be of the mind to do it, like Joe [Debbie's husband] is.

Debbie's selection seems to have been by mutual consent among all three daughters and their mother. Unlike some other caregivers, Debbie felt that her selection was appropriate, not forced on her by default.

Connie (Sharon's Caregiver)

Although we have described caregivers as "choosing" and "being chosen," such decisions evolve slowly in most cases. Seldom are family meetings held at which someone is overtly chosen to take on the primary caregiving role without having any prior involvement. Instead, small steps of helping and assisting increase over time to bigger efforts, as one family member volunteers to do more and more. Connie exemplifies this pattern. She began "running over" to help Sharon immediately after her own husband died, four years before Sharon's death:

She had an apartment with an upstairs bathroom. And so that made it really difficult for a long time for her. We were all keeping her going. She really hadn't been able to [care for herself]. I did her washing and took a lot of food over. And her daughter took food often.

This pattern of going several miles across town to help her sister on a daily basis continued for two years, with Sharon's daughter helping as well. Then Sharon's daughter and her family moved away from Missoula to a nearby state, just as Sharon began to realize that she couldn't live alone any more. At that point, Connie had been offering for some time to have Sharon move in with her.

From Sharon's perspective, her sister Connie—living alone in a large, comfortable home out in the Missoula Valley—was the logical choice to take her in. Sharon told us of calling her sister one day:

I had finally admitted what people had been telling me, that I really couldn't live alone. So Connie had several times offered to take me [laughs], and I didn't want to lose my independence. Finally I called her up and I said, "Is that offer still open?" So she said, "Yes!"

From Connie's perspective, having Sharon live with her made it easier at first:

When she first moved in with me, it was easier for me because I was trying to run over to her apartment all the time, and I was doing her laundry and taking her food because she was not able to be alone. So it really was easier having her here, under my roof. At first it was easier, that first year.

Again, Connie's selection as caregiver was by default and occurred more gradually than it might appear, if one heard only Sharon's story of "calling her up." Other potential family caregivers were less available. Sharon's two sons who lived in or near Missoula had complicated family lives, small homes, or teenage children still at home. Her daughter had moved away, and Sharon showed no interest in going with her and moving from the only part of the world she had ever lived. Her only other close family, a sister, lived in California. Although Sharon's children or her other sister might have "taken her in" if necessary, Connie had the fewest barriers and was already socialized into caregiving for her. Because Connie volunteered to take Sharon in, Sharon's sons who still lived in the Missoula area never volunteered any concerns in their conversations with us about not doing so.

Karen (Sarah's Caregiver)

Sarah explained how her daughter Karen had come to be the primary caregiver among her three children during the ten years she had had cancer:

Researcher:	Is there one daughter that's been particularly around to help take care of you?
Sarah:	Yeah, just one. The other one's working, and the other one is in Washington.
Researcher:	So the one that wasn't working got more time with Mom?
Sarah:	Yeah.

From Karen's perspective, there was resentment about the unequal burden:

I've got two sisters, but you'd never know it. I'm finding out that's the way it is in a lot of families.

As in most other families, the daughter who wasn't working and who lived nearby became the primary caregiver, responsible physically and eventually financially.

"The guys just can't deal with this"

In Missoula in 1997, caregiving clearly was still a "woman's job"; men were not spoken of or thought of as primary caregivers. In fact, one participant made the point very bluntly:

I think one of the things that I speak firsthand about is that with chronic and terminal illness, that if there's a couple dealing with it, depending on who is ill, I think women are greater caretakers than men are. And men will do it, but only if they freak out. And they'll hide their fear. And they'll find diversions. So they need help.

Another caregiver described the difficulty the men in her family had at the death of her mother—specifically, over having the Chalice of Repose come:

My husband and my sister's husband, well, they were most upset with this decision. They felt that it would upset Mom; it would not be fair to her to have to feel this withdrawal in this manner and be frightened by it. The guys couldn't deal with this. My sister's husband went back the next morning. He just can't deal with these things.

Value and Meaning: "I wouldn't miss this time"

Most of our families, caught up in caring for someone who is terminally ill, had difficulty articulating the value or meaning they found in this last time together. Value and meaning came to them later, as they reflected on it, rather than during the intense, arduous, emotionally charged period itself. Each person and family found their own kind of value in what they were doing. Our observations and conversations brought out very different kinds of values expressed by families and friends providing care:

- Being able to avoid nursing home care
- Family benefits and greater family cohesion
- Renewed relationship between caregiver and dying person
- Affirmation of church as a caring community
- Personal growth on the caregiver's part
- Doing one's duty.

Avoiding Nursing Home or Hospital: "Please don't ever make me go"

Avoiding the nursing home or rest home was a paramount value in most of our families with elderly members in 1997. Many had memories of parents or grandparents being placed in a "rest home" at the end of their lives and wanted to avoid that scenario at all costs. And most patients wanted to avoid hospitalization. So a major positive benefit of caregiving, no matter how great the burden, was that the dying person could be at home during their last months and days. The caregivers' pride in honoring their loved one's preference was evident in their statements:

I was thinking the other day that I don't know what else could work. A nursing home couldn't begin to give her the care that she really needs. And anyway, I'm glad to be with her day by day through this.

I wanted to keep him at home. He wanted to stay at home. He said, "Please don't ever make me go. I just couldn't, I just couldn't stand it." Walt clung to being here.

Debbie said of her mother, "She would never want to go to a rest home. I intend to leave her here until the end." When Roberta was admitted to the hospital with a broken hip, Debbie and her sisters debated whether to leave her there or send her to Hospice House or a nursing home:

> We brought her home. They said, "Do you want to take her to the Hospice House or a nursing home, or what's your choice?" And I said, "Home." I said, "There's no other choice."

Mabel's fear of a nursing home also motivated her daughter Bernice:

> I plan to keep her here. That's what she wants. She doesn't want to go into a nursing home. That's one of her biggest fears.

Debbie had placed her mother in a nursing home when she got out of the hospital, just to see if it would work for her. Her observations of the effects on Roberta strengthened Debbie's resolve to keep her mother at home and helped give meaning to their last six months together:

> Over time I saw her not responding to anyone. I saw her coming into a shell. I saw some strange interactions with her and the nurses, where I could tell that she had been causing problems. I could see that she was not happy, I could see her sitting in the corners all the time, hating to be in her room. And pretty soon I saw a lot of sadness, tears, whether we were there or not.

The assertion that most patients would prefer not to go into a nursing home may seem obvious. Many patients experience entering an institution as a kind of "social burial" (Seale 1998, 170) because it involves the rupturing of everyday social activities with friends and families. Although none of these families could have articulated this concept, it supports the determination of many families to maintain their loved ones at home as long as they were cognizant. From the caregiver's perspective, what seems to have mattered was keeping the promise made to the patient. On the most difficult days, when the burdens of twenty-four-hour care were (to an outside observer) overwhelming, what gave caregivers strength was the knowledge that the alternative would have been institutionalized care for someone still cognizant and resistant to the notion.

Family Benefits

"This has been an excellent process for my family"

For two families with grown children, grandchildren, and great-grandchildren, the value of family caregiving was that everyone could become involved—in caring, in being present as the person was dying, and in letting go. The experience of sharing in the dying of a family member created greater cohesion among the surviving family members and was regarded as a positive and lasting benefit.

Roberta's family was infused with an awareness of the reason they were caring for her at home as she was dying—of how important it was to all of them as a family task and a family experience—even while they were doing it. Two months before Roberta died, Debbie said:

> We have fun. We have enjoyed this part of it, actually. This has been an excellent process for my family, for the kids. For my family, I really feel strongly, absolutely, there has been some value. And for me, it's more so. I think it's an understanding of a full circle of life.

Three months later, Debbie described the family standing together in a circle around their mother/grandmother/great-grandmother as she lay dying:

> We were all in the room, holding her hand, telling her we loved her. We thanked her for letting us be a part of her transition, which was so beautiful—to see her peaceful, to hold her hand and feel this great powerful comfort of doing this. We felt so much love and warmth that time in the bonding that we all had with each other.

Learning to Let Go: "The entire family has to be willing"

Another caregiver, Dorothy, regarded her husband's final year of life as valuable and necessary for their family—despite his physical and emotional difficulties—because their children "weren't willing to let him go yet." She described herself as determined to get all five children to understand and accept Walt's impending death and to allow him to leave:

> I think the entire family has to be willing to let go. I think there has to be an acceptance all the way around. And that keeps the family going. It keeps them happy with each other. Afterward they can go on living.

When Walt was in the hospital a year before he died, the family had resolved not to intervene; they told the doctors, "don't do anything"—expecting him to die that night. According to Dorothy, however, at least one of Walt's children wasn't ready:

> My son sat by him and said, "Oh, Dad, you just can't leave now. You just can't leave now." And the following morning when Walt came to in the room, I said, "What do you remember?" And he said, "Well, I can remember just a real bright light in a tunnel. I could hear those boys, but mainly I could hear one of them yelling, 'Dad, it isn't time for you to go.'"

Dorothy described how she encouraged him to be patient after this near-fatal heart attack because his children weren't yet willing for him to die:

> His main thing was, he'd say, "Why do I have to go on? Isn't there just some way that I can leave?" I'd say, "Walt, when your time comes and your body and your spirit says it's time for you to go, you will go."
> So there was some struggle, that he wanted to go. And it's like I told him: It's good that you're still here because now your children are going to be happier when you go than they would've been otherwise. So he had to satisfy, I guess, he had to make his children be willing to accept it, so they could let him go. I think that was his main thing, that he had to get to the point where the children could let him go. And he realized that.

On Walt's last day, Dorothy sent their children into his room to tell him he could go, that the boys had his tools, the girls had his books, and his work was done. This process of building a consensus to "let Dad go" reflected this family's way of being. This family works together to help each other, even to the point of creating a legal family partnership among the five siblings to provide for their parents' last years. Their dad's dying had to be by mutual consent: As Walt's near-death experience a year earlier demonstrated, he couldn't just die until everyone was ready.

Others also spoke of changes in their family because of their awareness that this period was the end of life for one of them. Decisions that had long been avoided were made, when life was short—as Carrie, Dennis's mother, described:

It has brought an awareness to our whole family. And there's been a lot of good come out of this. It was almost like there was no other way that his brother would've ever gotten out of that hell hole in California. It's almost as though Dennis was the sacrificial lamb, that his suffering had to happen. Dennis always wanted his brother to come back, and his brother knew that, but he was stuck. What made him decide to do it was that death was close, that Dennis was getting worse. He called up and said, "Ready." So there has been an awful lot of good.

Researchers studying home caregiving have pointed out that for some families, lengthy caregiving has the positive benefit of bringing about a "pooling of family support" (Silverman and Huelsman 1990), as well as greater cohesiveness and a more unified system of care—which may benefit all family members. These two families appeared to have found the task of caring for a dying member helpful as a stimulus for more conscious and, in one case, formalized arrangements for mutual support among the remaining members to meet each other's needs as well.

New Closeness/Renewed Relationship

A mother caring for her son and two sisters caring for their sisters found new closeness in caregiving. It allowed them to restore family relationships stretched thin by adult lives separately lived and participate consciously as partners in dying.

"A privilege to be able to be present"

Carrie: I feel at times a privilege to be able to be present with somebody that's easy to be with. I didn't know it would be that way.

Researcher: You got to know him differently now?

Carrie: Yes, much better. How lucky I was to get to know him so well. He was always so lucid. His mind was good. We could have humor and family time.

For this mother, even with her physical exhaustion, the year of caregiving was a year of reconnection with her firstborn son as a new adult friend. They shared a new spirituality in Alcoholics Anonymous, holding "little meetings" in the car as they drove to the doctor; they shared the blessings of a sober mind, jokes, and the small pleasures of coffee in the morning; and they shared "living moment to moment." They both talked of being "joined at the hip"; by the time we met them, they seemed to have become truly each other's best friend. Shortly before Dennis died, his mother compared herself to a friend whose son had died rather suddenly of pancreatic cancer and who was filled with regret for things she hadn't said. Because of this year spent together, Carrie said, "I don't think I'm gonna regret, or wish I could say 'I love you' one more time." After Dennis's death, she said:

> There is no way that anyone who wasn't there could ever understand what goes on. I saw a phrase the other day I thought was so appropriate: Finding the real self of the other is like making a soul visible. The soul becomes visible. And that's what I felt like; it was like soul to soul with Dennis. It became that.

"I wouldn't miss this time"

Caring for Sharon was important to Connie for two reasons: her love and admiration for her older sibling and her hope that this death would heal some of the wounds left by her husband's recent death. Connie explained how she saw the situation:

> I'm glad to be doing it. I mean, I wouldn't miss this time. I'm glad to be part of the end of her life. And I was thinking the other day that I don't know what else could work. A nursing home couldn't begin to give her the care that she really needs. And anyway, I'm glad to be with her day by day through this.

～ ～ ～

> I really want to do this for Sharon and for all of us. It is very important for me to help her through the end of her life.

"I did everything I would want somebody to do for me"

Barbara's sister-caregiver Irene rejoiced in the opportunity to walk part of the way with her sister on her "journey to the other side":

> I told her, "I want to thank you for this opportunity to see through your eyes to the other side."

I love classical music, and she loves classical music. The music was really soothing to her. I fixed things that would look good. I knew her taste was not the best. I did everything that I would want somebody to do for me. I would say, "Barbara, why don't you just sit back and close your eyes, and I'll tell you a story. Just listen." I would tell her stories that had morals in them. And I'd talk about our grandma or our medicine bundle that we belong to.

Connecting the Church Family

For a local minister and a group of church members, the extraordinary effort to help one elderly parishioner stay in her own home, with her beloved animals, for six long months, was a symbol of their own connectedness to each other. This particular Missoula parish and its leaders—ordained and lay—have a tradition of active concern for the elderly, and their church events stress intergenerational ties. Thus, their effort to help Kitty was willingly begun out of an explicit tradition of caring for their older members—particularly those, like Kitty, who had no siblings, spouse, or children and who had made the church their family over many years. A member of the church described their tradition:

Cherishing the elderly has been a long tradition of this parish. They don't stop coming to church until they absolutely can't. But we started to notice that we lost them without knowing that we lost them. There was no way knowing whether they've decided to take the summer off and garden, or whether they're sick, or whether it's aging. So we thought, we have to pay deliberate attention to the elderly people. So we've had a whole series of programs, and one of our parish leaders spent two summers going from house to house visiting people, particularly older people. We spent a lot of time at that sort of thing. And so when Kitty started to pull away about three years ago little by little, and dropped out of Altar Guild, we knew.

The parish priest, who had orchestrated the system of care for Kitty, also spoke of the personal value to him of helping her in her last months:

I came here as a young priest. They took me in and taught me, and then they became my friends, and now I have to take care of them. It's that whole cycle of the child beginning to take care of the parent, and so for me it's been a blessing, because I know all of them.

Personal Growth for Caregivers: "What a privilege it is"

Several caregivers also pointed out that being with someone at the end became an opportunity for their own personal growth. Debbie mentioned the personal value to her of "learning to be sensitive" to her mother's needs, to "always try and put myself in her place." She said:

> It would be really easy to get wrapped up in what you're doing for them instead of how they're feeling about things. I had a hard time trying not to tell Mom what she needed, when actually she was fine. She could have told me what she needed, and I should listen to her a little bit more about some things. So I finally learned. I think it took me a while to realize that her needs were more important than mine.

Carrie, despite facing the imminent loss of her son, still spoke of the benefits— of being aware of impending death as an opportunity to understand death and to learn how to appreciate each moment:

> Other people would say, "What a tragedy." But in there, someplace, comes a knowledge of what a privilege it is. We're all going to die, but few people have the privilege of a dress rehearsal for my own death. That's putting it poorly, maybe, but it's a knowledge, an appreciation of life. . . .
> I think you really get to know your own soul and the soul of another pretty well. Nothing else carries the importance that it used to. In the midst of a lot of pain, suffering, and the knowledge of having a terminal condition, in the midst of that you find so much more to be grateful for. The things that are possible, the things that are enjoyable crop up. Whereas before, the mind would be on tomorrow, probably, instead of now. It's much, much deeper now. . . .
> Being told or given the time of awareness before death is an opportunity not everyone gets. Pretty soon you start to realize the pluses that there are.

Barbara's sister Irene spoke of what she had learned from being present at her sister's struggle, using the language of a warrior facing battle:

> Eventually you get to a point where the illness begins to teach you about yourself. Like we say in our language, you learn to dig

deeper, to really know yourself. To really know what your strengths are, what your limitations are, and then how you're going to go about attacking the challenge. You're never done learning.

For these three women, caring for someone at the end of life brought personal growth, and they recognized that the pain they experienced came from the lessons they needed to learn.

What Benefits?

Balancing this picture, some family caregivers—those with more financial difficulties and less family support, as well as those who themselves were struggling with personal issues, particularly other losses—did not speak with us of the "meaningfulness" of this time. Compounded losses and physical, financial, and psychological stresses may have made it more difficult for them to identify anything of positive value or meaning in this time of caring at the end of life.

Barbara's husband Dan had difficulty describing anything of "value" or meaning in Barbara's dying. His experience was marked by loss and fear. Dan and Barbara shared the hope that her remission would last a long time.

Dan:	What am I afraid of? Oh, not having Barbara around, of course. Barbara's my best friend. I don't have any specific plans. I hope that she gets better. That she beats this.
Researcher:	Well, I guess one of the things that we're interested in is what kind of things you're learning? From all this experience.
Dan:	Learning?
Researcher:	Yeah. What's different about your life? Insightful of anything?
Dan:	Heh-heh. [pause] . . . Oh man!
Researcher:	I guess it's providing an opportunity to see life differently? Or . . . [long pause]
Dan:	Yeah. There's a lot of things that you can't do [pause] together, like on trips and stuff like that we might do together. But we can't because if she's sick, somewhere when we're on a trip, the things to take care of her

> aren't there, so our kind of life together, to do things together, is not as much.

For Dan, the experiences and pleasures he and his wife had shared—camping, fishing, car trips to visit friends—were no longer possible. He could articulate his losses—of his best friend, of their times together, of his work—but could not find anything positive in this time as compensation.

Two other caregivers, Karen and Bernice—both caring for mothers with breast cancer that had spread to the bone—also never directly mentioned any positive values of caregiving or responded when the topic was brought up. From what they did want to talk about, however, we can infer that one value for both of them was in being the "good daughter." Each seemed to regard herself as the one who was willing to put her own life on hold to care for an aging parent—in contrast to siblings who did not. Each of them spoke of her duty and commitment to "care for Mom," despite the difficulties and disruption in each one's personal life.

Typical Difficulties

In this section we focus on aspects of caregiving that most of caregivers mentioned as most difficult or burdensome. We have made no attempt to judge or compare the degree of stress or burden; we simply report how caregivers described their difficulties. Among the issues caregivers identified are the following:

- Physiological stress
- Being "on a short leash"
- Living someone else's life—no privacy or time for oneself
- Scheduling, management of care
- Difficulty of setting limits
- Separation from other family
- Difficult symptoms
- Effects of a prior death.

From this limited sample, the identified caregiver difficulties appear to have as much to do with the cumulative physical and psychological burden of caring for someone who is chronically ill over a long time as with the existential experience of facing a loved one's impending death. Twentieth-century advances in medical technology and treatment mean that individuals with terminal diagnoses are surviving longer—sometimes much longer—than in earlier times. This longer survival increases the length of time prior to death that patients require daily care, in institutions or at home with family.

When we called to schedule visits, we quickly found that home care was a busy, sometimes exhausting experience for most families. Participants said, "Come back anytime; we're not going anywhere." In fact, however, caregivers did not find it easy to fit us into their schedule: Their weeks already were filled with nurse visits, other therapists, the hospice "bath lady," and visits from family and friends.

Most of our caregivers seemed not to have anticipated the all-consuming nature of twenty-four-hour care for someone who is terminally ill. The amount of help actually available to caregivers in this study varied greatly (see chapter 8). The remainder of this section discusses the difficulties shared by most family caregivers, regardless of circumstances or amount of assistance. The section that follows provides some snapshots of caregiving when adequate personal or financial support was not available.

Physiological Stress Reactions: Chest Pains

Some caregivers spoke openly about the "downside" of their caregiving. Months and years of caring for someone with a chronic illness had already worn them down. Now the final "push" was needed, and their resilience and strength were already worn thin. Connie had spent years caring for a diabetic husband on home kidney dialysis; after eighteen months of caring for her sister, she began having chest pains. When the pains occurred, Connie remembered that they had happened to her before:

> Before my husband died, probably in the year before, I began to have chest pains. And I had them thoroughly checked out, because sometimes I would faint. And the doctor told me that the kind where you pass out is the kind where you die. So I took that very seriously, and we had heart tests made, and my heart was fine. So it was always just a mystery what was causing those pains. But they started again for me now, before I had all this help. I haven't had any since this extra help. It was just stress.

The "extra help" was hospice care and services, which had begun five weeks before this conversation. Without hospice assistance, Connie recognized that she was at risk of serious physical stress reactions to the burdens of caregiving.

Connie was one of the "resilient," strong caregivers. She had a good deal of help from family and friends, as well as from hospice. Even so, she found the lengthy, unpredictable experience of caring for her dying sister difficult.

"I'm on a short leash"

One constraint that every caregiver mentioned was the lack of physical and psychological freedom because they could not leave the dying person alone, even for short periods of time. Perhaps because home caregiving has only recently (after several generations) become a part of family life again, most of the caregivers in this study had little or no previous life experience with long-term care at home—and thus had no basis for anticipating how constrained their lives would become when someone stayed home to die. There also was no way for them to know when their responsibilities would end. Connie described her situation this way:

> Because of the services we have, I am able to get out some, but it's hard. It's hard. I don't have any trouble getting out to do the errands I need to do because there's enough help for that. I decided some months ago that we just couldn't leave her alone anymore. She kept having these little fractures. And I could picture her on the floor, unable to move for a long time. And when you go out, it always takes longer than you think it will, just to do a quick errand. . . .
>
> I guess probably once or twice a week I go out to lunch with friends, or my daughter, but otherwise I don't. I do have a group of friends that I usually go to dinner with. And they usually go to a movie or something afterward. And lately I haven't felt like I wanted to do that. I just—I'm on this short leash. I have to hurry back home.

Another caregiver, Debbie, talked about her surprise at how "unfree" she felt while her mother lived with her:

> Another thing I wasn't prepared for, when Mom came to live with us, was losing the independence that my husband and I had. We found that we were limited; we couldn't go anywhere as we did before. We'd just pick up and go golfing, or just go, without thinking ahead or planning. I was not quite prepared for this. We tried leaving her alone a couple of times when we ran to the store, and we couldn't do it. . . . I couldn't just pick up and leave and do what I want to do and come back. And this went on for months.

Caregivers who had no other person living with them and no family or friends to call on had to develop specific strategies for surviving and meeting their needs. Sandy would struggle to get Ralph and his portable oxygen supply into the car to go with her to the grocery store if she needed something unexpectedly, leaving him sitting outside while she ran in. She counted on weekly visits from Ralph's sister or brother (who lived 100 miles away) and visits from her hospice volunteer to cut down on the number of times a week she had to do this. Even with two or three visits a week, however, Sandy's freedom to do anything else was severely limited during the 16 months she and Ralph lived in Missoula.

Bernice received no help from her family or friends in caring for her mother. Mabel disliked having anyone else take care of her (thus, Bernice had no help or respite from other family members or hospice volunteers) and did not seem to understand that she couldn't be left alone for long. So Bernice would leave her mother napping in the chair and rush to the grocery store or drugstore on essential errands. She felt she couldn't be gone more than twenty minutes. Bernice described how the situation affected her:

> The hospice nurse got me a volunteer, and I used her just once! Mom says, "I don't need nobody here." But she doesn't realize that for me to go out and hurry around and come home, it's stressful on me. Because nobody knows if one of her weight-bearing bones are gonna fracture.

In the six months we visited Bernice and Mabel regularly, Bernice talked about being able to leave their apartment for one half-hour shopping trip in any given week.

Another caregiver reflected on the loss of her hobbies during the last years of her husband's life:

> I used to belong to lots of things. I've taught flower arranging and landscaping. But even before he got so ill, I really couldn't do what I wanted to do.

"I'm living her life"

One of the caregivers (Connie) was very insightful and articulate about the constraints of caregiving, particularly in a newly formed household (i.e., a household formed by family members for the purpose of caregiving, in contrast to an existing household in which one member becomes terminally ill). Connie identified two areas in which full-time caregiving particularly affected her own life: interference with her ability to manage own needs and tasks, and the loss of her home and privacy.

> I guess one more thing I would say is how hard it is for me to settle down to the things I need to do, paperwork, to concentrate on my

own work. And I forget to take my own vitamins and stuff [laugh]; I'm just living her life! She takes every waking thought!

In the same breath that Connie talked about how glad she was to be sharing the end of her sister's life, she began to explain the downside: the loss of her own personal life. During their first year together, before Sharon "officially" became terminally ill, Connie had enjoyed having her sister live with her. They could play board games, go for car rides, and watch TV together. But the final months of Sharon's life were taken over by the demands of the illness, and the end-of-life "last things":

> What I'm feeling is that I'm really living HER life [laugh]. And my home is HER home [laugh]. I didn't feel I was living her life before. But from the time she moved in, I felt that my home became her home. I mean, I had expected to share it, but I hadn't realized that her kids come so much!

What posed an unexpected difficulty for Connie—besides having to become her sister's mind, think for her, and plan her care—was losing the privacy of her own home. This aspect of caregiving surprised her:

> Her kids do visit her, and it's wonderful. But, you know, when they're here, I like to give them some privacy. So it means I have to stay in my room or something. That was the surprising feeling to me. Because there's plenty of room here for the two of us, to have space and privacy. But when she has company—and she has a lot of it—then to give her any privacy I have to stay out of the way. And not only that, but I have to be hostess! [Laughs] It's not something I would have thought about at all.

The constraints of end-of-life caregiving, with its constant life-and-death aspect, affect even caregivers who do not have their family members at home. One caregiver, Karen, whose mother was at Hospice House for five months and then moved to a board and care home, described her difficulties in living her own life. Karen had constant responsibility to see that her mother received her medical care, except during the time Sarah lived at Hospice House.

> It's just been steady appointments. I finally got a perm myself. I felt so good yesterday [laughs]. I canceled three times because they would change her radiation or her appointments, so it's easier for me to change mine.

If these few families can provide the basis for a tentative generalization, we might say that more burden is felt by non-spouse caregivers, such as siblings or adult children, who bring a terminally ill family member into their home for an extended period of time. Spouses already are accustomed to "living each other's lives" and have developed patterns of privacy and of meeting their own needs within the relationship. A terminal illness may not be as disruptive to the life and needs of a spouse as to a non-spouse caregiver. In this regard, we stress that what matters is the perception or subjective experience of a burden. As with pain, each person has his or her own tolerance level. Exploring the differing needs of spousal and nonspousal caregivers—even though they appear to have the same degree of responsibility—may be useful for those planning support services and respite care.

Scheduling and Managing Nursing Care

Connie pointed out the difficulties of managing nursing care for a terminally ill patient at home:

> I really wouldn't be able to do this endlessly. She takes every waking thought. I have to keep track of. It just takes a lot of different things to keep her breathing; she has to have them. . . .
>
> Even though I do understand it, and I can do it, I still make mistakes. Sometimes I forget and miss, and she's an hour or two late getting a med or something. . . . After giving herself inhalations for years and years, she doesn't remember how to do it. You would think it would be second nature. I just can't believe that we have to instruct her each time. She has to take them exactly five minutes apart, and she has to be instructed again.

Family caregivers were required to perform some kinds of skilled nursing care and to be on call twenty-four hours a day, with only minimal training. If the patient has been referred to or requested hospice care, there was the additional support of a weekly thirty-minute nurse visit and phone assistance. Connie's assessment of this experience was stark:

> It's just all-consuming at the time you're doing it. If it went on for months, I don't think I could carry on at that level.

Other caregivers also mentioned how difficult it was to schedule every minute to sustain another person's life. Connie counted the number of appointments and visits she organized on a weekly basis: twenty-three, or three–four every day. This kind of schedule required a high level of management, as Debbie found out:

> I had to plan ahead, and I'm not a good planner; I'm not a good scheduler.

Setting Limits

Setting limits on care is one of the impossible tasks facing caregivers: With someone hovering close to death, every minute is precious; every cough can be significant.

> This uncertainty regarding the limits of one's obligation to render care is perhaps the greatest source of disruption in household organization. If one is always on call, always expected to do more, and never sure one is doing enough, it is impossible to plan for the future or maintain any interest outside caregiving. Caregiving in this case absorbs all household resources. (Albert 1990, 26)

Knowing when one has "done enough" was just as stressful and difficult for the caregivers in our study as the literature on caregiving describes. Even caregivers with extra help from family for respite care found they were limited:

> It is hard to balance. Because of the services we have, I am able to get out some, but it's hard; it's hard. Our cousin doesn't like to drive at night. So as it gets dark earlier, I'm going to be more limited in getting out. (Connie)

Another caregiver found that the psychological concerns for her mother became more intense as the time went on, even with a husband who stayed home and the resources to bring in a health care aide five days a week to stay with her mother while she worked. It was easier for Debbie to see in retrospect that she could—and perhaps should—have set limits on her personal caregiving and gotten more help:

> I think we needed to get different care people in here. I think it was too much for me to take care of her all the time. And Mom not being willing to adjust to people was a difficult thing. I think it would have been smart to have two or three people with a schedule. . . .
>   It got easier for me during the summer when I was home. I found it harder when I went back to work—wondering at work what was

going on at home, you know, having the need to be here and help her was very, very hard. Not just in worrying about it, but in not having a handle on things. It seemed like I was kind of out of control of the household.

We observed that some caregivers were not able to find any time for themselves, to set any limits on the amount of time and care they would provide. Their observable symptoms of stress—physical complaints, emotional instability, depressive reactions—were correspondingly greater.

The caregivers spoke about their sense of being exhausted as much by the unending and uncertain demands as by the physical care itself. Because of the great difficulty of setting limits when someone is dying, they tended to put off their own needs, and those of their families, until death occurred. Sometimes this feeling led to a new fear: that caregiving would never end, as one caregiver said:

I just don't know what to think about the future. Seeing her so well, this could be years, and I really don't want to do it for years. . . . I don't want to wish for, for her death, but it's the only way you have.

This ambivalence and internal conflict may be common among caregivers, even though most cannot articulate it so clearly. Once a goal has been set, a period of time for a task marked off, the human instinct to complete the task is strong, and this motivation provides energy. Finding that there is no end in sight can drain this energy away. So it seemed for these caregivers as we visited with them.

"I haven't seen my kids in three years"

For caregivers who were not caring for long-time spouses and therefore did not share children, one of the hardest part of caring was isolation from their own children and grandchildren. Two caregivers (Sandy and Bernice) were unable to visit their own children or grandchildren for years because of care for a mate in one case and a parent in the other.

Sandy had expected Ralph to die in the summer or fall of 1996, soon after they moved to Missoula. For two years, Sandy had put off leaving him to visit her three children in Colorado. As Ralph grew sicker, Sandy wouldn't consider going even for a short period of time. Missing holidays and the children's birthdays weighed on her, and she referred to it frequently in our conversations. In our first conversation, she said, "He knows I haven't seen my kids for going on three years, you know." Later, she amended that period to five years for some of her grandchildren:

Now my family, of course, they all live in Denver. And I've got, well, let's see. I've got five grandsons down there that I haven't seen for five years. It was Thanksgiving of '92—so five years I haven't seen 'em. One is going to be 16 the first of January. He's my daughter's oldest boy. I saw my daughter and her youngest one at my mother's funeral. That was three years ago September. And my son and his wife were up here, when was that? It was either the summer of '93 or '94 that they were here. And the following year I went to see my son and his wife. And I haven't been anywhere since. Because Ralph hasn't been feeling up to me leaving since then, so. And my youngest daughter and her husband and kids were up here a year ago June.

Sandy was bothered most by the uncertainty of Ralph's illness, which put her relationship with her children on hold while she faithfully cared for him.

What bothered Bernice about the seemingly endless task of taking care of her mother was the new granddaughter she had never seen, who was born in Minnesota after her son and daughter-in-law moved there from Missoula:

I've seen videos of this little girl, but I haven't been able to visit them. She said in her letter that little Kayla is starting to choose her words to the point where she can sound real grown up. She was born in December, so she is about 8 months old.

Just before Thanksgiving 1997, Bernice was still hopeful that her son might be able to bring his family out for a visit, but that proved impossible. At Easter 1998, she mentioned again her sorrow that she had not been able to go to visit them. Lack of money and the daily demands of caring for her mother seemed to have defeated her hopes.

Most Difficult Symptoms

Each illness exacts its own price on a caregiver's daily routine. For one, it was hygiene—struggling to keep her son clean as cancer spread everywhere on his skin, causing open sores and constant infections.

He had edema so bad he couldn't even stand in the tub and do it. Sometimes it was very hard to just raise his arms. . . . So we had to do what we could as far as washing. And it ended up the last washing we could do was a saline solution. I'd mix it up, and then

I'd take lap sponges. And he'd put his arms up, and I'd just run this salt water [over him]. He couldn't stand the shower. There was no rubbing. . . .

My big concern was in the end how would he be able to be kept clean. And nobody was able to help me on that. Of course, his disease is not common. I was the one who had learned as I went along.

For another caregiver, the most difficult aspect was waking up every morning at 5:00 to help her sister struggle for breath.

It's terrible, terrible. Her pattern now is she sleeps pretty well, but then she wakes up about five. She used to not wake up until eight or nine. But now she's awake every morning at five, struggling to breathe. And so we go through all the things she can have to relieve breathing. So the time is shortening between rest for her and for me. We go back to bed, we go back to sleep after that.

For two caregivers, the "most difficult thing" was not physical symptoms but when the person they loved became depressed:

What was it like? Well, it was much harder when he was sick than it is now. Because we went through days when he had terrible depression, lots of tears, and that was the hardest. It was for six, eight months, and it just got worse and worse. And I think that was far harder. We went through stages where he threw things and went through an angry stage. After he was gone, it was relief. He was free, and life could go on. (Dorothy)

The worst thing in the world is this part where he's suffering over something . . . and he does this to himself. It just agonizes me because I don't know what to say to him. I don't know what to do. It's hard. (Sandy)

The end of life can be accompanied by a loss of mental abilities, resulting from symptoms of the illness as well as from the medications needed to control symptoms. Thus, "dementia"—including subtle or pronounced impairment in cognitive reasoning, short- or long-term memory, and judgment—is a frequent syndrome. Families find this symptom particularly distressing in someone they know better, and who knows them better, than anyone else:

I think Mom's vacillating in her dementia was something that caught us off guard. I wasn't prepared for that. Like the time we were having some work done on the house here, and she told the gentleman when he came to the door that the people that owned this house would have to make the decision. It was just the divorcing herself from the fact that she was living with us. It did come and go. That's what caught us off guard. (Debbie)

Effects of a Prior Death: "I thought I'd get it right this time"

Connie was an emotionally strong, physically healthy, and intelligent woman who was close to her children and had many ties to friends in the community from years of working in the school system. Unlike some other caregivers in our study, she had as much support as she needed as she cared for her sister Sharon. Her description of her difficulties provides an in-depth glimpse, however, of the corrosive effect of a prior experience with dying that did not go well. Her emotional responses of guilt, anger, and sadness and her sense of feeling trapped were puzzling to her at first, when they came up in conversation, even though she confirmed our observation that everything was going well. Sharon's needs and wishes were being respected; the sisters were open in their communication and close emotionally. If Connie was "doing everything right this time," in her words, why wasn't she feeling better about it?

The subtext of further conversations with Connie and Sharon provided insight into their feelings about this experience and about each other. Connie was torn by two desires in direct conflict: hope that her sister would live longer and hope that she would die soon. In tears, Connie reflected on her sister's death in relation to her husband's death:

> [Crying] I've been thinking, I don't want to wish for, for her death, but—I felt that way with my husband too—it's the only way you have to get your life back, is when she's gone, and yet you don't want it to be. Hoping their life will be shorter so. . . .

The significance of comments such as this became clearer as Connie began to describe her husband's death four years earlier. He had suddenly chosen to speed his eventual dying by having his treatment stopped after seven years of home dialysis. He had not asked her advice or given her time to adjust: "What hit me was he chose to die."

Connie described her anger at his choice to hasten his death and her guilt that her secret wishes for his death during those seven years may have led to his decision to stop treatment, so he would not burden her more. She had never processed or shared these emotions with him or anyone else at the time of his death, and they resurfaced as she cared for her dying sister.

After the foregoing conversation, in which Connie found herself crying suddenly and unexpectedly, she wrote to her other sister by e-mail about the conversation and her feelings. Connie subsequently shared her e-mail message with us, as a way of explaining her ambivalence and conflict:

> Talking about caretaking for Sharon reminded me of [Connie's husband]. Sometimes I have thought that maybe I am supposed to get it right this time, but I have the same despairs.
>
> I get tired of the dependency, frequent calls or sirens, and the difficulty of getting out or even getting things done in the house. And feeling guilty here in front of the computer because I know she wants me in watching TV with her. Most of all I hate that the only way out for all of us is her death, and I don't want to be in the position of wishing it would come.

Connie added a written note to us about her e-mail:

> I really want to do this for Sharon and for all of us. It is very important to me to help her through the end of her life. Don't think that I am bitter or hostile about it—it is my choice. It just has a downside, too.

Connie's reactions to Sharon's slow dying were an unpleasant rerun of her experience with her husband's dying. Thus, in our first after-death interview, she said again, "I thought I was going to get it right this time." "Getting it right" meant that this time her emotions would be appropriate, that she would be able to manage the conflicting demands of home caregiving better, that she would have time to say goodbye, and that she wouldn't be overwhelmed by guilt afterward. A month after Sharon's death, however, Connie *was* feeling guilty—especially for having openly wished that Sharon would die in October, when Sharon had rallied and seemed to be doing better.

Sharon seemed to be aware of Connie's feelings. She mentioned to us in our first visit that she was "hanging on too long." Sharon knew that her life at times was a burden to her sister and said her major concern was that "[my] caregivers won't last"—that they will "burn out." Sharon also said that Connie, not herself, should be the subject of our research. To find the will to remain alive, Sharon needed Connie's reassurance that Connie also wanted her to live longer. Connie told us that she tried to provide this reassurance. For example, after they called hospice in, in June, and Sharon began making preparations for an immediate departure, Connie assured Sharon that her death wasn't imminent, and Sharon relaxed for a while. The paradox of end-of-life care for someone who is dying at home is that it can demand that someone else give up his or her own life for a while, to help the dying person go on living.

Both sisters were conflicted in their love for each other and their own needs. What each needed—her own life—was thwarted by what the other needed from her: They lived in a far too common caregiver paradox:

- To go on living, Sharon needed Connie's care and support, which Connie experienced at the loss of her own life.

- To go on living, Connie needed Sharon's death: "It's the only way you get to get your life back."

To summarize this discussion of typical difficulties, what seemed most difficult for caregivers in this study was being asked to perform the equivalent of skilled nursing care and to be on call twenty-four hours a day, with only minimal training and the support of a weekly thirty-minute nurse visit, for an indefinite but often lengthy period of time. A hospice staff person, in a reflective moment, said:

Part of the good work that we do is to make it seem not as scary, but maybe we're thinking that it isn't as hard as it really, really is because we're just more used to it.

Inner Resources

The inner resources that caregivers brought to their task, beyond the support that they may have had from others, was a major source of their success. Some brought religious traditions of caring and comfort; some brought more personal family traditions that helped them see even the most difficult days as meaningful. Others had an attitude of accepting each day or prior experience to help them through the difficult times. In this section, we examine their inner resources.

Acceptance: "You don't question the way the Lord works"

Sandy explained to us that she believed there was "some meaning" in all of this, although she didn't know what it was. Her straightforward, unquestioning faith in the face of adversity and the unfairness of illness and death was unswerving. (Ralph became ill with emphysema the month he retired, and they had never been able to enjoy being together in his retirement.) Sandy summarized her faith in these words:

> Yeah, I learned a long time ago that you don't question the way the Lord works. You just don't do that. You just go on your little way, and no questions. Because things are gonna be the way they're gonna be. You change what you can change, and what you can't, why. . . .
>
> All I hear now from him is, "I pray and I pray and I pray to let me die, and He won't let me." Well, I keep telling him, "You know, the day you were born, you were appointed a time to die." And I said, "Well, until you live to that time, you're not going to die."

Family Ethos

Each family has a particular ethos—a set of values by which actions of individual members are governed. Family caregiving is strengthened and guided by these unwritten and sometimes unspoken family values. Most family members probably could not readily state their unwritten rules that tell them what should be done. One of the families in our study, however, explained some of their hidden family history that helped shape their current actions.

Connie's willingness to care for her sister Sharon certainly came from a lifetime of love and affection between them. In an offhand comment, however, Connie revealed that the two sisters had another connection that further strengthened her resolve and saw her through the tough times, even with the stress of caregiving for a second long period right after her husband's death. The way she put it was simple:

> My son is coming, will be here for week. You know, Sharon's son gave my son a kidney. So we always like to get those two kidneys together.

Connie's husband had lived for seven years with kidney failure on home dialysis, and one of their sons inherited his father's kidney problem. Sharon's son, who was about the same age, had been the donor who gave his cousin a new and better life several years earlier. Connie and Sharon's children's lives were now physically interwoven; through this gift of life, the disease that had killed Connie's husband could no longer harm her son. Thus, gratitude toward Sharon's family gave Connie extra energy in caring for Sharon at the end of her life and made this time even more meaningful for her. Sharon's kidney donor son could not easily take his mother in because of his own living situation. Thus, Connie's willingness to take Sharon in without resentment, despite her own stress, became more understandable as an act of gratitude to her nephew as well as an act of love for her sister.

Dorothy and her family also spoke of a strong moral vision, which involved a "day-to-day" life of cooperation and continued support—not just while the children were young but as they moved into adulthood. This inner family ethos provided the basis for the strong external family support system they constructed to help their father during his last year of life. Dorothy was clear that their beliefs came from a personal family tradition, passed down from her mother, rather than from an external authority:

> The main thing was what you did day by day. That's just the way we feel. And I think our children probably feel about the same. I still feel that a minister can do nothing for you except comfort you. And if you've done your life right, you comfort each other.

"One day at a time"

Sandy seems to have brought her own inner resources to caregiving. She spoke of having to take it "one day at a time." Ralph worried about tomorrow, about whether he would be alive or not. Sandy's response was to focus on today and make each day a good one:

> We gotta take one day at a time, and then go to bed and go to sleep. And the next day we get up. If the next day is here, then we'll deal with that day. Because I think that dealing with one day at a time is enough.

This attitude, as much as any other factor Sandy could identify, helped her cope with sixteen months of living in an apartment in Missoula, away from friends and family in their small community, struggling to help Ralph breathe.

Carrie also had a "one day at a time" attitude, drawing on the teachings of Alcoholics Anonymous, to get her through the many difficult days she faced:

> Where we have been is living moment to moment. I think that we kind of realize that we really don't have the power we always

thought we had. A belief in a Higher Power can take an awful lot of burden.

"I knew from past experience"

Alone among the caregivers in our study, Dorothy had a long history of caring for terminally ill family members, including her mother and both of her husband's parents:

> I took care of Walt's folks, his mother and father. They had a woman in there, and when it got too much for her, I would go up and stay for a couple of weeks. . . . And then if she called me in the middle of the night, and his mother needed to be changed and moved to another bed, I would drive up in the middle of the night and take care of her and then come back to Missoula. So we worked this out for quite a few years. Twenty years ago was when I started taking care of them. I had five [years] with his mother, and then his dad.

These years of caring for Walt's parents, both of whom also died of congestive heart failure, gave Dorothy a wealth of practical knowledge about the disease and its symptoms, as well as a sense of competence and confidence about the difficult task of caring for her husband:

> I knew from past experience with his mother that when they get quite terminal that their taste buds aren't working right. Their bowels don't always work right. The kidneys don't work right. . . . When they're unable to do things, then you know that they're going down.

Dorothy had been with her mother as well as her husband's parents as they were dying; she wasn't frightened by dying and death. She understood the emotional ups and downs of the dying person, as well as their physical needs and their final readiness to go.

> My mother was afraid up until the end. At the very end, I was with her till midnight in the hospital, and she looked at me and she said, "You go on home." She said, "I'm ready to go. I've talked to all my family, and they're waiting for me." And before I got home, she was

gone. She was ready. And I think people reach that point. Walt's dad pulled all the tubes out of himself. They had him wrapped up with a straight jacket when he broke his hip. And he said, "I'm not living any longer." He got out of the straight jacket, pulled all the tubes out, and that was it. So I think people reach that stage: "This is it."

Sandy also had some experience caring for her own mother, also dying of emphysema three years earlier. She moved back home to the Midwest, but she found her step-father so resistant to calling in outside help that she could do little to make the situation better. After several months, she left her mother in his care and the care of her step-sister. In the months Sandy stayed with her mother, however, she came to understand what end-stage emphysema could be like and what kind of care is needed. When Ralph became ill, Sandy knew how difficult it would be for him and for her, yet she was determined to make his final days comfortable and meaningful. Knowing that Ralph's last year was better than her mother's had been provided Sandy with strength to continue and helped prevent her from feeling guilty when she finally could no longer care for him and transferred him to Hospice House.

The Caregiving Experience in the Subculture of Dying Persons

Families, especially the primary caregivers—as well as the dying person—found themselves participating in a new subculture. For some, the changes were subtle because home caregiving had been going on for a long time. For other caregivers, the terminal stages of illness brought marked changes.

Much of the tension experienced by family members providing end-of-life care arose from their dual membership: They still belonged fully to the culture of the living, but they also were living within a new subculture that surrounds those close to dying. Connie made the point most succinctly for us: "I'm living her life." Without necessarily being conscious of doing so, family caregivers had to struggle to maintain control over their own lives and connection with their social networks and the life they had led (and would lead again). As a result, they faced issues involving their own economic security, comfort, and sometimes health. Meanwhile, they were helping a spouse, parent, or child deal with these same issues, in the context of impending death—joining with them in the psychological tasks of life closure and saying goodbye. Having to bridge two cultures and maintain a foot in both added to their stress. The data also point to the difficulty for some caregivers of having experienced the effects of this subculture for years because of a chronically ill, dependent parent, without any of the extra support, however minimal, reserved for those who are obviously dying.

This view of caregivers as being required to straddle two cultures helps clarify the underlying reasons for two different approaches taken by families. Some families, particularly primary caregivers, had the attitude that their home was an "open house." They made us, as researchers—as well as their own friends and family—feel welcome, even as death drew very near. These caregivers also maintained some of their normal activities. Other homes were closed to most outsiders; outside activities and work stopped during this period, as the caregivers sacrificed their own needs and let go of connections to the culture of the living.

Caregivers whom we characterize as having an open house encouraged others from the majority culture to visit and to help with care. They appeared to be willing to let go of trying to control events; they neither avoided nor focused all their attention on the nearness of death. Letting others come to visit, to be part of the last months and weeks of someone's life, correlated very closely with an openness and acceptance of death by the caregiver and patient, which should come as no surprise. "Last" visits are difficult for patient and visitor if there is no acknowledgment that this visit may be the last, that life is ending very soon rather than later. An explicit and openly communicated acknowledgment of the dual nature of their situation—of this "bicultural" position—seemed to help these caregivers.

The Need for Preparation and Knowledge

Our observations suggest that the major need of all caregivers entering the subculture that surrounds persons who are expected to die is simply *knowledge*— about what end-of-life care involves; about the degree of help they need; about what to expect as the illness progresses; about managing the balance between the patient's needs and their own; about organizing medication schedules, respite care, and extra help; and about the process of dying itself. Caregivers such as Dorothy who came to their task with prior experience caring for others with a similar illness brought a schema that not only included relevant knowledge but prepared them for acquiring additional knowledge. Those who were confronted suddenly with this new world of end-of-life care at home had to learn a great deal of critical information and skills very quickly.

Even the most competent caregivers in this study had difficulty understanding procedures for an increasing number of medications. Other areas in which knowledge was lacking included signs that death was imminent and how to determine that death had actually arrived. Given that signs of impending death (i.e., that death is only a few days away) may be clear to medical professionals only in retrospect, it is difficult to know how much caregivers can learn in advance. In some cases, however—such as Carrie's, for example—more information and preparation would have been welcomed; she needed someone to answer her questions during the last few days of Dennis's life.

Recently, a new concept—"anticipatory guidance"—has emerged in studies of chronic illness in children. This concept refers to the entire process of providing the information families need when a child has a chronic illness or syndrome that requires long-term care (Battaglia and Carey 1999; Green 1999). Anticipatory guidance describes the process of providing information in advance about what the experience of caregiving for and experiencing the illness will be like, from the caregiver's perspective rather than the health professional's. Although receiving a list of medications and dosages to be administered daily certainly involves information, hearing from another caregiver's experienced point of view what the daily schedule of administering those medications will be like and what that process will require of a family caregiver is different. This kind of knowledge and guidance, in anticipation of need and driven by changing needs and situations during the dying process, is what our caregivers wanted when they spoke of needing more "information." Anticipatory guidance for family caregivers is an interactive process of information-sharing over time, driven by the amount of knowledge that individual caregivers already have and accessible at the time and in a format that meets caregivers' needs.

Many patients and families clearly prefer family caregiving, but it is a complex, demanding, full-time job. Families need opportunities to learn enough to do this job well. One fruitful avenue for further investigation is what kinds of knowledge, along the lines of anticipatory guidance, are needed to prepare families to take on this job, and who should provide it. Hospice staff can provide much of this information, but they generally are available to assist a family only for a short period of time each week.

The Paradox of Caregivers' Future Expectations

One assumption among persons seeking to improve end-of-life care is that caregivers who have the most support and provide peace and comfort to the person dying will emerge from this experience with a reasonable expectation that their own end of life can be similar: that they will be loved and cared for by family members during their own dying. The caregiving experiences we studied, however, did not always give caregivers the hope that the circle of giving would continue in the next generation of their family. For some participants in our study, the experience of caregiving led to very different expectations for themselves or did not change expectations that were based on earlier experiences. Five of the eight caregivers spoke of their expectations concerning their own life's end; the other three had nothing to say.

- Two caregivers (Debbie and Sandy) reported that they had begun conversations with their families about their own expectations and needs in ten or twenty years. These two caregivers appeared to assume that their children will want and be willing to provide for their care—in a home setting if possible.

- One caregiver (Carrie) doesn't expect her children to care for her and hopes to go into a hospital or institutional setting. Having taken care of her dying son at home for more than a year in accordance with his wishes, she now expects to start caring for her husband as his emphysema worsens.

- Two strong, competent caregivers (Dorothy and Connie) had long considered assisted suicide for themselves. Nothing about their recent caregiving experience had changed their views. Neither spoke of expecting that their own children/family will care for them. One talked of liking Jack Kevorkian. Her family plans to pay for nursing home care for mom "if she needs it" but did not speak of taking care of her themselves. The other has a DPOA and a living will, which appoint a friend to help her with suicide if she develops Alzheimer's disease, so that her own children won't be burdened. In her case, she fears the particularly debilitating effects of this disease more than she fears dying.

In this respect, research in Great Britain by Seale and Addington-Hall (1994) demonstrates that women in the last year of life were less likely to have people close to them who were emotionally dependent or invested in their existence—and thus were more likely to ask for euthanasia. Although both Dorothy and Connie appear to be years away from their own deaths, they may have been affected by the prospect of being without a caregiver such as themselves, rather than hopeful from their own direct experience of the value of the end of life. Ironically, Dorothy's and Connie's experiences as caregivers were among the best we observed.

Chapter 8

Support and Lack of Support for Family Caregivers

In chapter 7 we present the family caregiver's experience as she or he sought to assist a dying loved one. This chapter answers a new set of questions: What kind of support and assistance from others—families, friends, or community—did these caregivers receive as someone in their family was dying in Missoula in 1997? How did this support come about? What additional help, if any, did they need? What kinds of strain resulted from lack of support? What if there was no one to provide the extra help needed?

Support from Others—Family, Friends, Community

Chapter 7 illustrates that extended caregiving at the end of life can be a stressful, intense experience no matter how much support is available or given. The caregivers in this study can be divided into two groups: those who had good support from others and those who had little or none. Researchers on caregiving across the life span have used the metaphor of a "good musical ensemble" to describe a support system for caregiving. First, according to Schulz and Rau (1985), "There must be some stability to achieve a high quality performance." Schulz and Rau go on to describe a good support system as "consisting of different actors—friends, relatives, colleagues—each of whom has assigned functions and who together cover the full range of support needs" (145).

Some of the caregivers in this study clearly preferred not to divide responsibilities for end-of-life care, even if someone was available. Our observations and the available literature on home caregiving document, however, that a division of caregiving tasks does reduce the stress and burden to the primary caregiver and draws families together. When support is provided primarily by one person and other available family members do not contribute support, for whatever reason, tension is added to already difficult situations (Silverman and Huelsman 1990).

Table 8-1 illustrates the wide range of support available in our small sample of caregivers. Some primary caregivers had four or five people regularly available in any given week to provide respite care and help them, as well as hospice support. Others had no other family members providing such help but did have hospice, which could provide volunteers to relieve them for an afternoon. Some had little or no family support and no hospice support.

Orchestrating a System of Support

One caregiver's situation illustrates how a well-orchestrated system of care can be put into place to provide assistance to the caregiver and respite care seven days a week. In caring for her sister, Connie had organized Sharon's family to help out as well; she also had a great deal of support from nonfamily members, in contrast to some other caregivers.

Connie had an extensive network of family support:

- Sharon's two sons each came for an afternoon once a week to stay with their mother, to relieve Connie.

- A second cousin in Missoula, who was not employed at the time, was available to come over on short notice whenever Connie needed to run errands or wanted go out with her friends for dinner. This cousin didn't like to drive after dark, so as fall and winter approached he was less willing to come in the evening; he was available during the day, including weekends, whenever Connie needed him. This "on-call" assistance provided enormously helpful relief.

- Sharon's daughter, who had moved to another town several hours away, came back for long weekends twice a month, allowing Connie a more extended break.

- Connie's own daughter, who was very close to her, lived in Missoula and was available for emotional support. She took her mother out for lunch once a week during the last difficult months. When Sharon was dying, Connie's daughter stayed with Connie during the last 48 hours.

In addition, Connie had substantial nonfamily support:

- A hospice volunteer came for an entire afternoon each week during the last four months of Sharon's life, allowing Connie to go out or simply to relax at home without having to attend to Sharon's needs. This

Table 8-1 Supplementary Caregivers and Assistance Available Weekly

Caregivers and Approximate Terminal Care Period

	Dorothy (Walt)	Debbie (Roberta)	Connie (Sharon)	Sandy (Ralph)	Carrie (Dennis)	Karen (Sarah)	Bernice (Mabel)	Dan[a] (Barbara)	Church (Kitty)
Months of care	13	7	24	16	12	12+	18+	5	7
Support									
Total family [including caregiver]	5	4	3–4	1	1 (+3)[b]	1	1	1	0
Friends available weekly	0	0	1	1	0	0	0	0	5–6
Hospice[c]	13 mo	6 mo	5 mo	16 mo	0	4 mo[d]	14 mo[d]	4 days	7 mo
Weekly hospice volunteer	V	V		V					

[a]For the purposes of this table, we have used the experience of Dan, Barbara's husband and primary caregiver throughout most of the last year of Barbara's life, rather than that of her sister Irene's brief period of care.
[b]For the last month of Dennis's life, his father and brother lived nearby, and his sister came several times to help for a week, but only his mother could provide the care he needed daily.
[c]Hospice support includes weekly nursing visits, twenty-four-hour phone consultation, volunteers to visit and provide respite care if desired, and Hospice House if needed or desired.
[d]Still living at end of study period; no longer with hospice.

volunteer provided social companionship and a kind of "healing energy" therapy that Sharon found very helpful.

▪ The hospice "bath lady" came twice a week for Sharon's bath.

▪ A Senior Companion from Missoula Aging Services—fortuitously, someone Sharon had once known and liked—visited weekly.

▪ Connie arranged to pay someone to do housecleaning once a week, to free her from concern about the house when Sharon's care was "taking every waking thought."

The additional family caregivers had to become as competent as Connie at giving Sharon her timed doses of medication to help her breathing. As Sharon found talking more and more difficult, they also learned to keep up a running conversation without requiring much response from her.

Characteristically, Connie had become proactive in arranging for more help, beginning more than six months before Sharon's death. The system existed because she had created it, as Connie's own comment documents:

I decided some months ago that we just couldn't leave her alone anymore. . . . That's when I talked to the kids and told them they need to give me some support time because I had to get out. I would have to get out for air, at least. And so that's when they set up a regular schedule.

As welcome as this support was, it meant that Connie was scheduling twenty-three different appointments each week. After Sharon's death, Connie summed up her experience:

I think we did about as well as we could. We had a lot of support.

In contrast, Bernice—who cared for her elderly mother who was totally dependent on her—made only minimal arrangements. She had no family support on a regular basis. Bernice's sister visited from out of town for two days, three to four times a year; her son and daughter-in-law provided no regular help. Her nonfamily support consisted only of a weekly visit from hospice nurse—until hospice had to terminate service.

Family support: "You comfort each other"

Walt's family provided the strongest example of caregiving that everyone planned for and participated in. Dorothy's did day-by-day caregiving for twelve months and was supported by the four of their five children, who lived in or near Missoula. Dorothy summed it up:

> The kids always have participated in everything in our family. No matter what goes on, all five of them know it. My daughter in D.C. calls me at least twice a week. Lots of phone calls. The kids have always called; they always drop in, we go out to lunch, we do things together.

Walt and Dorothy's daughter who lived next door gave her mom a day "off" each week by staying with her dad; the two sons came several times a week and spent time with Walt, visiting and keeping him company. Until Walt could no longer get into the car, their older daughter took him for rides, especially in the nearby Bitterroot Valley where he had grown up:

> I tried to come in several times a week and even oftener toward the end. And last winter to early spring, I started taking him on rides once a week. Our last ride was down the Bitterroot. Down to Hamilton to a funeral for one of his relatives. So he got to see a lot of his relatives that day. After that, there was no taking him out of the house anymore.

This family's closeness and cooperation during Walt's illness came out of Dorothy's mother's strong religious tradition. Dorothy explained how her faith came about and how it had become her family's moral vision on a daily basis:

> My mother was into church, and we were raised very religious. And even through all that, she always felt like church was not the main thing. It was what you did day by day. That's just the way we feel. And I think our children probably feel about the same. My children went to Sunday School and to church. But I still feel that a minister can do nothing for you except comfort you. And if you've done your life right, you comfort each other.

A Family Team: "Everyone just pitches in"

Debbie also organized a great deal of supplementary support from her family when she brought her mother Roberta to live with her. What is striking about this family's caregiving was the willingness of Debbie, clearly the primary caregiver, to share this responsibility with others—and the willingness of other members of her family to join in. During the six months Roberta lived in her daughter's home, she could not be left alone; she required increasing attention and care as her heart failed. Unlike Walt and Dorothy, Debbie and her family had not made explicit preparations for this time, but she described how they quickly developed a flexible team system:

> I didn't know before Mom moved in that I would need so much help. I did not know. When we first entertained the idea of Mom coming in, I thought, "Wow!" I didn't know what to do but I just knew we could do it. Whatever we had to do, we'd deal with it. If we needed to look at something else, we'd look at something else.

Debbie emphasized that "it wouldn't have been possible without Joe" (her husband). When Roberta began failing visibly at the nursing home in the spring and they decided to move her into their home, Joe quit his beloved summer job working outdoors at a local golf course so that he could be around during the day while Debbie was at work. She explained:

> Joe has just been really wonderful with this whole thing. I tried to encourage him to continue working because we were going to hire someone to stay with Mom, until I could do it. But he felt that we needed the support, and I do need support.

Debbie and Joe understood that Debbie would worry too much about her mother if she had to leave her at home without a family member there while she was at work and that her mother was going to be difficult with anyone else, unless someone in the family who knew her was home as well. Debbie's grandson summed it up accurately: "[Roberta] gets fussy [and] really does like to cause a hard time, with the nurse, the bath lady." Debbie spoke about how making this kind of caregiving work "takes a family":

> It does take more than me; it takes a family. It wouldn't work if everybody else didn't pitch in.

So they formed a family team: Debbie, Joe, and two others: their grandson and one of Debbie's sisters. Debbie's grandson, who was nineteen years old, was already living with them while he attended college. He also became a companion for Roberta when he was home, sometimes fixing her breakfast and talking with her when others were not around. Debbie's younger sister, who lived in another Montana city five hours away, came over regularly to stay for the weekend; she was the one person Debbie and Joe would allow to take over Roberta's care for an extended time, so that they could both leave. Debbie put it this way:

The support that I appreciated so greatly was my sister coming over and giving me a time to get away comfortably. If I were even going to go to the stores or somewhere or go with my husband, knowing that Mom was fine with this. She wasn't fine with everybody. To get away and know that she was comfortable, I felt great support in this. I recommend highly that people have various people come in and help.

In addition, Debbie arranged and paid for a private home health aide to come in five days a week while she was at work, even though Joe was now also at home. Debbie continued to have this aide come during the summer, even while she was on vacation and home full-time, so that she could have the same person beginning in the fall, when she went back to work in the public schools. This home health aide, who was a stranger in May, soon became part of the family and stayed with Roberta until her death; she spent Roberta's last day and evening there as part of the family.

Debbie described her approach as very open and flexible: "If we needed to look at something else, we'd look at something else." This flexibility helped make their home an "open house," where visitors—even strangers doing research on end-of-life care—felt welcome.

Making Use of the System

Sandy was one of the caregivers who had no regular weekly assistance from friends or family—mostly because she and Ralph had "moved in town" from a rural part of Montana 100 miles away to get hospice care. Sandy made more extensive and intentional use of hospice services than some other caregivers; she used hospice volunteers extensively and even the two MDP researchers to get extra assistance and respite.

The other great resource supporting Sandy in her caregiving was the apartment she found. It stood on the banks of the Clark Fork, close to a grocery store, with a view of the cottonwoods along the river, the Missoula valley, and the mountains to the west.

I couldn't believe it when I found that apartment right there on the river. I told him, "Now I've found an apartment on the ground floor that's all set up for wheelchairs and handicapped people." And I said, "It's right on the river. It's going to be pretty nice."

Being forced to move from their home to a strange city, to find care for what turned out to be a long, slow dying process (sixteen months), could have been a terrible experience. Instead, their apartment, with a wheelchair-accessible bathroom, easy access to a walk along the river, and the beautiful picture windows in the front room and the bedroom, brought them joy every day and made Sandy's caregiving far easier.

The apartment complex had been built with federal housing funds to provide housing for disabled residents of Missoula, although the complex's planners probably did not envision end-of-life needs when they planned the complex. Its design and accessibility were central to the relative lack of stress we observed in the end-of-life care Sandy provided. The apartment reduced—to a degree—her need for assistance and support. What would have been a very difficult experience for Sandy and Ralph, because of the lack of family members or community links, became instead a time of sharing and moments of joy.

Our conclusion is that even with hospice services, and with family and friends to help, caregiving for someone who is dying is likely to be stressful and difficult for a primary home caregiver. Good palliative care may inadvertently exacerbate caregiver stress by prolonging life beyond what was expected or predicted. What a caregiver expects to be an all-out, intense effort for three to six months can turn into more than a year of all-consuming care. And when either hospice services or other family are not available to help, the difficulties of providing care and the resulting stress were correspondingly greater. Some of the caregivers had neither other family members nor hospice to support them at critical times.

Lack of Support for Caregivers: Causes and Consequences

Along with the record of substantial help from family, friends, and professional caregivers, there were several caregiving situations that lacked support from family, the kind of palliative care hospice provides, or both.

Caregiving at home for terminally ill persons can be thought of as a three-legged stool: To remain stable, caregiving requires a strong and competent primary caregiver, additional assistance from family members and friends, and adequate palliative care. The caregivers described in the preceding section—Dorothy, Sandy, Connie, Debbie—had orchestrated this support from family, friends, and community resources. Other caregivers either chose to have little assistance or through circumstances had little or none available. For some, family members and friends were potentially available, but no "family team" had ever formed. For others, using hospice services conflicted with the patient's personal struggle for a return to health, or at least remission. The caregivers' situations described in this section illustrate the complex interaction of individual attitudes and expectations, the caregiver's relationship with the dying person, and external circumstances.

Interaction of Patient Preferences and Caregiver Sacrifices

This section describes the experiences of caregivers who seemed to have less support than they needed. The existence of support was related in part to roles that the caregivers took on for themselves, which seemed to fall along a continuum of sacrifice and self-preservation. Some sacrificed their own lives entirely to provide care at the end of life; others (described in the preceding section) were "self-preservers" who obtained extra help and assistance, thereby ensuring that their own life and health would be maintained during this difficult time. Two of the caregivers we discuss in this section, Carrie and Bernice, seemed willing to be sacrificers for the sake of the person who was dying. Two others, Karen and Dan, fall somewhere between in attitude: managing to preserve some of their own life but doing so without asking for more help (see Figure 8-1).

In the cases of Carrie and Bernice, lack of support appeared to come from the patient's preference for a single caregiver available twenty-four hours a day, as well as from the caregiver's willingness—or even need—to provide that care personally, refusing other help.

"Doing it all myself"

Carrie was required to give intense and demanding care for almost a year, and she was the caregiver who had the least outside help or support. She had neither hospice nor regular family assistance for most of Dennis's last year. She exemplifies caregivers who "do it all" by themselves. By the end of Dennis's illness, Carrie seemed worn out physically as well as emotionally. A month after Dennis died, Carrie admitted how difficult it was for her with no professional or personal support at the end:

Figure 8-1   Continuum of Self-Preservation and Sacrifice

Self-preservers		Sacrificers
Dorothy	Karen	Bernice
Debbie	Dan	Carrie
Sandy		
Connie		

It was so hard on me. The third time they upped the Fentanyl, the nurses in the chemo over there, and the doctor tried to talk him into going into the hospital. And he said "No." And I was on their side, trying to ease this to him. He refused. I wanted to say, "Who do you think is the one that suffers through this? You're out of it." It was the first time I ever wanted to say, "Me, me. I need something."

In addition to providing twenty-four-hour care for Dennis, Carrie was the only one close to her mother, who was more than ninety years old and living in a nursing home 100 miles away. Whenever Carrie had a break—generally when her daughter could come from long distance to stay—she would drive to see her mother for a day. In August, as Dennis approached the end of his life, Carrie's mother broke her hip, and Carrie spent extra days with her.

Because Dennis's home was in a rural area of Montana, an hour's drive from Missoula, the location certainly reduced the choices of services available to him and to his mother. According to Carrie's account, however, her lack of assistance appeared to be related as much to his preference for her care over anyone else's and his total refusal to go to a hospital as to their rural isolation. Carrie had become so expert at taking care of her son that he preferred her to anyone else—even other family members:

He would say to me, "Oh, you are so gentle when you put on the Vaseline." He said [his sister] just rubbed, the nurses rubbed. He says, "I feel like a big baby."

Carrie was aware of her need for extra help but described her own frustration in finding the kind of help she needed in their setting:

The social worker constantly made her token visits. She'd say, "What can I do for you?" every time. And I got so I had enough to do to be innovative for myself without having to tell somebody, today we're doing it this way. It was doubling my load to have these people. I was training them. I finally told her, "When you go out and find another Carrie—better yet, two Carries—then you come back, and you will have done exactly what I need. Otherwise, stay away from me."

Carrie found the task of explaining the care her son needed and "training" home health care nurses too draining on her:

I realized how impossible it was for anyone to help me because they had to be taught. This was trial and error and innovation. And they marveled at what things we came up with. I think you'd have to be with somebody as much as I was.

The only nurse from their local home health service who was really "good," from Carrie's perspective, took an administrative job with the service, and her replacements came in on an inconsistent, rotating basis. By the time we started visiting, they did not appear to have any extra nursing care, even on a weekly basis; they were relying solely on the outpatient visits to Dennis's doctor for medical care, with Carrie doing the rest herself. Later in Dennis's illness, he received IV therapy at home from a different home health care provider. They apparently never pursued any assistance that hospice could provide, however. Carrie said only this:

> Hospice care was brought up, and there was some reason why it wouldn't work out. It was because of the changeability of the schedule. Night or day meant nothing to us.

This difficulty connecting with hospice probably reflects Dennis's desire to fight for every extra day of life and to pursue the chemotherapy that provided some extra months of life, even at great physical cost. When chemotherapy could no longer help, his reluctance to accept palliative care continued.

"I got some days where I tell Mom I just absolutely can't stand it anymore."

Bernice represents another example of the stress placed on family caregivers when they have no support or relief available during a protracted terminal illness. The almost complete absence of daily/weekly support for Bernice in caring for her mother was distressing to observe, even for researchers making brief visits.

Bernice's daily schedule was controlled by her mother's needs. Besides the major medical tasks, Mabel made constant "little" complaints and was seldom comfortable: She was too cold, she was unable to sit comfortably, nothing tasted good anymore, and so forth. Mabel's pain patch schedule punctuated their lives. Mabel also was on oral medications, particularly to control less severe pain. She often was uncomfortable taking them or refused them outright because they upset her stomach. Bernice had to work continually to keep her mother comfortable.

Bernice's description of her experience in brief, matter-of-fact statements reflected her own "day-to-day" approach—characterized by sheer endurance, with little planning or reflection. During the times when Mabel was in pain and more uncomfortable, Bernice was even more depressed in appearance and behavior. As she put it: "When she goes down, it puts me in a bind."

Bernice and Mabel did not have strong social networks within their family or within the community when Mabel's serious illness came. Although Bernice had one son who lived with his family on the outskirts of Missoula and another son and daughter-in-law who had lived in Missoula until recently, neither of them participated in any regular care for Mabel or assistance to Bernice. Their one means of involvement seemed to be visiting occasionally on Sundays:

> They both work. And they're pretty active with the kids after work. I mean, they're into everything and church and they were coach and assistant coach for the Little League ball teams. But they remember birthdays and Mother's Day and Christmas and Thanksgiving.

Similarly, Mabel's other daughter, who lived two hours away in northern Idaho, visited every few months, staying for a couple of days. Bernice and Mabel regarded these visits as purely social and something of a burden, rather than for the purpose of helping Bernice in any way:

Bernice: On top of everything, my sister and niece are coming over today. They have to leave Saturday.

(after that visit)

Mabel: Yeah, my daughter came over for awhile. But they don't stay only about three days, and back they go.

The family visits, especially from Bernice's two little grandchildren—Mabel's great-grandchildren—were the most joyous moments in these women's lives. But they did not relieve Bernice's unrelenting caregiving responsibilities. Some of her tasks, such as getting her mother transferred from her wheelchair into a car and out again (to go to doctor's appointments or to Wal-Mart for new reading glasses), seemed beyond Bernice's own physical strength and enormously stressful for her and Mabel:

> It's a big effort to get her to the doctor, and the car the way it is. . . . Mom and I used to go down [to see Bernice's children] when I was working, but since Mom's got this bad cancer, no. The way my knees are, that fibromyalgia, in my knees and just pushing her up and down in the wheelchair aggravates the knees, and the stress, that makes it worse.

Bernice could identify no regular social activities or interests to meet her own physical, emotional, or social needs, and her mother apparently had few in her own life:

Bernice: Well, Mom, she's always been, uh, she doesn't socialize much. And after my divorce, moving in here to Missoula, well, I got to working, and I'd come home tired, and I just really didn't make any friends of my own, either.

Researcher: I wondered what kind of social life she's been able to keep. You don't have a club or church or any kind of group that you were part of?

Bernice: No.

The lack of support or assistance for this family from community resources was puzzling at first, particularly because they had chosen hospice care early and therefore had access to volunteers and other services. As we listened carefully to Bernice's explanations for why getting help was so difficult, we began to understand.

Researcher: You said you hadn't had much luck getting a hospice volunteer to come in yet?

Bernice: Oh no. I started with them, but Mom, she didn't like anybody coming in. And with her losing so much control of her life, I backed off, even though it would've made me feel better. And well, I also told the volunteer that I really don't want to take advantage of them, and I don't want to make myself feel that I'm taking advantage of another person. I told the volunteer that when I absolutely had to have her, so there is an appointment that I had this week, last week, that I had to meet. So I called the nurse up and asked if D_____ was still my volunteer, and she says yeah; so I called D_____ up and talked, and got the recording machine. And here without me knowing it, D_____ had quit volunteering through the summer. Well, I told my hospice nurse what had happened, that I would like to have a volunteer to come in and let Mom get used to her.

The hospice nurse later confirmed to us that hospice had tried for months to get volunteer help for Bernice and Mabel but had been defeated each time by the combination of Mabel's refusal to let anyone else besides Bernice help and Bernice's depression and inability to ask for help for herself. Over the next six months of visits and phone calls, Bernice continued to talk about plans to get a volunteer in; but as far as we know, that never happened.

Bernice gave evidence of being without any hope for herself. She had lost her job and was put on disability because of stress. This loss of work—and the loss of identity in the community that work provided—coincided with her mother's increasing debility. Bernice complained that keeping their small apartment clean was hard because her time was taken up with caring for her mother and, even more important, because she lacked the energy to do it.

There's sometimes where I'll go in and lay down too. Those are days where, I mean, I got some days where I tell Mom I just absolutely can't stand it anymore. I've got to go lay down. And then she'll go lay down. To clean house, it's kind of hit and miss, just do it when you can. Then there's times where, the mood I'm in, I just sit and look at it. I mean, I could care less!

Later in the fall, when Mabel's pain from bursitis and her unexplained neck pains had subsided a bit, Bernice mentioned her relief and described how difficult it had been for her "just sitting here watching her in pain." Our field notes capture the difficulties we observed in this home:

Bernice shows signs of chronic depression/high anxiety. She complains of not sleeping well, has many small aches and pains, no energy for daily tasks, and few daily pleasures. She reports rising relatively late in the morning, another sign of not sleeping well. Her voice is flat and without emotion; she frequently looks close to tears. There are two bright spots in Bernice's life—"hospice hugs" from the nurse who comes once a week, and the daily TV soap opera "General Hospital" at 1:00. Bernice is addicted to the soaps again, and isn't too pleased about this, but it is the one "bright spot" in her day [field notes, July 25, 1997].

Mabel's health and needs remained relatively stable during the period of our study, and hospice finally stopped providing care, although there was no change in the terminal diagnosis. This development left Bernice with only a monthly visit from a nurse to check medications and required Bernice to take her mother, wheelchair bound, to her physician for any medical care.

"I didn't realize the stress it puts on the caretaker's family"

Karen's experience with her mother Sarah illustrates the difficulties of managing end-of-life care for someone with a terminal illness even when the person isn't living at home. In Karen's case, the ongoing demands on her time and energy for many years, growing financial strains, and lack of active support from her two siblings combined to make her feel overwhelmed, even though she was not providing daily care during our study. Again, Karen fit the profile of the chosen caregiver: She was not currently working, she lived in close proximity, and she was not as burdened with other caregiving. Karen's younger sister, who also lived in Missoula, was employed outside the home and still had minor children to care for.

Karen began actively caring for her mother ten years prior to when we met them, with the first diagnosis of breast metastases. Karen has remained her mother's "case manager" during Sarah's advancing bone cancer. In the year they participated in our study, Karen helped her mother move from a senior residence to Karen's home, then to Hospice House for four months, then—after her cancer appeared to be growing slowly—to a small board and care home.

During the brief time Sarah lived with Karen (after she could no longer stay at the senior residence), Karen described becoming even more distraught:

> I was to a point where I was ready to just drop. Because she was up all night, just climbing walls and everything. When she went to Hospice House, it took me two weeks to get so I could start sleeping at night again.

The stress and difficulties for Karen and her own family were compounded because she had to manage her mother's care at a distance and pay the extra medical and care bills. Keeping her mother in her small home in a rural valley outside Missoula proved impossible. Moving her mother home would have been only temporary in any case because Karen and her husband, now retired, planned to sell their home and travel south during the winter:

> You know, I don't have a room for her. So I was scared to death to bring her home [from Hospice House]. I could've just brought her home until I found another place, but I thought, if I bring her home she's not gonna want to leave here. And I can't do that. I've pushed my family back for 9 years now, and I've gotta start, I've gotta get back with them.
>
> My husband is about ready to divorce me [laughs]. It's been hard. He's been great, but we're going on 11 years now since I moved back and started taking care of Mom. He's been retired for

6 years now, and he had bought our fifth-wheeler and worked like the devil to get it paid off so when he retired we could go have some fun. And we haven't gotten to yet. Every time we plan something, Mom gets bad. It's almost funny.

Even though Sarah lived independently or in a senior residence for eleven years rather than with Karen, Karen described continual responsibilities to see that her mother received appropriate personal and medical care, except during the time Sarah lived at Hospice House. She also visited her mother almost every day, driving twenty-five miles round-trip each time:

It's just been steady appointments, by the time I get her eyes checked, her teeth cleaned, her toenails clipped. It's just something steady. The biggest problem that I ran into is that Mom isn't bad enough to be in a nursing home, and yet she needs help with some things. The home health service is coming out and helping her with her shower. And, boy, that was a relief because I knew she was okay with it—with me helping her—but I could tell it was kind of embarrassing for her. She has no problems with them.

Karen also had to manage her mother's numerous daily medications. She "fixed boxes" of medications weekly, and the board and care home put them out for Sarah in a little cup at her plate at each meal. The difficulties of managing Sarah's life and her own led to situations that illustrated the difficulty Karen had in meeting her own needs while taking care of her mother:

I finally got a perm myself. I felt so good yesterday [laughs]. I canceled three times because they would change her radiation or her appointments, so it's easier for me to change mine.

As in some other families, Karen could find no bright line separating the care she gave her mother for the preceding decade from the care she provided to her mother in her last, terminal illness. The length of time that Karen's own life was put on hold made this last period much more difficult for her.

"I'm a person that stays to myself"

In addition to direct help in caring for someone who is dying, caregivers need social and emotional support from colleagues and friends. Barbara's husband Dan faced two kinds of loss: the impending loss of his life partner and the loss of his work identity because he had to quit his job to take care of her during her lengthy illness. Being unemployed for a sizable period of time—particularly for a healthy, able person—creates significant stress. In losing his job, Dan also lost his work identity and social connections to others. He always had been a loner; the loss of work left him more socially isolated, as he explained to us:

Dan:　　　　　I got friends, but I'm picky and choosy. I got one, two friends.

Researcher:　　Are they helpful to you?

Dan:　　　　　Yeah, well, one friend is bugging me. They're always asking how things are going and always there to talk to me about how it is. I'm a person that stays to myself. And like I've said, I've only got two other friends. Barbara's my best friend.

Barbara's concern for her husband was that there was no social or emotional support for him as he dealt with her terminal diagnosis and the daily effort to provide her with food, comfort, and care. She was far more concerned about the lack of support she perceived for him than he appeared to be, when we talked with him separately. She became very emotional as she spoke of the difficulties they faced as a couple and the isolation her husband experienced:

> I think women are greater caretakers than men are. And men will do it, but only if they freak out. And they'll hide their fear. They need help. . . . It's very painful emotionally—for the couple, the family. . . .
> I just am a firm believer that he's got to find some way to air what he feels or what his experience has been. We went to a caregiver support group, and he was very apprehensive. "Are there going to be a lot of people? Do I have to say something?" I almost had to grab him by the hand and drag him in there. I told him that I felt like it was very necessary for him.

This support group—the only one meeting in Missoula at the time —had no one in it even close to matching her husband's situation. Dan also described their one visit:

Dan:　　　　　You know, we went to a support group; it meets on Tuesdays, I think, and we went in there. I was the only guy. And there wasn't any men in there. I mentioned in there that my perspective is gonna be different from a woman's side. I felt very uncomfortable. Barbara was

with me. Good thing she went with me because I don't
think I could have sat there.

Researcher: So, would you like to be involved with a group of
people like yourself who are men, who are husbands of
patients who are terminal?

Dan: So, yeah, I would be interested in something like that!

Barbara agreed with Dan's description of their visit:

Well, we got there, and it was all women . . . two facilitators and six
older women who were taking care of elderly parents, or a spouse
that might have Alzheimer's or some other condition. So he felt
like he couldn't relate to all women, and none of them named
something that was familiar to him. They were very nice ladies, but
at the same time, Dan told them, "I just need to see more men that
might understand how I feel, or I won't come back."

Throughout the period when we visited Barbara, she continued to search for
social and emotional support for her husband and children as well as for herself, but she could never find the help she perceived they needed.

Dan and Barbara's emotional dependence on each other apparently was so
great that when they both needed help from others, it was difficult for others to
break into their relationship. This situation may not be uncommon in couples
facing physical illness and impending death. The cohesiveness that holds a
couple together can prevent them from being flexible enough to adapt to
changing circumstances—especially allowing others to help them both.

Employment/Financial Strains

In chapter 5 we described the financial picture of the study participants and discusses how their finances affected and were affected by terminal illness. We now
examine the financial picture from the perspective of caregivers, to make clearer
the interrelatedness of support, planning, and financial concerns or problems.

Three of the eight primary caregivers had little assistance with direct caregiving from other family members and were still actively employed when illness came. This lack of available family support, combined with the demands
of end-of-life care, had direct effects on the primary caregivers' employment
situations and financial resources. Again, the snapshots of two of these caregivers, in their own words, illustrate the systemic, interdependent factors that
affect end-of-life care.

"This is my job, because I don't have a job"

Barbara's husband Dan exemplified the extreme stress placed on a family when a wife and mother faces an untimely death and the family becomes more and more isolated during an illness that extends across years. Barbara's family was a younger, nuclear family with a husband and two children from a previous marriage still living in the home. Her illness and death interrupted the normal family life cycle, in which parents are able to raise and launch their children into adulthood, socially and financially, before dying.

Some patients and families begin their journey with many connections to community—school, work, clubs, churches—which can be sustaining even over a long period of illness. This family, however, had few connections in Missoula, outside of Barbara's work colleagues. Dan and Barbara had moved to Missoula in the early 1990s, shortly before she was diagnosed with cancer. Her six-year illness and her husband's decision to give up his job to provide care for her through several serious episodes further isolated them.

There is likely to be an impact for family finances when the terminally ill person is still needed to ensure the family's survival, either as breadwinner or as the family organizer and manager. So it was in Barbara's family. Barbara was accustomed to being the one in her family who was responsible for managing family finances, as well as working full-time to provide income. Her illness and incapacity to fill these essential roles created a void that no one else in the family could completely fill.

Barbara's family differed markedly from other families in the study with regard to the timing of death in the family life cycle and the family role played by the person who was dying. A young family's loss of a parent is likely to place greater stress on the family system because there will be no time to adjust to the changes.

Dan saw caregiving as his full-time "job," particularly because the demands of his wife's illness had caused him to give up full-time work:

> You know, I don't have a job. I'm just staying home and taking care of Barbara, when she is sick. And this is my job, because I don't have a job. This kind of keeps me busy.

> ≈ ≈ ≈

> I've been doing this already for six, seven years. You know, sometimes it's hard to get her to eat, a lot of time it is. With these treatments it's hard to find the right things that she is gonna eat, even after six years.

As Dan made caregiving into his work, he found that he resented the help offered by Barbara's teenage children—his stepchildren:

You know, they try to help, but that's not what I'm looking for. I don't want help that way. This is my job. Like yard work, I don't want him doing yard work. That's *my* job.

"I don't know what I'm gonna do"

A significant part of Karen's continuing stress comes from her worries about how to pay for her mother's care. Karen describes how her mother had limited finances—Social Security, Medicare, and a small Medigap—that no longer covered the costs of Sarah's care after she left Hospice House:

I'm getting a little panicky. I don't know what I'm gonna do. Her cancer benefits just ran out, and she isn't able to get any more till August [this in March]. We're paying for her medicines, plus the 200 she's short on the rent. We haven't told Mom. I'm just debating. Every day I sit and I keep trying to figure out what I'm gonna do. I'm about out of my money that I've been using.

Apparently, insurance benefits for medication might have been available once but no longer were, so the financial stresses were even greater as Karen struggled to pay for required medication plus the extra costs of the board and care home where her mother moved after she left Hospice House.

Those benefits have run out for the medicine and her insurance. That's a long story, but they messed her up on that, and she has no coverage on medicine.

Karen, in her early sixties and with a husband who had retired, found that the constant demands of caring for her mother prevented her from working. Of course, this situation only increased the financial stress on her.

I thought about going back to work, but with all the appointments nobody's gonna let you take off every day. It amazes me; I don't know how some of these people do it that are still working and running their folks. I'd think a lot of them would just have to quit their jobs.

Karen's situation probably is typical of many families. Where the nature of family relationships is such that one caregiver is chosen and others do not participate, the consequence can be that the primary caregiver eventually will sacrifice work opportunities and income to continue to provide care.

When There Is No Family: Orphans

"We knew we were Kitty's family"

Kitty represents terminally ill persons in Missoula who are effectively "orphans"—with no living family members to provide any care. Kitty had lived independently as a single professional in Missoula for almost fifty years. She had cared for her mother in her home and then lived in Missoula into her eightieth year with no husband or children, no nieces or nephews. Her church became her family, and members of the congregation tried to provide enough support that she could remain at home until she died, as she wished. Kitty's story is particularly instructive as an example of how difficult home care really is and how much primary nonfamily caregivers may have to do to make it work.

The experience of Kitty's church in trying to help her stay at home by providing daily visitations and other kinds of help is a paradox: The longer they were able to meet her wishes and help continue to live alone in her own home, the more conflict they felt about whether this approach was the right choice. One church member said:

> [One of Kitty's friends] saw us as neglecting her because Kitty had diarrhea, for years, and it was uncontrollable. She hid it very well, but her friend picked up on this, and told other people that Kitty wasn't being taken care of.

In fact, the people who were caring for Kitty weren't sure they were doing "the right thing" by helping her avoid the inevitable move to Hospice House for six months. Kitty's priest described how the church got involved in helping her stay at home:

> At that point [last spring], her doctor had talked her into going to Hospice. She was in the hospital, ready to go to Hospice. She was ready to go because I think she was afraid she couldn't take care of herself anymore. Then she got a burst of energy that morning and said, "I'm not going." And so her doctor and I got on the phone. "What should we do?"
>
> So we said to her, "Somebody's got to see you every day." And she agreed to let Home Health do that. And I thought for weeks that was happening. It wasn't. So then I called four parishioners— two of them nurses. And they would try to visit her each once a week. And then the assistant priest would call her five days out of the week to make sure. And we just started. As things turned up, we started plugging it in.

Kitty's priorities were to stay in her own home and to have her dog and two cats with her. Apparently she sometimes believed that she could take them to Hospice House, although at other times she appeared to understand that they could not go. Staying in her own home was of paramount importance not only for Kitty but for her pets' sake as well—which may have strengthened her resolve even more. So for six months, Kitty's church sent in visitors during the week, made daily phone calls, had lay ministers visit on Sunday with communion and flowers from the altar, and stayed in contact with Hospice staff and Kitty's doctor. When Kitty developed a serious foot infection in October—another sign that her body was failing—friends from church drove her each morning for two weeks to her physician's office for IV antibiotic treatment.

The commitment by Kitty's church family to honoring her preferences was impressive. But in our conversations with those involved, Kitty's caregivers warned against thinking of their effort as a "model" for other churches—or even for the many other elderly parishioners in their church. The priest spoke of the intensive effort he had to make to set up and monitor the system, which fell to him to do:

> How do we make this work? Well, that's a tough one. That's really the tough one—how much time do I have to put it together? We know this is our next need. We've got a body of people here who are about to hit that age. And we're gonna choke on them. I can't do it all. So we just don't do it. . . .
>
> If we had ten Kittys, we couldn't do it. We'd have to re-create a social work staff here. We simply can't. I think if you were to go around town you'd find that most every church, if they'll tell you honestly, feel understaffed. At least the clergy do. They don't have the folks to do that.

Unmet Caregiver Needs in the Subculture of Dying Persons

Among the group of caregivers we studied, several unmet needs were common, regardless of the amount of support. These unmet needs related to comfort and mobility: adequate respite care, better transportation assistance, and housekeeping assistance.

Respite from Twenty-four-Hour Care

Having someone who can be trusted to come in and take over caregiving for even a few hours is a rarity. The level of care required at the end of life means that only a trained volunteer or a family member who has been provided with some hands-on coaching can stay with the patient. Having respite care available is essential for lengthy terminal illnesses. Meeting this need is not always a straightforward matter, however, even setting aside considerations of cost. As Bernice and Mabel's situation illustrates, some patients will not accept hospice volunteers. Adult day care settings require the patient to leave home, which generally is not an option as life draws to an end. Some patients are reluctant to have other family members come in, even if they are available.

Transportation

Caregivers in this study needed help with transportation as patients—wheelchair bound and tethered to oxygen—became more difficult to get into and out of regular cars. Even a short ride to a family gathering or for a necessary doctor's appointment was difficult. None of these caregivers knew if any transportation assistance was available to them, other than ambulances for emergency transportation.

Housekeeping

One of the first difficulties with full-time, twenty-four-hour caregiving is that keeping a clean, orderly house becomes more essential—and much more difficult. Before the period of full-time caregiving, the person who is now ill or the primary caregiver would have handled these chores; now neither can do the housekeeping well.

When we asked Carrie what she most wanted, she answered:

> I'd like to have somebody who could come and go, with their own key, who could come at their own hours, to just know what needs to be done. I said the next one through that door is gonna have their work clothes on, and I'm going to put my feet up and say, "There's the kitchen."

Connie admitted that as caregiving demands grew, she finally decided to hire a housekeeper at her own expense:

> You know, I'm seventy. Another thing I've done for myself is I've arranged for somebody to come in and clean the house once a week.

Recently there has been a movement at some political levels to look toward churches to become the new social agents of care for welfare families, unwed mothers, and elderly persons. The one clergyperson we spoke with, who had helped orchestrate the system of care for Kitty, was emphatic in his refusal to regard the church as *the* answer to the unmet needs of dying persons and their caregivers, particularly given the numbers of elderly people in our society in the next few decades.

We end this chapter by reemphasizing that a complete, orchestrated system of caring is required to support family caregivers and preserve opportunities for them to experience this time as having meaning and value. A break in any link of this chain can ruin the chances for caregiving to be more than a burdensome, stressful obligation. Participants who subjectively and objectively succeeded at caregiving had the strongest, most complete chain of comfort and support available to them throughout the period of our study.

Chapter 9

Personal Growth, Meaning, and Spirituality

The idea that personal "growth" and meaning-making occurs at the end of life may be surprising. In fact, a person's spirit and mind can keep growing and making meaning despite—or sometimes because of—imminent bodily death. For some people, confronting their own dying helps bring about this kind of growth. People facing death may feel compelled to accomplish tasks in their work or worldly affairs or relationships. They may even find new meaning to their lives or to their illness. They also may choose to ignore their dying and find meaning by clinging firmly to their past life.

This chapter focuses on the different ways participants discussed and reported what was most meaningful to them, beyond their everyday care and experience. The participants in this study evidenced varying types and degrees of personal spiritual growth, including meaning-making during the periods that their bodies were deemed incurably ill and objectively failing. We reported some of these experiences in chapter 7, in terms of what participants found enjoyable in their daily life. This chapter draws in part on the same data, in a framework that stresses its significance and meaning.

Finding meaning, personal growth, and spirituality at life's end are among the most profound and powerful events in any culture. C. F. Seale, a British sociologist who studies cultural constructions and responses to death in modern life, reminds us that dying and death are constructs that have different meanings within different cultures. As we observed and explored the perspectives of the participants in this study, we were struck by the power of one common thread, despite their differences: the effort to look for and construe a connection or continuity with some aspect of existence beyond the death of the body. They and their families made this connection in a great variety of ways, but the common thread of continuity appeared again and again.

In addition to the unique ways that participants found to maintain their connection to others and to affirm the social bond in the face of its dissolution through death, the research study itself provided another avenue—the opportunity to engage in conversations that helped participants reconstruct their life at a symbolic level through telling their life stories and sharing their meaning with a new listener. For at least some of the participants and their families (Dennis, Barbara, Sharon, Ralph, Walt, Sarah), the research process itself created a "resurrective practice," in Seale's (1998) terminology, through which they could construe the continued existence of the things that mattered to them, beyond their own bodily death, and affirm the importance of their social bonds. When we realized the importance to the participants—including the families—of the conversations we were having, we created a special "legacy book" that recorded the words of the dying person as a gift to them and their families.

In exploring these different approaches to death, another of Seale's concepts is of value. Seale (1998) points out that all cultures provide some kind of cultural narrative or "script" for understanding and making sense of one's life in dying and knowing what one should do. Traditional scripts have been provided by various religious traditions, and they remain powerful. But for many people, including some of these participants, those religious traditions no longer provided a meaningful path. One new type of script is biomedical, offering membership in an imagined human community of other persons with the same illness. Cancer patients and AIDS patients have found such scripts appealing, allowing them to become members of an vast army, bravely fighting the same disease and going toward brave and honorable deaths. A second kind of cultural script now circulating is what Seale calls a "psychological" script, which depicts the dying person as being on an inner adventure of personal growth.

Neither the biomedical script, which focuses on a particular illness and its trajectory, nor the script that emphasizes psychological-personal growth may be satisfactory, however—especially for elderly patients with chronic illnesses. Emphysema and congestive heart failure, in particular, do not provide the dramatic trajectory and "last battle" allure of cancer. Byock (1996) has expanded the concept of an "inner journey" to suggest that the last stage of life can involve new opportunities to complete important life development tasks and to make meaning out of one's worldly, bodily existence and history; he also suggests that completion of these tasks provides a sense of meaning for individuals facing death. Byock's conceptual framework describes the developmental tasks or challenges that are particularly characteristic of the process of dying. In the last section of this chapter, we summarize how the participants' experiences in this study contribute to validating this developmental framework.

These different scripts or constructs—religious/spiritual, biomedical, and life task completion—were potentially available to these participants. The accounts of what they found meaningful illustrate how they chose to make use of one or more of them.

The question of spiritual experience at the end of life comes up again and again in discussions of death and dying, outside of any particular religious belief system. There may be a primary human instinct to believe that some connection continues to life, despite the apparent finality of death. But this experience is the most difficult to define or talk about.

Modern psychology increasingly regards spiritual and religious practices as reflecting an inherently meaningful human motivation toward connection with others—a motivation that is more primal and broader than any specific religious belief or system. This concept encompasses necessarily subjective experiences of "communion with a larger whole"—a primal sense of participating in something that is larger than the self, beyond one's current physical existence (McAdams 1993).

We have broadly defined the concept of "spiritual growth" at the end of life as the process of making meaning of one's life through relationships to oneself, to others, to nature, or to a transcendent realm. Thus, we include as evidence of spirituality and meaning-making whatever beliefs, orientation, or experiences we observed or the participants described that brought them comfort through a sense of connection or meaning. This generous perspective is grounded in what religious traditions provide: a belief in the connection of the individual person to a larger-than-self Reality—one's family, a Supreme Being, the spirit of oneness in a fellowship or community of faith, or rejoining the oneness of creation and nature in some nonspecified way.

The diversity in these participants' understanding of and stance toward spiritual questions and meaning is impressive. They found their own individual paths to meaning and, in most cases, to the kind of spiritual connection that met their needs. These diverse paths of developing spirituality and meaning included organized religious faiths, traditional Native American beliefs, family, nature and animals, and alternative modern spiritual paths such as Alcoholics Anonymous and Unity. Each of these approaches provided one or more of our participants with a framework or "script" for understanding and expressing the meaning of their life and/or death.

Meaning and Connection through Religious Faith

Ralph developed a spirituality during the last year or two of his life. He had not been a very religious person during his life, by his own admission:

> To tell it with honesty, there's a number of years that I seemed to kind of let stuff slide as far as this religion went, you know. It was more fun to go fishing and hunting than it was to take and go to church. You know, you could think of a reason to go out fishing, but it wasn't so easy to think of a reason to go to church.

But with the onset of his terminal illness, Ralph began to turn toward the religion of his childhood:

So I mean that came back, when you get to the shape I was in. I've been this way seven years, so you think and you look the situation over. When you read the Bible and when you hurt as bad as I have, if you see a chance to better the situation that you're in, I believe you're going to take it. It's a little easier to think of it the other way now.

Ralph's mate and caregiver, Sandy, read the Bible to him regularly, and Ralph took comfort from occasional visits from the new pastor of the same church he had skipped so often in his youth. Ralph also enjoyed a Sunday morning church broadcast on television. Ralph's faith was not well conceptualized, nor could he develop a sense of certainty about his covenant with God. He once expressed great anxiety over a brief slippage into profanity and told Sandy that he might be in "deep trouble" with God over what he had said.

Ralph's view of life after this life was concrete and specific: He could get back to doing some useful work, as Sandy recalled:

Ralph said, "It isn't the pain. I can bear the pain. It isn't the discomfort. It isn't the choking or that. It's this uselessness, this not being able to do anything." He can't hardly wait to die and go to heaven so he can go to work. That's all he talks about: "Oh, I hope they got somethin' for me to do when I get there."

Dennis, who was dying of cancer at thirty-nine, also talked about his spiritual development as a consequence of his incurable illness. His growth had little or nothing to do with organized religion, to which he remained somewhat indifferent. He received visits from "a pastor who likes to drop in." He noted that even though this pastor "stayed too long," he did manage to offer some comfort:

We've had quite lengthy discussions on dying, etc. He's one of the ones that told me that this is just completing the cycle. You have to understand that everybody will face it at one time or another, and you're just kind of ahead of the game right now.

Despite his discomfort with the organized church, Dennis gave evidence of developing a strong faith in God through his participation in Alcoholics Anonymous.

For Sarah, making meaning at this time in her life did not seem to be very important. From all we could observe, her meaning had been clearly made, and it did not seem to need revisions just because she was terminally ill.

Sarah reported that her church had always played an important role in her life. She looked forward to her pastor's visits to Hospice House and made excuses for him when he was too busy to visit her. She was proud of the fact that the church brought communion (and sometimes flowers) to her. When we asked if she believed in life after death, her response was, "Sure"—but with no elaboration.

Sarah did not initiate topics about religion or faith issues. When we brought them up, her responses were characteristically brief. Faith seemed to be a given in her life, not a topic to be expanded, developed, or elaborated. When we asked if communion was spiritually uplifting, she replied, "I don't think of it as every time. It is and it isn't." When we asked if her church and God provided her with spiritual strength, her response focused on the fact that visitors from the church brought her flowers from the altar.

Because Sarah simply accepted the religious aspects of her life, at this stage in her life she also simply accepted life's meaning. She had spent her life helping people—particularly children. To her, this behavior was not unusual or outstanding. It was not something that she sat down and planned to do with her life. It was simply what one did.

Sarah was still alive at the end of our study period; her illness had not progressed to the stage that characterized other participants—a stage that may well call forth clearer statements of spiritual well-being. She did not speak of fearing death but neither did she dwell on it. Like Saint Paul, she seems to "have learned in whatever state I am therefore to be content" (Philippians 4:11).

Of all the study participants, Kitty had been the most deeply involved in a church community throughout her life. Her spirituality at the end of life was focused on the tangible care her community gave her, not on theological beliefs. Her mental abilities also were more and more diminished by her illness, and she had lost the ability to discuss abstract topics. Kitty's friends told stories about her lifelong quest to understand theological mysteries, but at the end of her life she was content simply to allow her church community to nurture and care for her, and she did not spend time raising such questions. She had cared for elderly parishioners over the years; now that it was their turn, she knew her church would care for her. One friend at her memorial service remembered her this way:

For years after I moved from Missoula, Kitty saw to my grandmother's every need: doctors' appointments, grocery shopping, financial paperwork. Above all, the church manifested through fellowship was *her* church. Her beloved local community of folks from the parish was the fulcrum of her life, and it gave her life.

Kitty focused not on belief statements or life-after-death concerns but on the tangible experience of being part of a faith community that had always surrounded her with love—and was doing so at the end of her life.

It's just a—not a *belief* in God, but a reliance on a God, just knowledge that I can't put into words. I think because of that, I'm not afraid of dying, you know. I'm just not ready yet! [Laugh]

Although Kitty said she wasn't afraid, she spoke of dying in very realistic and stark terms. When we mentioned that we wanted to understand what was most helpful to her during this time, she replied:

What's most helpful? Just personalized interest. You know, to care about how the person is doing and just a sort of interest that somebody cares, and you aren't left alone, hanging. Because, after all, dying is a personal and lonely thing. You have to do it by yourself. But it'd be kind of nice to have somebody around watching you go.

At the end, when Kitty had to leave her home and her animals to go to Hospice House, she was never alone. Somebody always *was* around to care and, at the end, to watch her go. Kitty's parish priest described her last days:

She had to give the care of her last days over to complete strangers. And what a blessing it was. Kitty kept having pain, and the nurse came in and took her face in both of her hands, and she held it close, and she whispered in her ear. "Sweetheart, I won't let the pain get the best of you." And she stroked her forehead and gave her a kiss and got a syringe and gave her an injection. And I thought, "That is the definition of mercy."

Much like Kitty, Roberta was too affected by her illness at eighty-seven to talk with us about her own spiritual understanding or concerns, past or present. Roberta's family helped us understand her past experience better, however, and gave us their perception of how she came to terms with the end of life.

She was a Presbyterian as a young girl growing up. In fact, she was one of the congregation of Reverend McLean, [author] Norman McLean's dad. And she used to fall asleep at his sermons because that brogue was so heavy. Anyhow, she had her great faith in God as far as she herself went. She prayed, and she believed in God. She did question things, though.

Two months before Roberta's death, her daughter indicated that she was aware of Roberta's lifelong anxiety about dying and her aversion to the topic:

She never really had any kind of faith in her life. What we're seeing with her right now is a lot of fear. We're seeing fear of passing on.

A month before Roberta died, however, her daughter perceived her as moving beyond her customary anxiousness.

We were kind of concerned about her spiritual health and how she was feeling about things. She was very frightened. She'd go to bed at night and would be frightened, just scared to lay down. I realized then that she had a great fear of dying. Then the last part of October, I saw a change in her clarity, and she seemed more cognizant of things that were going on. . . .

She told our minister that she did question some of the things. And for the first time she was able to think about things and maybe assimilate some of the things that he was saying. It surprised me. It surprised [our minister] too. She used to be standoffish if she didn't want to talk about something. But now she wanted to talk about it. And she listened to him and shared with him, which surprised me. . . .

I felt that she knew that this was the time. Actually, when she hurt her hip that night, I could see a change in her then. She wasn't frightened. She was calm, and she was describing her pain very clinically—something she would never have done in the past. And she held my hand, and waiting for the ambulance she was very calm. She was not frightened.

Roberta's daughter was not hoping that her mother would have a deathbed conversion or awakening but simply that she would not be afraid. Although the foregoing observations are not objective proof that Roberta experienced a sense of peace and connection at the end of her life, they demonstrate that her daughter's concerns were satisfied.

Spiritual Connection with Nature and Animals

Ralph's lifetime personal spirituality was not based directly on organized religion. His communion with God's creation of mountains, rivers, creeks, animals, and fish was the major focus of his life, and it provided him with a sense of value, integrity, and, at this last stage of life, redemption. His more religious, church-oriented spirituality—which developed during his illness— complemented his spiritual communion with nature but never transcended it. He came to the experience of illness with a strong sense of meaning about his relationship to Creation, symbolized concretely in his Swan Valley home, and this connection grew even stronger in the last months of his life.

Like Ralph, Dennis found spirituality through the beauty of and connection with nature. Ralph was a woodsman; Dennis was an athlete. Both wanted nothing more than to spend their remaining days in familiar, outdoor settings. Ralph found the many trips to Missoula too burdensome and reluctantly moved away from his natural paradise for the last year of his life. Dennis would not make this sacrifice. He insisted on staying in his own home, with his view of the mountains, no matter how difficult it became for him and for his family at the end:

> I don't find my Lord in the church. I find Him out in the beauty of nature. . . . And fishing—I love to fly fish. I love the different smells and sights and sounds. I do take evening strolls if I can, because I just love this area, the mountains; nor would I want to die in a more beautiful place than this.

Barbara's highest priority during her last summer was a trip to the Oregon coast. Despite the difficulty of traveling and her fear of getting sick in a strange place, she persisted; she wanted to see the ocean again, perhaps for the last time. Kitty also dreamed of another trip to Oregon in the spring with a friend and her dog. Talking about this trip, even though her increasing debility made it unlikely, seemed to be an effective way of remembering the first trip she had taken, the previous spring.

Our conversations with some of the other participants, who expressed no interest in being out-of-doors in nature, also revealed a strong connection at the end to the natural world through animals. In particular, Kitty's pets were a strong symbol of her own life and values. They had all been rescued from certain death at the Humane Society, but her dog seemed to be the closest to her heart:

> I've never been without a dog, and I can't imagine living without one. The cats are just angelic, but it's not the same.

Kitty's friends said at her memorial service that "her animals were her life," and her connection to her dog Beau seemed to sustain her and give life meaning. Shortly after our first visit, Beau began to lose weight, and Kitty worried about him intensely. A home visit from a veterinarian led to a different diet, and for a while Kitty reported that he was "better, just fine." But Beau continued to lose weight, and Kitty finally had to admit that he wasn't just fine. In fact, he had cancer, and she finally agreed to have him put to sleep in late October. Not only was Kitty's tie to Beau her strongest connection to another sentient being; her acceptance of his dying in some way seemed to have presaged her own.

Beau may have been the last cord keeping Kitty in her home because she knew he could not go with her to Hospice House.

Roberta, who was eighty-six, had never liked dogs or cats, but her two important daily experiences in her last months were her bird, Waldo, who sang for her daily, and looking out the window at Mount Sentinel. Mabel, who was living in reduced circumstances in a small apartment, had few meaningful experiences she could articulate. She took special delight, however, in the wild animals that came up onto the lawn outside her patio window to look for food. Watching them transformed her lined, anxious face into an expression of joy.

Meaning and Connection through Family

In Walt's last days, his family provided him with the meaning and comfort to help him accept his death and endure the physical difficulties that come in dying. Walt's family found deep meaning in caring for their father, and he experienced a year of being loved unconditionally in very concrete ways by his wife and children. For example, when he grew too ill to get out of bed, one son often stopped by to take a short nap with him, without a lot of talk.

There was no evidence of a concern with or consciousness of religious or spiritual affairs on Walt's part. In an after-death visit with one of his daughters, however, she explained her discovery of Walt's early religious experience and her acceptance of his way:

> Dad wouldn't even talk about religion or anything like that. But I had his old Bible at home. And I drug it out and I took it to the house here maybe two weeks before he died, asking who the people were that had given him this book. And he got all excited that I even had his Bible. And he admitted he'd been baptized and that this aunt had taken him to church when he was in high school and all this stuff. I had no idea. I was struggling with "Is he saved or is he not saved?" And it was something that I didn't know how to approach him to talk about. But I had a clear conscience about it all after lots of my own prayer on it. And I think he was. He didn't want to admit that he wasn't manly or cool or something like that.

In our after-death interview with Walt's wife, Dorothy, she explained a bit more how she and her husband had viewed death and the comforts of religion:

> We had always said, "If you're religious, you should have a religious funeral." But why have a religious service if he never went to church? And so we both decided, why have a minister that didn't know you? Because his spirit goes on.

Walt and Dorothy were both brought up on religious principles and values, but neither seemed to have a church connection in their married life. If their daughter's explanation is accurate, for Walt religion "wasn't manly or cool." Dorothy, by her own admission, apparently learned to live the spiritual life without ongoing involvement with an organized church or faith community. Yet this family clearly had deep and strong spiritual values. Describing Walt's death, Dorothy said:

> The spirit and the soul tell you when you're going to go. You have to be able to be released, I guess. And I think that's part of what your spirit does. It releases you. I've had friends from all types of religion and gone to all types of churches. And we all actually have the same belief. We just believe it in different ways.

The advantage of Walt's and his family's religious background was that it may have taught them consideration for each other, hospitality for others, the ability to willingly share, and a sense of peace. Perhaps these qualities at least in part were the product of Walt's and Dorothy's early religious training. Interestingly enough, these family characteristics also were what made meaning in their lives.

Alternative Spiritual Paths: Alcoholics Anonymous and New Age Spirituality

Dennis, like Ralph, moved from a "God in nature" spirituality toward a more religiously oriented spiritual experience during his last days. Dennis found his sense of meaning through Alcoholics Anonymous:

> I think it's a personal relationship with a Higher Power in my life. There's so much spirituality in AA and in fellow recovering alcoholics. . . . I don't have to attend church. Church has become people to me rather than the ritual or the laws. We get settled on our "don'ts" and forget that there's some "do's" out there.

Dennis had joined AA about fifteen months before his death. Although he never directly mentioned a connection between dying and this decision, at another time he said that he was glad to have the time at the end of his life to complete some important life tasks, or loose ends:

> I'd rather it be this way. Because it gives you a chance to tie up any loose ends that you may have. And believe me, we all have them.

There's a lot that has to be done. There's a lot that has to be thought of.

The spiritual path offered by AA provided Dennis with a meaningful framework for meeting the challenges of dying, as he explained in terms of his new sobriety:

The tragedy in death is the suddenness and the unknown. The car accidents, accidents that happen. When you're given a time element to think about it, it's a lot different. You have the chance to rectify anything that's in your power to do so. You know, I have to think that Serenity Prayer a lot. You know, because I want to change the world. I want to be so right and so complete. Well, I'm never gonna be that way. But as long as the important things are taken care of, how wonderful. And sober. And I'm gonna be sober hopefully that day, or that night, or whatever. And I remember reading in the Bible where it said, "Don't be drunk." I just remember reading that passage. "Be sober when that time comes." I think it's a personal relationship with a Higher Power in my life, you know.

Other evidence of Dennis's deepened interest and sense of spiritual understanding can be found in his retelling of a conversation he had with his nine-year-old daughter:

My daughter is having more of a tough time. She wears her emotions on her sleeve. One question she had for me that was really interesting was, "Why is God so mean to you?" And I said, "Oh, He's not mean to me. He's giving me strength to put up with this disease. And that's what God does. He's there for you when you need help." And I hope that set her straight. I've thought, you know, how can this be allowed? I haven't done anything, you know. It goes back to the thing that, well, if there was something very wrong with my life, I suppose I do deserve this.

Sharon had grown up in a fundamentalist Protestant church whose strict rules of behavior lead her to rebel as a teenager by smoking and going to movies. Part of her development in later life involved seeking out new spiritual directions, including the writings of Edgar Cayce and Unity teachings. Her move to Missoula, when she was fifty-nine, was partly for her own spiritual growth because it enabled her to learn more:

When I lived in _____, I met with a group that started there to study Edgar Cayce. I've always been interested in church, and the impact of religion, and I thought I'd do some writing in that regard. I knew nothing about Unity Church, except it was a New Age church.

After Sharon moved to Missoula, she was able to pursue her interest in spirituality through Unity and other spiritual groups meeting in Missoula. Sharon's beliefs were not centered on a church or faith community, however:

That isn't an ending place, to my way of thinking. Usually people's religion hasn't really much to do with churchgoing.

Reflecting her exploration of Unity and Cayce, Sharon seemed to have a belief that her spirit would endure—and perhaps even come back for another life. She seemed unwilling to discuss her own beliefs directly with any outsider, but comments such as this provide some indication of her thinking:

I missed [learning] the computer. I'm sorry about that. I'm gonna have to come back and do that again. And I'm gonna come back and get an earlier start on it. Maybe I will get into some of that one of these days.

Sharon's trust in the existence of a spiritual life beyond this life was deep and secure, and it helped her meet death with equanimity. Two months before she died, even though she was having more difficulty expressing conceptual thoughts, she tried to explain her understanding of life and spiritual life:

I just kind of take fears and pass them on to heaven.

∽ ∽ ∽

I think there's got to be more than just this actual life experience, or there wouldn't be so much interest in life after death. I feel that all these things that you never finish, they go on. How they do it I don't know. I don't know how much you carry of your identity from one phase to the next. I just figure whoever's running it has been doing a pretty good job.

∽ ∽ ∽

I think all you have to do is ask the Universe. And the Universe answers. It does, if you pay attention and make notes, do whatever you need to capture it. Because a lot of times we pray for things or wish for things, and then when they happen we just go on without marking it or paying any attention.

Very close to her life's end, when thoughts were difficult to express, Sharon still found words to describe her own change in thinking—particularly learning to accept total dependency, brought about through her experience with progressive illness and dying.

> [Long ago] I decided that being hit by a truck was what I wanted. Not to be dependent on anybody. That's one thing I always wanted, not to be depending on anybody for anything, and here I am almost totally dependent. And I guess it's a good thing because you'd be kind of supercilious about it. And when the time comes that somebody else needs help, well, you need to be able to remember the time that you needed it.

Sharon talked as if these life lessons she was learning would be important for her next stage of existence. She conveyed a clear sense that some part of her would continue to exist, and she seemed confident that what she was learning would be useful to her in new state—without needing to know what that state would be like.

Native American Spiritual Traditions

Although two of this study's participants had some Native American heritage, only Barbara had been raised within a Native American culture and traditions. At the end of her life, Barbara found the practices of her Native American heritage and her lifelong Christianity equally meaningful, and she brought them together to help her understand her illness and how she should respond. In particular, the Native American tradition offered her a script for a heroic quest that would benefit her people. During one visit, she explained how she had come to honor and practice both traditions:

> Indian people historically had what was a pure belief style. If you want to connect to spirituality, symbolically the sun represented a greater power. That's why we say the sun dance, praying to the sun and all of this; it's just symbolic of the Creator. With Christianization and education, Indian people were forced to almost become culturally schizophrenic, spiritually schizophrenic. One day they're this way; the next day, they're this way. [Our] particular cultural beliefs were outlawed at one time. People were being hung, put in jail for practicing sacred ceremony. . . .

So therefore they started saying, "Okay. We'll dress like you, we'll act like you, we'll pray like you, whenever we see you. But when we're alone, and we have that opportunity, we're going to slide back into the way that we were, the way that we've been taught." So now, what you have is this generational habit of being baptized in whatever faith it might be, but at the same time, something inside telling me there's more to me than church on Sunday, confession. I shouldn't have to wait once a week to say, "God, I'm pitiful. I made a mistake today. Forgive me." You know, save it all up for the priests and wait for absolution. . . .

And I think that the [Native American] spirituality and the value system are going to revive. The two are not divided. They're not separated. It's one and the same. I don't mean to sound disrespectful, but I think Indian people in particular have just decided, "I'll do both." I feel comfortable with both. They give me a vehicle for expression. And that's where I'm at.

Barbara's years of illness had been marked by spiritual development and support from spiritual powers in both faith traditions. Native American remedies given to her by her family provided tangible, physical communion with her traditional culture:

From the very beginning I know that I was taken care of spiritually and emotionally. When I left for Seattle for surgery, that very first weekend they held a sweat for me, and they prayed for me, and the spirits told them to bring me raspberries. If you look at herbal medicine, they prescribe red-raspberry leaf tea for women's afflictions for labor or for uterine [problems], and here I was being given a jar of raspberries to eat on the plane on my way to Seattle. So from the very beginning it has been part of me, and I have not separated myself from it.

In a similar way, Barbara's personal faith in a Christian God provided a sense of hope and healing:

But I know that with me in particular, the ability to know that God exists and that Jesus is alive and well and is an intervenor is amazing. Because I was really on a skyrocket with my blood tests since April. The CA jumped up to 375, and then they started the medicine when I landed in the hospital, and it came down 12 percent. And then I just finished my second treatment. They did another blood test, and it showed over 50 percent drop. Really amazing.

As Barbara grew more ill, the traditional ceremonies of her own people provided her with meaning and, at the end, helped her pass over to the other side. She described her reluctance at one point during the previous year to make the long trip home—because of pressures of work, having just gotten out of the hospital, and so forth:

> And we got there and then made the decision to go over for a ceremony. And so we did, and it was very good, and so I was glad that I did that. It gave me a lot of energy. It's a sacred ceremony called the Medicine Pipe opening. I was included in the prayers. I got painted. [Shows her hand and wrist] That's what this is— markings they paint on your wrists and face. And I just leave it on there until it wears off. But all that connection for me is really critical. And I need it. . . .
>
> We believe in long-distance healing. You don't have to be present. Because there are numerous, uncountable people that you don't even know that know a relative of yours and who have heard about you, and they honor you and they offer prayers or something for you. All the way out in Maine, or over in Australia, or up in Canada. They go to a ceremony, and they mention you. One of the ways of healing through ceremony is that I have contact with several people that [are going] to a ceremony, and I can give them tobacco to take. The question becomes, what is your belief in God all about? If He is the Be-all, then why is the church, the building, the only place where God lives?

Barbara described a mystical encounter at a Native American sacred ceremony early in her illness. This event helped frame her growing understanding of the essential oneness of her Catholic faith, with its emphasis on sacrifice and atonement, and the Native American Sun Dance, which has at its heart suffering and sacrifice for others. At the end of her life, she looked back on this experience as central to her understanding of the spiritual as well as physical battle she was engaged in. This experience provided her, early in her illness, with a relevant "script" for her dying, grounded in her own cultural tradition. Here is the story as she told it:

> In 1991, I was doing some work at the Pine Ridge Reservation and the Rosebud Reservation. Pine Ridge seemed very lonely, but at the same time it struck a curiosity in me. As if I had known it or was

very familiar with it. So I found myself getting in the car and driving out for miles by myself and looking around and feeling like, you know, where am I? What is this land? This isn't mine. . . . I'm not Lakota Sioux. But here I am. . . .

Then when I was on my way to Rosebud, I saw two poles—white poles, long and tall tipi poles—and they had various colored cloth on them. And right away, the message to me was, "There is something holy going on here." And I immediately pulled in here, and two men were standing at the gate, and they asked what I was doing, and I asked them, "Well, what is going on?" And they said, "Elmer Running Sun Dance is just starting. We'll mark your car." And they tied some cloth on my aerial so that I could come and go and they'd know that I wanted to be there. So I drove over there and got out of the car. The dancers were being instructed by the medicine people, and they were going to get up early the next morning to put the center pole up to begin the dancing. And I told myself, "I want to be there."

So I made a note to myself to get up very early, before sunup, and drive up there. I was there, and I watched them and watched the sun come up. And then I had to go to work at nine. When I got back up to the sun dance, about three in the afternoon, they were in full dance. It was an amazing visual, sensual sight, to see over 200 men and women dancing around that pole, sun dancing, praying for people. . . .

And then I noticed that several of them had pierced, like they did in the old days. And there was a man at the east end of the arbor that was piercing. He was dancing back and forth, and his skin would stretch out, and I was standing there watching him, watching him suffer, for relatives. And when he broke loose, there was such a shock of energy that went around that arbor that it came around and it struck me right in the heart center. And I immediately burst out crying. I was so overwhelmed. I stayed as long as I could.

Throughout her conversations with us, Barbara found meaning in the imagery of herself as a warrior, fighting fiercely against her illness; she finally envisioned her own suffering as redemptive for others. This encounter with the Sun Dance was, for her, a calling into battle:

I know now I was called there in preparation for something greater to come—which means the battle with cancer. That is my cultural belief, that we *are* given opportunities to prepare us.

Alternating with this language of a warrior and the imagery of a battle, in the same conversation Barbara spoke of learning to let go. These alternating visions characterized her mood through the summer months:

I was telling a couple of students the other day that I'd truly reached a point where I was not in control. It was out of my hands. Whatever was going to go on, it was no longer up to me. It just basically was whether the body was gonna hang in there, whether it was my time or not.

Finding a Connection to Something Larger than Oneself

The common thread among the participants who were dying, independent of their expressed spiritual or religious orientation, was the search for some tangible evidence of continuity with ongoing life after their own death. The implied question—"Will something that I valued and cared about most in this world continue to exist and to be valued, after I'm gone?"—often formed the subtext of their conversations with us, when we asked what was meaningful to them at this time. Participants in their dying months actively sought to affirm a personal continuity that in some way would transcend their physical death.

Finding this connection was important, regardless of whether the person had a religious faith in a spiritual life after death. A tangible connection was assurance that what they valued most in life, something of their essence, would not end but be continued or remembered by others. At its most basic, this need for continuity can lead to providing a tangible legacy on earth. For our participants, these tangible connections were the most meaningful and satisfying: passing on one's tools, being assured that animals rescued from the shelter would be cared for, having a sister complete one's writing, seeing and affirming the connection to grandchildren and great-grandchildren, preserving the land. At the higher or transcendental end, this search for continuity is part of the human need for communion or connection to a greater whole.

In discussing the developmental challenges, Byock (1996) includes developing this sense of connection to something enduring as part of the task of accepting the finality of one's existence, of one's death. And so it seemed to be. Finding some kind of connection beyond their own physical existence appeared to help participants in their effort to achieve a sense of meaning and of completion or closure in dying. Thus, it helped them "let go" of life with peace. Some developed it more easily; others struggled, holding on to life itself as they sought ways to continue their connection with life beyond their own death. For some, their lack of any connection to a tangible legacy seemed to make the acceptance of their dying more difficult.

D. P. McAdams—a psychologist who studies life stories—theorizes that each person's life (at least in Western culture) is built around the twin motivating drives of gaining independence or mastery and developing and keeping connection with the human community. He labels these opposing motives or tendencies "agency" and "communion," respectively (McAdams 1993). Using McAdams's framework, this section examines the importance to participants of gaining a sense of meaningful connection. Finding some connection was a crucial step in helping them make the transition from independence to acceptance of the finality of their existence, as well as the total dependence on other people that characterizes end-of-life care.

Aiding the Transition from Independence to Dependence and Letting Go

Because achieving this sense of continuity is important to persons who are dying, we examine some of the ways that participants found or were aided to find a connection that would be meaningful to them. In Sharon's case, for example, we can see how her story changed during the three months we visited her—from a focus on losing her valued independence to a realistic acceptance of her final days as totally dependent and helpless and a willingness to "let go." On our first visits, Sharon spoke of her fears of being helpless:

> I sure don't want to be laying around absolutely helpless, being taken care of totally.

In telling her life story, the major theme was gaining independence from her family, the Pentecostal faith, and her home town—through smoking, going to movies, and an early marriage. Sharon also spoke repeatedly of her regret that she hadn't pursued her interest in writing. At times she seemed very depressed by these thoughts:

> I've spent my whole life saving things to write about when I got old. I never did do it. And now I've stopped saying it. I guess if I really had a whole lot to write about, I would have done it.

By the time of our last visit, three months later, Sharon gave every evidence of having accepted her total dependence on the care of others—her sister, her children, caregivers from Hospice. What stands out as helpful to Sharon in making this transition was her sister's promise of continuing her writing and ideas. On her last visit home, her younger sister promised to take Sharon's writings back to California to finish them and possibly use them in the family history book she was doing:

Researcher:	I was impressed when Connie showed me the big book of all your family newsletters. I didn't know you were such a writer.
Sharon:	I never published anything, but I did a lot of writing.
Researcher:	Well, I think you're great—the family historian.
Sharon:	Well, not really, because I didn't start soon enough, and I quit too soon. My family's all interested in it, and I think my younger sister, the one that's been here, will probably get into it. She wants to.

Sometime later, Sharon explained that her family newsletters contained family history and news, as well as some of her own stories and essays. Apparently, these family newsletters gave her the outlet to develop and share her views and her life philosophy. These stories and "stuff" were the pieces she regretted not having published. But her sister's commitment to continue working on Sharon's writing brought Sharon visible relief that her ideas would continue beyond her own death:

I'm sorry I didn't have more years of it. It was good while I was doing it, and I brought in extra things as I could. It did really hold the family all together real well for a while when it was needed. I wish I'd started sooner and continued longer. But it's better than nothing. I think my sister in California will probably pick up a lot of that because she's very interested in it. . . .

I was always going to write. I didn't ever get very far. We've been going through a lot of the old papers, and I've been surprised: I did leave a lot of scraps and notes that my sister was interested in. I gave her those. She'll copy them and send them back. But she'll do something with it. I've got a lot of stuff—got a lot of short stories and stuff that I've done through the years. We did enough talking now so that I think she can pick up on the things she was interested in.

By giving some continuity to Sharon's unfinished lifework of writing, her sister enabled Sharon to let go of any further needs for achievement or mastery and to accept her helplessness and dependence with more peace and equanimity. Six weeks before her death, Sharon spoke in a way that indicated a sense of peace and completion and a focus on each day: a cup of coffee, a cigarette, her seventy-fourth birthday party. She no longer expressed any worries about being dependent on Connie, and she no longer mentioned any regrets that she hadn't done more with her life or her writing. With her sister's help, Sharon had found a way to accept the finality of her life and her total dependency on others. Byock's framework points out that finding ways to transmit one's knowledge and wisdom to others at the end of life is a key developmental task, and doing so alleviates one kind of suffering.

Ralph came to the end of his life with a religious faith, but his religious belief in an eternal life for his spirit wasn't necessarily sufficient to help him accept his dependence in this life. He also struggled with losing his independence and sense of agency, or mastery. He focused on his success in protecting his land through the Land Reliance after his death. This focus appeared to help him as he faced total dependency and dying:

> There's people that's just wanting to subdivide and all that stuff. Because that's where the big bucks are; but like with me, the big bucks don't interest me. I can't take it with me. I've got this Reliance. It's an organization and it's got people that belong to it and they put their land into this. The Reliance makes the rules, what they want done. We got everybody up there, [who] hadn't gotten really into subdividing and selling in the last four or five years.

For Ralph, ensuring the continuity of his land was the visible symbol of his connection to a larger whole—to his neighbors in the Reliance and to the land itself, which after his death would be preserved as he had known it.

Unlike Sharon and Ralph, Walt was too ill by the time we met him to talk in such terms, but his family was sensitive to his need for continuity in what had mattered to him most: his family and his work. Walt's wife Dorothy told us how the family helped him let go of life at the end:

> The children talked about his wishes after he was gone. The boys told him how they would divide up his tools. The girls told him which one would get his books.

Passing on a set of tools may seem more mundane than placing property development rights in a land trust, but the meaning of the act is the same. All three of Walt's sons had become skilled workers in various construction trades, like their father. Passing on his tools was a symbol of the work Walt had loved doing, which he lived to see his sons honor as well.

> I came to Missoula through a friend who sent me out to help a plumber. And I was getting pretty discouraged. Then a few days later they sent me out to work with a swell guy, a swell fellow. And

he says to me, "My gosh, we got to hurry if we're going to get up to Eureka." We had two truckloads of stuff, you know. It was a refrigeration job. . . . I was only supposed to take the load up there and then come back. I was just a helper. Well, it turns out that he hands me a torch and told me to go soldering. "By gosh," he says, "I didn't know you could solder." I said, "I can't. I'm just learning." When I got back, I determined that I was going to be in refrigeration instead of plumbing. And those old fellows, they took care of me. Oh, lots of fun. Lots of fun.

Thus, something of what mattered most to Walt would live on with his children, and he was assured that they would care for and treasure these gifts. His son remembered it this way:

Dad wanted to make sure that I got his oxi-acetylene tanks. So I did. . . . His stuff really wasn't that valuable. Mainly the thing both of us wanted was a piece of him. . . . One thing Dad wanted me to have was a dust pan that I made in seventh-grade metal shop. He kept that dust pan over the years and wanted me to have it back.

In contrast to Ralph, Sharon, and Walt, Kitty seemed to have had much more difficulty in her last year withdrawing from her past life and developing a connection to something beyond her life. Mabel also appeared to have no framework, or any assistance from her closest family, in finding meaning in her past life in a way that would help her accept her own dying. "Letting go" of life appears to be more difficult when there is no ritual or symbolic way to experience one's connection. (The "Implications" section at the end of this chapter pursues in more detail the opportunities families and friends have to help those who are dying find these connections.)

Validation of End-of-Life Tasks or Challenges

A conceptual framework elaborated by Byock (1996) suggests that dying can be considered a stage of life and that human development is a lifelong process. Byock examines dying as the last of a continuum of developmental stages—such as infancy, childhood, adolescence, adulthood, and advanced age. Like the other stages of life, dying has "characteristic challenges, or developmental landmarks" that "may develop a sense of completion, satisfaction, and even a sense of mastery within areas of life that are of subjective importance" (Byock 1996, 247). Byock's framework offers a way to recognize opportunities that may otherwise be obscured by the person's distress. Providing assistance to individuals to confront any uncompleted tasks can be part of the assistance dying persons welcome, and doing so, in Byock's view, helps alleviate the emotional and psychological suffering of those dying.

These landmarks can be summarized as follows:

1. Sense of completion with worldly affairs

2. Sense of completion in relationships with the community

3. Sense of meaning about one's life (through life review, telling of one's stories, and transmission of knowledge and wisdom)

4. Experiencing love of self (self-acknowledgment, self-forgiveness)

5. Experiencing love of others—being able to express love and gratitude

6. Sense of completion in relationships with family and friends

7. Acceptance of the finality of one's life, including total dependency through finding a connection with some enduring construct

8. Sense of new self beyond personal loss

9. Sense of meaning about life in general

10. Letting go, including for some surrender to the Transcendent.

The findings of this study suggest that not every dying person works toward or achieves all of these landmarks. Although Byock arranged them in a logical sequence, he viewed them as a means of understanding issues that persons who are confronting death may find are most salient and necessary for them to work through. Some participants in this study had long since accomplished some of these tasks, such as putting worldly affairs in order or saying goodbye to the community and even family members. Others—especially those who confronted death at a relatively younger age—may have been acutely conscious of many of these developmental challenges and the need to accomplish them in a very short space of time, and thus spoke to us about them openly.

Table 9-1 shows the extent to which Byock's developmental landmarks appeared to have been acknowledged or realized in each participant's situation, based on direct evidence from participants or their families. In two cases (Barbara and Kitty), we were not in contact with them or family members during the last month of life, so we have less solid evidence on which to base our judgment. (In all cases, this summary represents only the researchers' judgment, based on the data available. It does not represent conclusions verified by the participants themselves.)

Table 9-1 Observations of Participants' Completion of Developmental Tasks

Task	Dennis	Barbara[a]	Ralph	Kitty	Sharon	Sarah	Walt	Roberta	Mabel
Sense of completion of worldly affairs	Yes	No	Yes	No	Yes	Yes	Yes	Yes	?
Sense of completion in relationships with community	Yes	?	Yes	Yes	Yes	Yes	Yes	Yes	?
Sense of meaning about one's life	Yes	Yes	Yes	Yes	Yes	Yes	Yes	?	?
Experiencing love of self	Yes	?	Yes	Yes	Yes	Yes	Yes	Yes	?
Experiencing love of others	Yes	?	Yes	?	Yes	Yes	Yes	Yes	?
Sense of completion in relationships with family and friends	Yes	No	Yes	No	Yes	Yes	Yes	Yes	No
Accept finality of life, total dependency	Yes	No	Yes	No	Yes	Yes	Yes	?	?
Sense of new self beyond loss	Yes	?	Yes	No	Yes	?	?	?	?
Sense of meaning about life in general	Yes	Yes	Yes	Yes	Yes	Yes	Yes	?	No
Letting go	Yes	No	Yes	No	Yes	Yes	Yes	?	?

[a]Based on conversations with us three months before her death.

A "yes" indicates that we found clear evidence that the person had come to terms with that particular "landmark" or challenge; "no" indicates that there was direct evidence to support a lack of resolution or rejection of that challenge, and "?" indicates that we could not tell, from our data, whether the landmark was ever achieved. For the purposes of this comparison, we have used only the data we gathered directly from Barbara three months before her death (see below).

We base these estimations on what the participants brought up in conversations with us and on reports of family members about the person's concerns. If the dying person expressed no concern about worldly affairs, seemed at peace most of the time, or talked about life as having meaning, we accepted that as adequate evidence that he or she had dealt with that task. If a participant continued to bring up worries, such as concerns about his or her relationship with family members, we accepted that as evidence of a continued struggle to bring those relationships to a good close.

Byock asserts that the suffering that accompanies dying can be alleviated by identifying and paying attention to these psychological and spiritual challenges and facilitating the person's struggle to complete the tasks involved. Our data clearly indicate that Dennis, Ralph, Walt, Sarah, and Sharon had confronted many of the developmental landmarks that Byock describes and dealt with the challenges to their satisfaction. The case of Roberta is less clear to us because her dementia increased rapidly after our first visits, and she generally was reluctant to discuss any of her personal life.

Three other participants—Mabel, Kitty and Barbara—appeared to struggle more actively with several of these challenges. Their struggles contrasted with those of the other participants, reflecting a range of persistent distress and suffering that can accompany dying. Because of Kitty's growing dementia, discussing her concerns was more difficult, and Mabel lived on long after our study period ended, even though she was considered close to death when we began. Barbara—an articulate, very self-aware individual—provides us with a in-depth look at the suffering that can accompany dying when the person is unwilling or unable to master critical developmental challenges before death.

Struggling with Challenges of Dying

As we have noted, many of the older participants had already struggled with and achieved several of these developmental landmarks before we met them. Barbara, however, who was dying at a much younger age than most of the other participants in this study, had many more challenges presented to her all at once. At forty-six, she had had the fewest prior opportunities or need to put her worldly affairs in order, to close relationships with her work and professional community, or to engage in a review of her life. When we talked with her over the summer, she was in the midst of dealing with several of these developmental tasks, and her emotional struggles and suffering were acute and evident.

Irene's account of Barbara's death offers evidence that Barbara's struggles finally came out well and that Barbara indeed had met more of the challenges in her dying, so that her last weeks of life were more peaceful for her. We use a developmental framework to interpret her struggle.

Barbara several times referred to her strong need to complete her life affairs, particularly involving her children.

My daughter coming on Saturday is going to be a real gift to me because she is going to help me go through things and give them away or throw them away, donate them. I will feel much better when this is done. Because one thing that was one my mind is when I die, so much goes on. I'm Indian. That complicates things.

Barbara worried about her son and daughter having the legacies they needed, and the treasured artifacts, including portraits of each of them and of Barbara that were hanging on the wall of Barbara's house. Barbara was feeling herself growing weaker and needed her daughter's help to accomplish this task. But characteristically, she also realized the necessity of doing it while she still had strength.

Barbara also brought up the difficulties in finances that she and her husband continued to experience and her worries about the difficulties he would face in managing them. This area also remained unresolved for her.

Much of the conversation with Barbara involved a kind of life review. She was very articulate about her life's story; she found meaning in her individual achievements and her lifelong dedication to helping Native American people—her own tribe and nationally. Our assumption is that her ease in telling us, as relative outsiders, about her life was evidence that she was able to do this with friends and family and that they acknowledged and listened to her telling.

Barbara appeared to be struggling most with the task of accepting the finality of her life. Byock notes that this task of accepting one's dying, depending on the individual, can involve several different steps:

- Acknowledging the totality of personal loss
- Expressing in some way the emotional depths of tragedy that dying represents
- Withdrawing from worldly connections and emotionally connecting with some "enduring construct"
- Accepting the totality of one's dependence.

Acknowledging the Loss and Expressing the Tragedy

As Barbara talked at one point about the lessening of pain she was experiencing, she began crying softly, asking, "What does that mean? Am I healing more, or . . . ?" She seemed most upset not about the pain, which was under control at that point, but about the chaos of not knowing whether her death was certain. A few minutes later, she brought up her grief over her young daughter's emerging adult life, which she would not live to see or provide guidance for:

> My daughter, she's nineteen now, and she's at a stage in her young womanhood where I'd want to give her a lot of information about her health care. She's very much aware of taking care of herself and of being at risk for ovarian cancer. She now has that history and has to be aware of it. . . . That's a concern because she still is a child. Just because she turned eighteen doesn't mean that she is an adult.

At various times, Barbara brought up her perception that there wasn't any support for children whose parents were dying, until after the death. This reflection was her way of indirectly anticipating and acknowledging her dying and death and her inability to continue to be their mother. Losing her self-identity as mother was far more painful to Barbara than losing her identity in her professional life. During the time we visited with Barbara, her suffering over her personal loss came up often as a recurring theme in many of her comments.

Struggling to Find an Enduring Connection

We have already noted the relationship between finding a connection with something that will endure beyond one's personal death and becoming able to accept one's dependence and let go of this life. By her own account, during the summer Barbara was still working on this task. The connection that appeared to be growing in her life and offering her hope was the connection to the traditions of her people. We have already seen her account of how Native American traditions had helped her: the Medicine Pipe Opening ceremony she attended in the spring before her death, her memories of the raspberry tea her family gave her when she first discovered her cancer, her visionary experience of the Sun Dance and its central sacrifice of the dancer for others. Barbara saw in her illness a final "sacrifice" for her people, akin to the Sun Dance, in which the personal physical suffering of the dancers, voluntarily chosen, purifies the entire community.

Struggling to Accept Dependency on Others

During the summer, Barbara continued to describe herself as independent and able to continue working from home. She had weekly nurse visits from a home health care service, but she wanted no other assistance from anyone but her husband and children. Barbara's sister later commented on Barbara's struggle to accept her eventual dependence on others, affirming that during the summer she had not accepted much, if any, loss of control or dependency:

> Barbara is stubborn, you know. That's something I can say, and, stubborn in a good way, but stubborn in a way that, um, she never wanted to be dependent on anybody for anything. And that kind of stubbornness, what it created was, um, "Well, I won't really deal with that until I have to."

According to Irene, Barbara finally acknowledged that she could no longer manage her life just three weeks before her death. Barbara called from the hospital to ask if Irene would take care of her; and from then on, Barbara allowed her family to love her and care for her "like a baby," no longer expecting to be independent and in control.

One reason for the many "no" and "?" entries under Barbara's name in Table 9-1 is that Barbara was actively struggling with most of these challenges during the time we met her; therefore, she brought them up over and over in conversation. Only reflected through the eyes of her sister, describing her dying, is there any evidence that Barbara confronted and acknowledged these tasks and came to some sense of peace about them.

The Legacy Book

Without realizing at first that we were doing so, as researchers we created another visible assurance of continuity and meaning for at least some of our participants. When we could not visit Dennis during his last month of life, we put together a booklet of his thoughts and reminiscences and sent it to him and his family as a record and report of our conversations with him. He had time to read it and to share it with his parents, sister, and brother before he died. The family then displayed it prominently at his memorial service and thanked us afterward for providing them with a powerful legacy. Their appreciation encouraged us to continue doing this for the others in our study.

Subsequently, for each of our participants, we selected from the transcripts of conversations the passages that seemed most meaningful to the family and most representative of the person and typed them. We eliminated false starts and vague phrases but did not change their words or rewrite their oral speech into more standard written forms. We wanted to capture the living presence of the person we were encountering, which required using their exact words and narrative style. We chose the statements to reflect the meaningful and honest reflections and thoughts of persons in whatever place they had reached, knowing that their illness was terminal and the end was near. Thus, we left out the more negative comments and included instead what was most true about these people—what they would want to leave with their friends and families.

These "legacy books" differed from other types of end-of-life books, which often consist of pictures and stories about past life, written in monologue form. The legacy books we created deliberately tried to capture each person's perspective at the end of his or her life.

In some cases, as with Dennis, we completed the book and gave it to the participants before their death, if the participant remained alert enough to appreciate it (Sharon, Sarah, Ralph). In other cases, we were able to provide the book only after the participant's death, as a gift to the family (Barbara, Walt). Our intention was simply to give back to each person or family some tangible evidence of the valuable information and wisdom they had shared with us. The legacy books also became one additional means of creating a sense of continuity for the person with the others who mattered most in their lives, however. The legacy books made tangible for the participants a narrative reconstruction of the aging, dying body and self through everyday talk (Seale 1998). Each legacy book affirmed the person's continuing connection to their social community and became a positive benefit to them and/or their families of their participation in the research. One family made many extra copies (after we had given them six or seven), so that each member of their large extended family could have something of the person who had died.

Similar efforts, sometimes called "memory books," have become more common as a way of capturing favorite stories of elderly relatives in their own words and including pictures and mementos. These books can be created well before the final months of life and shared with family and friends as a way of honoring and recognizing the person's contributions (Stone 1996). We stress that each person's narrative voice is unique. Such efforts gain their power and meaning only if they use the person's own words and are not retold in another's words.

These legacy books were intensely personal and revealing. Thus, we have not included them in this book. We have chosen instead to include a portion from just one, Sarah's, as an illustration of the format and style that proved meaningful to participants and to their families (see box).

ALWAYS HELPING:
The Legacy of Sarah

Easy Going

I guess I'm funny. I don't let stuff bother me too much. I've been trying to think up any concerns I have. I haven't found any. . . . I must have lost mine. I can't think of any. Not much use of doing anything else but smile. . . . I'd rather not be grumpy.

Real Good for Hospice

The doctor called Hospice House and asked them if I could come here. He said that he thought I would be real good for the people here. I thought that was a nice way to say that's where you're going, because I'm not down in bed like most of them are. And if they need the bell or something like that, I could help them. Well, I left the rest of it up to him.

Had It All Figured Out

I read that book . . . on death. I had it figured out just about the way the book did. I read the book to see if I was right.

Music Memories

My dad and my uncle and I all played by ear. I played piano, guitar, and banjo. I got chased out with the banjo. They would't let me stay in the house. That's too loud. You can't play that thing quiet.

We used to have a jam session every Saturday night, and one time on a Sunday afternoon . . . my dad picked up the violin and we started playing and looked outside, and here's a whole block full of cars. They had all parked on the street listening. . . . Oh, we had lots of fun.

Helping Children

We would take kids in for foster care until they could find a place for them. All the way through we had some, boys and girls, mostly boys. One time we had six newborns. We had bassinets lined up. Our house was the center for all the kids that had to come in, you know, to move to this one special place. The last one that left was four years old. We got him when he was a baby. It was hard when he left, but they're so glad to have a place of their own that you can only be glad they're going.

I had a day care at the church and I helped at Sunday school—age three to five. I was always into something like that.

Caregiving
I took care of my husband for eight years. It was hectic. But when you get there you can take it because, you know, it was impossible not to. They keep you so busy you don't have much time for guilt.

You just done it because it had to be done. We kept him as long as we could, but it just got to where he was too bad.

A Fighter
You gotta keep fighting. . . . Well, I've been fighting. Believe me, 'cause this last siege was something else. That radiation stuff's rugged. . . . They gave me a choice, and I thought, "Oh I don't want any more chemotherapy. I want to stay away from that if I can so I chose the other. I'm not sorry I did because if it does what it's supposed to I'll be good for another forty years."

Having Fun Now
You know, there's a husband and wife and grandma and grandpa that run this place. And they're just nice, just nice as they can be. They kid me all the time. You know, "Don't give Sadie that. That's too good for Sadie." Stuff like that. Then I have to watch myself 'cause I can answer him back. I don't get mad but I can kid back too, but sometimes it's better not to.

Friends Help Me
My doctor's just like a friend. I had him four years before, and now it's been a good five or six years.

Helping Friends
I enjoy helping people. Well, I feel like if I'm able, why not, you know? I had three friends visit last night. One little lady, she's blind, and when I lived at the Manor we were real good friends. And she's blind, and I helped her a lot. And then when I moved, why she said it was just not right anymore that she didn't have me. So they came last night to see me. Another lady there had a bad foot and leg, and she still calls me. Whatever would happen to her, I'd run and get help.

Another one [a fellow patient] wasn't with it, and she'd start to crawl out of bed, you know. And I could always get her to stop. I mean it was nothing much on my part.

Implications

Among the study participants, we perceive a correlation between their assurance of some connection with something they valued most and their degree of acceptance of the finality of their own life. Even though Ralph and Sharon had strong religious faiths and believed in some form of life after death, the need to create a connection with the life they had lived, some sense of continuity, was equally central to their preparations for death. Walt and his family experienced a sense of closure through his children's act of honoring his tools and books; this act allowed his spirit to depart. Creating a sense of connection seems to have its own value at the end of life.

The families in this study seemed to be aware of the dying person's need to experience connection to a larger whole, and thus continuity with life, and found ways to demonstrate that the person's values or important concerns were meaningful and would be continued within the family or in the community. This effort to contribute to the dying person's sense of connection may be a central task for family or friends to take on for someone who is dying. Families can actively seek ways to assist anyone who is seriously ill, even before death is near, to identify the legacy they want to pass on and to do so in some meaningful way. For some, this sense of connection and continuity can involve a memory book—like the legacy books we created—that records recollections of a life well lived and advice that the person wants to pass on. It can involve honoring decisions about who will take favorite things and treasure them. Such actions contribute to creating a tangible sense of continuity and meaning for the dying person.

Chapter 10

The Final Days of Life

We relied on after-death interviews with caregivers to learn about the last days of the participants in this study. With one or two exceptions, the families of our participants drew close and cut off contact with others during the last days of life, and we respected their privacy unless they specifically invited us to visit. In each case, we had seen the person who was dying within the last month; as their conditions grew more and more critical, in most instances we could keep in touch only by telephone. In many cases, caregivers had no time or energy to return our calls. After death, however, the doors to our communication with the caregivers were again open. Families welcomed the opportunity to talk about their experiences. We learned about the last days of the patients' lives through the caregivers' accounts.

Table 10-1 provides a summary of the context in which the patients died.

Home clearly was the preferred locus of care and dying for most of the patients in this study. Ralph, Barbara, and Kitty transferred to Hospice House near their very end of life, but the others died at home. Also of interest is that on the whole, family caregivers were well informed about the physical signs that would indicate the last hours of life. The notable exception was the case of Dennis and his family. They had no hospice support or other health care professionals to assist them in understanding what was happening during his dying.

Final Days

In this section, we present the narrative accounts provided by the closest care-giver of each patient, to provide a window into the last days as those close to

Table 10-1   Summary of Patients' Last Days

Patient	Location	Hospice care?	Family/caregiver knew death was imminent
Dennis	Home	No	No
Barbara	Home/Hospice House (12 hours)	Last 4 days	Yes
Ralph	Hospice House (3 days)	Yes	Yes
Sharon	Home	Yes	Somewhat
Kitty	Hospice House (2 weeks)	Yes	Yes
Walt	Home	Yes	Yes
Sarah	Hospice House (9 months)	Yes	Yes
Roberta	Home	Yes	Yes
Mabel	Home	Yes	Yes

the patient experienced them. We present these narratives without interruption or analysis; we have analyzed much of this information in other chapters.

"It seems it wasn't finished right": Dennis

Dennis, a younger cancer patient, continued to insist on remaining at home as his condition grew obviously more critical. His mother reported:

> The doctor could see through me that it would be better to put Dennis in the hospital for a few days when they were going up to this Fentanyl again. They were trying to talk him into going to the hospital so that he could be monitored. And I told him, "Dennis, just to be monitored." He said, "I am not going to any hospital." And I never wanted it to come to that. I always wanted to be able to have him where he was most comfortable. And he looked at me and said, "We'll talk about this later." And I said, "I wish we could talk about this now in front of the professionals." And he repeated, "We'll talk about this later." But anyway, we went home, and he tried really, really hard—just broke my heart—to do things even, you know, above and beyond. All he took was water for about the last two, three days. Always if he heard somebody talk about

hospital he'd say, "No." And then the last time I gave him a pill, he blew instead of swallowing.

In our minds, we didn't know how imminent death was. His brother left for work, and after work he was going to come here and help us discuss with Dennis again about taking him to the homestead.

I'd been up since about two. And about seven I told my husband, "I'm going for a little walk." I took the dog. When I came back I ate a little bit of leftover from last night. And it just stuck. And I had to go to the bathroom to throw up. Then I laid down, and that kind of relieved it. My husband was with him, reading the paper. And the next thing I knew, he came in and said, "Carrie, I think he's dying." And I went in, and he was dead. But that made me mad. Because all the time I invested, I wanted to be there.

And I've wondered over and over if Dennis made some indications of any kind. I could have talked. I would never have left him if I would have known he only had two hours. I really missed the opportunity to say to Dennis, "How do you feel differently now?" I thought it was the legacy that in the long run he might have wanted to leave. I don't know; we don't always want to leave the way we feel at a particular time. So I felt that he might say it.

And I did not recognize the signs of near-death. It would have helped if somebody would have told me. Now, some people might not be able to take it. They would either deny it or not want to hear it. But I think the nurses knew me well enough over the years to know that I was resigned.

If someone would have told me, "I think the end is pretty close now." It would have helped to know that the hearing is the last to go. It seems it wasn't finished right.

Passing Over to the Other Side: Barbara

The story of Barbara's final days comes from her sister Irene, who cared for Barbara in her home during the last two weeks of her life. Irene was able to provide Barbara with comforts from both cultures in which Barbara lived so successfully: the "white man's world" and her own Native American traditions. Irene found great meaning for herself and for their extended family in helping Barbara "pass on" to the world of her ancestors.

She came to my home from the hospital, two weeks before she crossed over. We very seldom use the word "death." We say "crossed over" because it means that we are going to see them again. She rested that night. The next day she was up cooking fry bread. She was making Indian tacos for her son and her brother who was coming to visit. She had a load of laundry in the washer, and she was pushing the vacuum around my house.

I made it comfortable. In February of '97 she called me and said, "Can you come home and help me to die with dignity?" And I reminded her of it, and she smiled at me, and she knew that we had come to fulfill what she asked.

I had help from the home health care people. They knew Barbara from before, and one of the nurses was married to a Native American, so she really felt comfortable. I've never been a nurse. I was a greenhorn.

I brushed her teeth, I combed her hair. I put makeup on, I painted her fingernails when she wanted them done. And I kept her in clean pajamas every day. I put lotion on her, I gave her foot massages. I did everything that you do for a baby. I read to her. I played music for her. She loves classical music. I have a CD player that plays continuous CDs. I went out and got plants that would be very soothing to look at.

I fixed things for her—I knew her taste was not the best, but I fixed her things that would look good in the beginning. She watched me cook. I baked. I never bake. I baked things, and I made soups. I just would put a little for her, and she'd maybe take two bites. And then I was beading these moccasins for a friend of mine.

I fixed her a real soft bed. She was always kind of a little bit chilly; I put flannel sheets on her bed, and then I put a silk pillow, you know, because she was losing her hair, you know. I bought her flannel pajamas and I got her little foot things, and I had a lot of pillows in her room.

You know in our, in our culture we like smudge. She was on oxygen. But we'd open up my back door and we'd light the smudge outside and we'd let some of it come in, and then we'd close the door. We didn't know if she was smelling it. But then I knew she was. And she responded to it.

And her friends came to my home, and all they'd do is they'd just come in and just stand at the foot of her bed. They would just stand there, and all they want to do is just see her. And then people brought food. Although she wasn't eating, she could see us eating. She talked on the phone a few times, but often I would say, "Well, she's sitting right here, but she can't talk. She's doing okay." And I would tell them a little bit about how she's doing, and she would listen to me, and then I'd tell her the news that they were saying. So she didn't have to hold the phone and talk. She could just listen to what I was saying.

We also had a baby there. We had a little four-month-old baby. Barbara couldn't talk any more. But she could see the baby. This little baby did something for her. My sister would lay her right by Barbara. I think that a lot of times at that point, people are afraid to touch 'em. But this little baby would just kind of grab at her and was just laying right on her. And it did something for her. It would calm her.

The day before we took her to Hospice House, our parents came, and Barbara had stopped eating and stopped drinking water. And she had this faraway look in her eye. And I'd call her and she'd look away, and then she'd focus back on me. And asked her, "Barbara, have you started your journey to the other side?"

And she looked at me, and she just smiled so big. And I told her, "I'm here with you. I'm not going to leave you. You don't have anything to be afraid of. I want to thank you for this opportunity to see through your eyes to the other side."

In our way of life, you know, we believe that our ancestors come to get us. We sensed, we felt my house was full of those many relatives. We got all kinds of little warnings that it was that time. My back door opens out to the golf course. And the last night that she was with us, we stayed up and talked. And we had the back door open. We sat there with the door open all night. And it was just like, you know, it was just like people coming and going, you know.

Toward the end, I fixed a little couch that makes into a bed in the living room, and she was in the living room with all of us. And we sat and visited and talked about her life. I mean, this is what we do. And she gets to hear it. We talked about when she was real young, and we talked about when she had her first child, and we talked about the landmarks in her life. We also talked about her, and it was also very sad. We all took turns crying.

And I read the Bible to her and played a flute music tape for her. Barbara had one foot in what we call the white man's world. But she also had her other foot in our Indian world. She always went toward what we had in common. I always read her the Psalms— Psalm 23—and then I would burn smudge for her. I hung my eagle fan above her head because our belief is that's the dream world. And that when you lay down to rest, that eagle spirit is going to help you to have good dreams.

I did everything that I would want somebody to do for me. I would say, "Barbara, why don't you just sit back and close your eyes, and I'll tell you a story. Just listen." And she would do that. She'd just close her eyes, and I'd talk about our grandma or I would talk about—she loved to hear about our medicine bundle, that we belong to. I would tell her stories that had morals in them.

I think that her passing was so peaceful. Because we all wondered what is it going to be like? And we all worried: Can we handle this? And my mother, she would go into the bathroom and she would cry, and she'd tell me, "Why don't you call the hospital and have them, you know, come and get her?" She was worried whenever Barbara would start coughing, and then I would reassure her, "Mom, we're doing everything we can for her, and they're going to do the same things that we can." And I started worrying about my mom: Can she handle this? And I would just let her cry.

The last day, I would always say, "Barbara, can you close your eyes? Rest your eyes, Barbara." And then she'd close her eyes. She knew my voice, and I felt good about that. Pretty soon her eyes would be open again, and I'd go over and tell her who I was, tell her what time of the day it was, what kind of weather it was outside, who was all there.

We thought Barbara was leaving us several times. Her breathing was just really getting erratic, and she'd hold her breath. We thought that she was leaving. And then all of a sudden, I told my mom, "You know, I think Barbara's waiting for something. I don't know what it is, but maybe she doesn't want to leave here at my home." Because she knows I have to live here. So then Hospice called, and Mom answered, and said, "The hospice (house) has an opening. What do you think?" I said, "I think we should take her. We've done as much as we can do. And I think that we need a little bit more skilled people that know more about the end." And so we agreed. And so they said, "We'll send the ambulance." So we started getting her ready. We bathed her and changed her pajamas and everything, and then we all went out there. We took her there at 1:00 in the afternoon, and she passed on that night at 11:30, 12:30.

And I called for the harp, the people that play the harp—the Chalice of Repose. They had come to my house when she was there. And it not only helped Barbara, but it helped us. My mother didn't care for it because she felt it was too morbid [laughs]. They came [to Hospice House] at six o'clock, and I just felt a real peace, peace for her.

I was tired, and I told my mom, "I'm going go home and rest. I'll come back in the morning." This was about maybe 7:00. We were talking in her room, and so Mom said, "We'll stay for awhile. We'll see how she's doing." We had been up for the last five days. Then the nurse came in and said, "We're going to turn her. Can you all, you know, step out for a little bit? We're going to change her and turn her." And so we all went into the front room, and I told mom, "Well, okay. We're going to go into town." We were all getting ready to leave. And the nurse came, and she said, "I don't think you guys should leave. I think it's time."

We all went back in, and then her breathing came back again. Then that's when we all started laughing, and tears were just coming to our eyes. We were laughing because we were saying, "She's just keeping us here. You know, she doesn't want any one of us to leave." So that was about 9:00. Then I said, "Well, I'm going to go home at ten, because really I am just beat." So she heard us say that again. So we went into the front room, and then the nurse came back, and she said, "I hate to keep doing this to you, but I think you need to come back."

So we went back, and that was the first time I felt her hands. They were cold, and the back of her legs were cold. Right there I just knew that it was close. But yet I really didn't know. Then my aunt came and went in to see her. And her daughter went in and was holding her. And she left us.

"Now you can go see your kids": Ralph

Ralph, an older emphysema patient, was rational up to the last week of his life, when he finally became too much for Sandy, his caregiver, to handle alone. The hospice nurse had made Ralph and Sandy aware what the signs of his last days would be:

The hospice nurse has been telling him for months that this is what's gonna happen to him. That eventually he would just get sleepier and sleepier and sleepier, until one of these days he'll quit.

Two weeks before Ralph's death, Sandy told us that Ralph often prayed to die:

So all I hear now is, "I pray and I pray and I pray, let me die—but He won't let me." It's gettin' so he hates to get up in the morning now: another day! I can't leave him alone. He's too weak. Now he's gettin' quite a few cold—the bogwobbles, he calls it. It's something horses get. They get wobbly on their feet, and so they call them bogwobbles.

The week of Ralph's death, Sandy reported to us that Ralph had been "in kind of a little half-way coma" and had lost three pints of blood. He wouldn't take his medicine; worse yet, oxygen deprivation caused him to distrust Sandy and even to accuse her of trying to kill him. Sandy finally called the hospice nurse at 4:00 in the morning. The nurse came quickly, sedated Ralph, and made arrangements to transfer him to Hospice House immediately. Once Ralph was there, his awareness faded in and out: Sometimes he remembered things, but mostly did not, as Sandy reports:

He had a couple of moments when he was conscious and could talk. He told me, he says, "You know, this is just about over with." And I said, "Yeah." He knew he was dying, you know. And he says, "The first thing you're gonna do is go see your kids, aren't you?" And I said, "Yeah, okay." That's what he wanted me to do first— was to go see them because I had gone a long time without seeing them so that I could be with Ralph. As sick as he was, I wouldn't have left him.

Sandy did not feel guilty about giving up her constant care of him at the very end:

I couldn't do it. There was no way I could do it. You know, with the pump and everything, I just couldn't do it. It's so hard to see him gasping for air that way. He didn't even know I was there today. He never even asked for me. But he knows that I know that what he's saying to me now he doesn't mean. I can pray just as hard at home.

The next day—the day before Ralph died—Sandy had a long visit with him:

He looked at me, and I asked him if he was still mad at me. He said, "No, no." He was just so confused about everything, and that was the main thing that he was angry about, you know.

That night, Ralph had another episode of internal bleeding. He died the next day. Sandy observed:

They called and the Hospice chaplain came and got me, and I went out there. But I—by the time I got there he was gone. I wasn't there when he died, but I don't think he woulda known it anyway.

Following Ralph's wishes, within a month after his death Sandy flew to Colorado to visit the children and grandchildren she had not seen for three years.

"Twelve hours to make the transition": Sharon

Sharon's last day came very suddenly—less than seventy-two hours after her last visit with one of her sons and a niece. Even her daughter, who lived several hours away, was not able to come back in time. Sharon died at her sister Connie's home. Connie tells the story of the sudden "turning point," which no one in her family quite expected or recognized when it came.

The turning point was very sudden and very dramatic. Her hospice nurse said there'd be no question. We'd know when that came. . . .

Terry, her son, was here Saturday, and that's the day my daughter came. I picked her up at the airport and we went shopping, and we were gone a couple of hours. When we came home, Sharon was still fine. She and my daughter hugged and visited a little bit. But she was tired, which is normal after visiting a lot—first with Terry and then with my daughter. She went to lie down, and then it was hard to wake her up. She was just so deeply asleep. And the next day it was still that kind of thing. She would get up to use the commode. She'd wake up enough to that, then she went right back to sleep again. . . .

I guess I didn't call her kids right away. I was confused because she said that night that her stomach was upset. And I told her that we could do two things. She could either take a pill, which made her very sleepy, or she could take food. And either of those would help her stomach. And she chose the pill. So I wasn't sure all weekend if she was reacting to that. . . .

I called hospice. But it was a weekend, so I talked to the other nurse. She didn't know Sharon that well and just gave some general advice, but she didn't come out. But when the nurse came on Monday morning, she knew that she had pneumonia. She recognized it.

Sunday night, she fell in her room. She got out of bed herself, and I think that she collapsed as soon as she put her feet to the floor. I didn't find her until I got up early morning. She'd been there awhile because her feet were cold, but the rest of her was warm because the house wasn't very cold and she was in the warm nightie. She was deeply asleep that time. My daughter was there, so together we were able to get her back to bed.

Sometimes she'd come to, kind of half-conscious, and talk a little bit. But she didn't make sense. I wondered if she'd had a little stroke, too. Because she would either just repeat a phrase over and over or else say nonsense words. She didn't stay awake at all. She'd just emerge a little bit and then sink back down again. She had one drenching sweat. . . .

When the hospice nurse came Monday morning, she thought Sharon probably would be with us 2 or 3 days. She knew that she had turned that corner. She kept talking about that corner. . . .

She ordered the hospital bed and the catheter and morphine pump. And we settled her comfortably in bed, and she just never moved again. We moved her, turned her over once, but she didn't ever wake up again. It was during the night that she died. My daughter was here with me.

Don [Sharon's other son] came after work on Monday. I don't think Terry was back again. I called and asked them if they wanted to see her. Don was here, too, when the mortician came. . . .

She died in the early morning Tuesday, and we kept her until mid-afternoon. I read that you want to give a person twelve hours to make the transition. With my husband [who died at home four years previously] I felt I had to call the mortuary. We'd washed him and had fresh pajamas on, and he looked so nice. But we had agreed that we'd call Five Valleys when he died, and I just seemed to think that I had to do it. And they came in 20 minutes! I could have waited until the kids came to see him.

Getting Permission to Die: Walt

Walt had suffered through many heart attacks and hospitalizations over the previous eleven years. During the most recent one, about a year before he died, he apparently hung on mostly because his family was not ready to let him go quite yet. His wife and caregiver, Dorothy, told us:

I guess he had to make his children be willing to accept his dying. They were very close to him, and at the end they had to let him go. That was his main thing. He had to get to the point where the children could let him. And he realized that. I don't think people realize how much they have to do this. And you're lucky if you can go on long enough for the family to release you. The entire family has to be willing to let go.

Dorothy described how the family managed to release Walt:

The children came in, and they talked to him and told him everything was all right. They all talked about his wishes after he was gone. The boys told him how they would divide up his tools. The girls told him which one would get his books. So everything was discussed, and the children did not feel bad about taking the things. I think that people close themselves up too much when someone is ready to pass away, until there's too much confusion.

One of Walt's sons elaborated a bit:

Dad wanted to make sure that I got his oxi-acetylene tanks. So I did. Which was not a problem for my brother. He took pretty much all of Dad's wood tools, and I took pretty much what was metal. We assured Dad that there wouldn't be no fighting over nothing. I mean, we both told him we loved him. His stuff really wasn't that valuable. You know, mainly the thing both of us wanted was a piece of him, personality wise. One thing Dad wanted me to have was a dust pan, believe it or not, that I made in seventh grade metal shop. He kept that dust pan over the years and wanted me to have it back.

A Gift to Her: Kitty

Kitty's final days were spent in the place she had worked so hard to avoid: Hospice House. She was taken there at the insistence of her Hospice nurse, after the nurse found her disoriented, incontinent, and clearly no longer able to care for herself, on a Monday morning one month before Kitty's death. During the first two weeks at Hospice House, Kitty was able to eat in the common dining area, visit with others, enjoy her tapes in the family room, and read "all the time." She said to the staff, "This was a good move for me."

During her last week she declined rapidly and became comatose. She struggled to make some last changes in her will, with great difficulty. At one point, she roused out of her coma and said to a nurse and visitors in her room, "I have an announcement. We're all equally alive." The staff who reported this statement inferred that it was a sign of her movement toward death with comfort.

During one visit, Kitty's priest saw that she kept having more pain, and he finally said to the hospice nurse, "She really does seem to be uncomfortable." The nurse came in and took Kitty's face in both of her hands; she held it close and whispered in Kitty's ear, "Sweetheart, I won't let the pain get the best of you." The nurse stroked Kitty's forehead, gave her a kiss, got a syringe, and gave her an injection.

In her last days, Kitty was in and out of consciousness. She recognized friends, but she was on heavy medication to control the pain from an infected foot.

Several friends from Kitty's church, as well as the woman who had cleaned her house faithfully for several years, visited her regularly during the last week. All three priests from her parish came out to be with her. Kitty was seldom alone during this time. One friend brought her dogs out to visit, so that Kitty could have animals around her in her final days. On Kitty's last day, the assistant priest visited her twenty minutes before she died, and another friend from church was there sharing a letter from a friend who had moved away.

At Kitty's memorial service, the parish priest summarized her end:

> This fiercely independent woman in the end had to do exactly what she didn't want to do. She wanted to die at home, and she did not. She had to give the care of her last days over to complete strangers. But it was a gift to her. Hospice took the things she feared most and made it a blessing. They gave her a feeling of safety and compassion. She died with dignity and peace and grace.

"We were all in the room": Roberta

Four days before Roberta's death, her hip fractured sometime during the night. She had been able to get up and dress each day until this point, and she was conscious and able to interact. After Roberta was admitted to the hospital and prepared for a hip replacement, her kidneys failed, she became comatose, and the family and her physician agreed that she could go home to die. She was transferred by ambulance back to her daughter Debbie's home late in the afternoon on the day before her death. Debbie narrates the story of her mother's last twenty-four hours:

> The day we took her home, before the ambulance ride, I said, "Mom, you're going home with us." And she had a big smile on her face, and she had a twinkle in her eye, and she was so happy. She knew that she was coming home. I'm glad we brought her home. We had everything set up, thanks to our hospice nurse. We had the bed set up when she got here by ambulance, and her nurse was waiting for her. She had a new morphine pump for her.
>
> We sat and visited for a little while with Mom, and we talked about Chalice of Repose. And my sister and I kind of decided that we would try the Chalice. We decided to do it right then. So we called and made arrangements for them to come over that evening.

My husband, and my sister's husband, were upset with this decision. They felt that it would upset Mom. That it would be a signal to her that she might be dying, and they couldn't deal with this. But we went ahead and decided yes, we could try this. The Chalice people assured us; they told us exactly what they would be doing, and we were very comfortable with this. They assured us that if she was in distress with this, they would leave.

So we set them up, and they started playing. And Mom was quite shocked, I'm sure. She jumped, and she was making very strange hand gestures. But as time went on with the music I could see her relaxing, and I could see this transition in her, and it was very, very soothing, very lovely for all of us. . . .

And all of a sudden her bird decided that he likes this music. Now, he never sings past 6:00 at night. And he was just out here singing up a storm while the harps were playing in Mom's room. We had a house full of people, too. My two sisters were here, and my grandson, one of our sons, and our husbands, my sister's daughter and her children. Everybody was here. And Betty [Roberta's day care nurse] came in. They were all in the room. We were all in there, and it was just beautiful. And then our minister came and listened to the last part of it. Someone had called him to let him know that Mom had come home. . . .

So when they left we sat and visited for awhile, and my sister and I kept taking turns and checking on Mom, and there was a great peace about her. . . .

Then that night I got this harebrained idea. I thought, "Why do we think that her kidneys are failing? How do we know this for sure? Why don't we give her an IV? Why can't we give her some kind of something to make sure that she's, you know, not shutting down?" I really wanted to do everything I could to help sustain some more life in her. And I was having a real difficult time adjusting to this possibility that she wasn't functioning, that I'm not doing anything to help her. It was hard. And I worked with this all night. My sister and I took turns and sat up all night with Mom. . . .

And I thought, okay, I need to ask hospice about this. So when the nurse called the next day and said, "How are things going?" I said, "She seems to be fine, she's comfortable, but I need to talk to you," I said. So she came about 6:00 to 6:30 in the evening. I said,

"Come on, I want to visit with you." And I shared with her my thoughts. "Can we give her an IV? Can we try and make sure that her kidneys haven't shut down? What can we do for her?" And this dear person said, "Yes. Yes, we can do that." Not telling me no, we couldn't do that. I knew that this was the answer. But she said, "Yes, we can do that. But let me tell you a little more about what's happening to her." So I listened to her, and she carefully explained things to me for 15, 20 minutes that made me understand this process that was happening to Mom and why it was so important for me to let go of her. And I told her, I said, "I'm having a hard time letting go. I can't let go of her." And she says, "Well, this is difficult for your mom, too." . . .

And she was very, very kind, and I felt a lot of compassion from her and from her explanation of what was happening to Mom's system and everything and medically why it would be harmful for them to start giving her fluids. And how if they started pumping fluids, her system wouldn't absorb it and she would get all this fluid back into her again, and it would cause more problems and I . . . I could understand that. . . .

I couldn't even begin to relate the dialogue. It took about 15, 20 minutes. I looked over to my sister, and I said, "Okay, I can let go of her now. I can let her go." I asked my sister, "This is okay with you?" And she said, "Yes." And I said, "Okay, how much time do you think she has?" And she said, "I've seldom known people to live like this, dehydrating, for very long. I would give your mom through the weekend maybe, at the most." I felt better knowing that I could release Mom. . . .

When this conversation ended, Deanna went in the bedroom, and she came out and she said, "Oh, we're losing Mom. Come quickly." And we went in there, and the hospice nurse could not believe the change in her breathing. I mean, it was just incredibly different. We had just been in there a half hour before and she was fine. She had intervals of breathing, holding her breath, and then would start breathing again. . . .

And so we realized then that it was a change. And then my niece showed up. She has four children; two of them were with her, one of them is a little 2-year-old, and one is 3. And they came in and held Grandma's hand. And the little girl cried a little bit; the little boy held her hand and said, "Bye-bye, bye-bye." We don't know why. . . .

And it was just an incredible thing that was happening. And we knew right then we were going to be losing Grandma. And so I called my sister at the lake. She had left that morning to go back to the lake and get things, and [that] was an amazingly good thing. Because I don't think Mom wanted her here when she died. Because my sister just lost her husband a few years ago, and the pain—it was so painful. . . .

So then the hospice nurse suggested we could call my sister and let her talk to Mom. And so we did this. I called her at the lake and told her that we were losing Mom, and—and would she like to say something to her? And we put the phone to Mom's ear, and she talked to her on the phone. It was wonderful. Then we called Rick in Kentucky, and he talked to Grandma on the phone. And then we called her other grandson in Texas, and he got to say good-bye to Grandma. She definitely had made a decision to leave us. . . .

And our other son wasn't here yet. He lives in town, and he called up and wanted to know how things were going. And I said, "I think you should get over here now." So he was here. He got here 5 minutes before she died. . . .

We were all in the room, holding her hand, telling her we loved her, telling her, thanking her for letting us be a part of her transition, which was so beautiful—to see her peaceful and to know that it was okay to hold her hand and feel this great powerful comfort of doing this. It was—it was beautiful. We all felt this; every one of us felt this. Every one of us were so touched, celebrating and thanking her for her life. And it was truly most beautiful. She was so light there, just like a little feather on the breath. . . .

And we felt a great peace for her, and we felt so much love and warmth that time in the bonding that we all had with each other. It was just incredible. . . .

So we stayed with her for a few minutes, and then this wonderful hospice nurse said, "I need to do some things here, some work. Would you like to stay with her, or would you like to wait till I'm done?" And I said, "You go ahead and do your work, and we'll be back." And she came and got us, and we went back into Mom's room and she had fixed her up so beautifully. She had her hands folded, and she had her bed made up. It was just a beautiful gesture, the things that she'd done. She made Mom look so nice, and we were so happy that the nurse could be here with us and be part of this.

Debbie: It was beautiful, a beautiful feeling to be with Mom and to be . . . be a part of her passing. It was about 9:30 at night. We kept her until 1:30 in the morning.

Researcher: You didn't feel the need to call the mortuary right away and rush her out? How did you know that?

Debbie: I just felt I could do anything I wanted to do. I just didn't want them to come until we were ready to let her go. We talked, we visited, we went back in and visited with her.

Final Days and the Subculture of the Dying

Of all the features that characterize the subculture that surrounds terminally ill people, issues of control, social networks, comfort, and growth seem to be most salient during the final days of life.

Although dying people do not have much control as life ebbs from them, their caregivers and families—who have teamed with them throughout this period—still struggle with an effort to maintain their choices and control and to honor the wishes of the dying. The eight caregivers present different pictures of this loss of power and control.

Carrie, who had been "joined at the hip" for a year with her dying son, Dennis, expressed her sense of loss because she was not present with Dennis when he died. "With all the time I invested, I wanted to be there." Missing this last moment affected her deeply for months after Dennis's death. She had been in control up to that time and now felt that she was not.

The only other caregiver who was not immediately with the patient when he died was Sandy, Ralph's mate; she had returned to her own home from Hospice House, although she knew he probably would die that evening. Unlike Carrie, Sandy had no regrets about not being with Ralph in his last moments, noting that he probably wouldn't have known her anyway. Sandy appeared to feel no loss of control from missing Ralph's last breath. She felt she had said her goodbyes earlier and could do nothing more.

The other dying patients were surrounded by family or friends at their moments of death. The shrunken social network that often accompanies terminal illness suddenly expanded in each of these cases. Barbara, Sharon, and Roberta were surrounded by loved ones of all generations. Walt, who had a close family throughout his illness, continued to have them with him to the end. Kitty, who had no family, was attended to by her many church friends. The decreased social networks of terminally ill patients were reversed, in a sense, as people came deliberately to gather round the dying person.

One aspect of the social networks surrounding the participants who were dying is worth mentioning: They deliberately included children and pets. In addition to close family, several of our participants spent their last hours in the presence of young children and beloved animals. Irene describes how Barbara was transformed by having a baby near her; Roberta's great-granddaughter was brought to visit with her the night of her death; Walt's grandchildren lived next door and were there during his last days. A friend of Kitty's brought her own dogs to visit Kitty at Hospice House a day before she died, knowing Kitty's deep love for animals. Walt's dog stayed in his bedroom until his death. And Waldo, Roberta's pet canary, burst forth with song when the Chalice of Repose played for her.

Personal growth is apparent in caregivers and patients in these accounts. Barbara's sister Irene explicitly describes Barbara as finding peace after the long struggle and enjoying her last days of being cared for as she waited to go over to the other side. For others, growth at the very end toward accepting death and finding meaning is more evident in the family itself. Descriptions of the final days of Walt, Sharon, and Roberta offer evidence of growing family unity and the making of meaning. Some families—notably Walt's and Roberta's—said good-bye openly as the person was dying, even calling children and grandchildren on the phone to be part of the farewell.

Chapter 11

Memorials at the End of Life

This study paid special attention to how families and friends created meaningful symbols or symbolic interactions at the end of life. One definition of the human species is that we are beings who create funerary symbols or rites, acknowledging the personal existence of individuals. Memorials are symbolic, condensed expressions of meaning through events, objects, or interactions. For this study, we were especially interested in how families and friends created or found personal—even unique—symbols for the life and death of someone they loved. In this chapter we describe some of the deliberate choices families made to personalize and make meaningful their received cultural or religious traditions.

Sociologists beginning with Blumer (1969) have put forth the concept of symbolic interactionism to explain the meaning-making propensity that characterizes humans:

1. Human beings act toward things or events on the basis of the meanings those things have for them.

2. These meanings derive from the social interaction that one has with one's primary group.

3. Meanings are handled and modified through an interpretive process used by persons dealing with the things they encounter.

At the end of a life, those still living turn to traditional symbols, or create unique ones, that can convey the meaning of the dying person's life. These symbols or symbolic events and interactions provide a source and representation of continuity for family and friends. At the beginning of this new millennium, when traditional cultures, ceremonies, and rituals often retain little of their original sacred meaning, families from traditional religious and nonreligious backgrounds find their own personal ways to memorialize, symbolically celebrate, and let go of the person who has died. In this chapter we report our observations of how families and friends found personal ways of saying goodbye, expressing their grief, and acknowledging the beliefs that were meaningful to them.

Funerals and Memorial Services

We attended memorial services for eight of the participants who died during or after the period of our study. (Mabel remained alive for another year, and we were not informed of her death.) Of these eight, none had a traditional funeral with the body present, followed by a graveside rite. Three had memorial services in a local funeral home or other location after cremation (Dennis, Roberta, Sarah); three had memorial services in a local church after cremation or burial (Ralph, Kitty, Barbara); one family took the ashes to the cemetery and personally interred them without a service (Walt); and one family had a private family dinner and informal service for family and friends some days after the death (Sharon). The only war veteran, Ralph, also had graveside rites for some of his ashes. All of these participants had an obituary published in the local paper.

The choice of cremation seemed common and noncontroversial among this population. In the MDP study of local funeral practices, the cremation rate for Missoula was 64 percent in 1995 and had increased steadily during the 1990s (Blandford et al. 1999). Part of cremation's popularity in this area can be attributed to the choice it allows for a final place for remains. Several families followed their loved one's instructions to scatter their ashes in beloved outdoor spots: the Bob Marshall wilderness, a favorite camping spot, near a wild river. Cremation also eliminated the problem of making a single choice about placement: Some of Ralph's ashes were interred at the Missoula Cemetery, with American Legion graveside rites befitting his service in the Korean War and creating a place for the veteran's grave marker; the rest of the ashes were scattered in the wilderness area near his home. The summary in Table 11-1 illustrates both diversity and uniformity among this small group of participants.

Symbolic Interactions and Personal Symbols of Meaning

From our conversations with the families and from the field notes of our experiences as participant-observers at the memorial services, we have marked the events, formal or informal interactions, or objects of remembrance that were clearly meaningful and intentional. As we note above, all but one of our participants had some kind of memorial service—either a public service or simply a private family ceremony. In this chapter we describe what families did that

Table 11-1   Committal and Memorial Decisions

Disposition of body:	Cremation	8 of 9 deaths
Type of service:	Church memorial service	3
	Funeral home memorial service	3
	Senior residence memorial service	1
	Family interred ashes privately, open house for friends	1
	Family and friends service	1
Places for ashes (some ashes were divided):	Park	1
	Outdoors/wilderness areas	4
	Family homestead	1
	Local cemetery	3
	Husband's coffin	1
Meaningful symbol or symbolic event:	Ceremonial potluck	
	Thanksgiving dinner for family and friends	
	Hospice tree lights	
	Visit of caregivers to home place	
	Community potluck	
	Memory table at memorial service	
	Private interment by family members	

made standard rituals or funeral services more personal or in some other way celebrated the uniqueness of the person and created meaning out of the experience of death.

Thanksgiving Dinner and Informal Service

Sharon had specifically instructed her children and her sister Connie that she was not to have a funeral or memorial service. The family fully understood and intended to abide by her wishes. Connie asked Sharon shortly before death, however, if the family could "get together" after she died, as long as it wasn't public; Sharon agreed that such as gathering would be okay with her. Sharon died relatively suddenly, and the family finally decided to have a small family gathering at Thanksgiving (a week later) because one of Sharon's grand-daughters had already bought a plane ticket to fly to Missoula to see her. As the week went on, the small family gathering grew, and when Connie called to invite us, she said:

> There are a few more people than we thought there'd be, so we can't do it at home. And I'm not much into thinking about a dinner. So we've reserved a conference room at the 4Bs [a local restaurant, motel, and conference center]. We'll have a Thanksgiving meal at 2:00 and an informal memorial service about 3:00.

Even though this get-together was meant to be only a "small gathering" for family, Connie also made phone calls to invite the MDP researchers, Sharon's friends in Missoula, and the hospice staff and volunteers. No public notice of the gathering was printed. About twenty to twenty-five people were there for the dinner, and perhaps ten more came in before the informal service began. The setting was a fairly sterile hotel conference room, with round tables and a buffet dinner setup at one end. As people gathered to eat and talk, however, the room grew warmer and more home-like. Several families from Sharon's faith community were there, with teenage children for whom Sharon had baby-sat in earlier years. Young grandchildren of Connie's and other family relatives played around the tables and went in and out of the room.

After the meal, Sharon's minister and friend from her faith community led a time of remembrance. He began simply by having everyone introduce them-selves briefly and tell how they knew Sharon. Then the minister offered his reflections on Sharon's life and personality. He said that although her "bodily expression" was gone, her spirit and soul were present. He then played some music, read a letter from Sharon's other sister (in California), and led everyone in a guided meditation to close the service. None of Sharon's children, or her sister, spoke except during the introduction time.

This memorial time focused on the continuing presence of Sharon's spirit in the room. There was no sense of ritual or religious mystery; instead, it all seemed matter-of-fact and obvious to most of those present. This shared spirit of understanding may have been one reason Sharon and the family did not want a more public or traditional memorial service. For those who were pre-sent, there was little need to explain what was going on.

Memory Tables at Memorial Service

Two of the families who chose memorial services at the funeral home created memory tables for the service. A memory table holds photographs, awards, hobbies, and treasured objects that reflect the departed person's life and values. These displays can be extraordinarily powerful evocations of a life.

Dennis's table held his special putter, a golf pro cap and golf shoes, a baseball mitt, a fishing hat, and pictures of Dennis with his kids. Tied to the table were balloons from his sister's children. On a bulletin board, the family also displayed artifacts from some of Dennis's medical treatments, such as a certificate for having endured numerous radiation treatments with a good spirit. The legacy book that we created for Dennis from our conversations with him was open for people to read. Dennis's engagement with his illness had been a vigorous and prolonged battle, and these artifacts were meaningful to his family as evidence of that time.

Roberta's memory table, representing her eighty-five years of life, was even more of a revelation: She had been a state champion archer in the 1940s, and the table contained a picture of her shooting, as well as her trophy. The table also held a Smokey the Bear doll (representing her years working for the U.S. Forest Service), a stylish fur hat, a crocheted shawl, some costume jewelry in a Victorian jewelry box, and a bird sculpture that symbolized her love for birds. There were photographs of Roberta from the time she was a young girl through her married life and as a very vibrant-looking woman in her sixties.

The memorial services for Roberta and Dennis followed a traditional order: A minister offered a sermon; family members read scripture and poems and presented some prepared remembrances. The memory tables helped personalize the more conventional aspects of a memorial service.

Hospice Tree Lights

Ralph and Roberta had Hospice Tree lights donated in their honor. The Hospice Tree is lit in the memorial park in mid-December. Both died in November; Sandy went to the lighting of the tree—to which all families who have lost a loved one are invited—and found it meaningful.

Visit to Home Place and Community Potluck

Two weeks after Ralph's death, his family held a memorial service at the small church in his home town for all their friends. The hospice nurse, chaplain, physician, and volunteers who had been with Ralph and Sandy for sixteen months were especially invited to come, as were the MDP researchers who had met them in the last four months of Ralph's life. The fact that all those who had been most involved with Ralph's life at the end made the 100-mile trip for the service is a reflection of his spirit.

The service itself, led by Ralph's minister, followed a traditional order of worship, with hymns, prayers, and a sermon focusing on Ralph's firm faith that he would be given some good work to do as soon as he got to heaven. After the service, Sandy arranged for the ten people who came from Missoula to see the homestead, which was about a mile from the church, on a back road off the main highway. The 160-acre ranch lies along a creek in a mountain valley, with the Mission and Bob Marshall mountains on either side; even in December it looked beautiful, with pine trees and a pasture for visiting elk herds in the winter and feeder calves during the summer.

This visit became a symbolic way of saying goodbye for everyone who knew Ralph only in Missoula. It provided them with assurance that Ralph had indeed "come home" and that what he loved most in life would endure. For Sandy, the visit provided a private time of saying thank you and closing a momentous chapter in her life. After the visit to the homestead, everyone joined Ralph's community for a potluck luncheon for about 100 in the town community hall, heated by a large forty-gallon oil drum stove. Sandy and Ralph had met at a dance in this hall eighteen years earlier, and holding a banquet in his honor there seemed altogether fitting.

Private Interment by Family Members

Walt's family had planned to have no funeral or memorial service—just an "open house" for family and friends after his death. Walt had been at home, dying, for so long that the family had done their grieving and letting go well before his death. Walt and Dorothy had talked often about their experience of dismal funerals, often conducted by a minister who had never known the deceased. Because Walt during his adult life had no church connection, having a religious service "didn't make sense." Dorothy recalled:

> We had always said, if you're religious, you should have a religious service. But why have a religious service if he never went to church? And so we both decided, why have a minister talk that didn't know you? And we wanted it simple because if there was any money, there were people that needed it, there were children that needed it, and it was foolish. Because his spirit goes on. So what was the point of spending lots?

∾ ∾ ∾

> We have always laughed, Walt and I, about when he was a pallbearer for some good friends of ours. One man got up and testified for him, and he talked about his horse more than about him. We got so tickled.

With this perspective, the family decided to take Walt's ashes from the crematory out to the cemetery and have a private family time, placing his ashes in the niche. This ritual turned out to be a time of a few tears but also laughter, as Dorothy recounted a week later:

It was really all so funny. Because my two sons, of course, were in the same trade that their dad had been in. And so they didn't let them close it up [the niche for the urn]. They said, "No, we'll take the screwdriver and we'll put that plaque on. That was our dad." It was quiet, and we had some laughs, and even the man from the funeral home was delightful. Because we got the little vase that goes onto the, uh, the door. And we said, well, we didn't bring any flowers. And he said, "Well, I might steal these over here and put them in for you." Sooo, we had a good laugh over that. So it was quite pleasant, all in all. My daughter had brought a bunch of balloons to take and put out for the kids and grandkids.

This private time, just before the open house, was the family's time to gather and say goodbye. Walt had been a skilled construction worker and had given his tools to his sons as their legacy. So the simple act of placing the plaque on the columbarium niche was fitting for this family, as a symbol of their cohesiveness in death as well as life.

The family then held an open house with food that afternoon at Walt and Dorothy's home. The open house was announced in Walt's obituary; friends as well as family were invited to come. About sixty or seventy people came to see Walt's wife and children. There was no ceremony as part of this open house; people greeted the family informally and then sat and talked in the yard on a warm, sunny day.

Ceremonial Potluck and Memorial Service

When Barbara died, her family took her body back to the reservation homeland for a funeral service in the local parish church and burial. Because of the long distance from Missoula, this service did not include most of the people she knew and worked with during the previous decade. So Barbara—anticipating her death and the traditional burial—thought there should be some way to have a ceremony in Missoula that would include both of the worlds she had lived in. Sometime before her death, she had written out instructions for a memorial service, including hymns and readings, that honored her Native American beliefs, her Catholic faith, and her work at the university within the same ceremony— "so that others could grieve, and heal," in her words. The decision to hold a ceremonial potluck and feast of celebration at the university immediately after the service came from Barbara's friends and family. The service and potluck were announced in the newspaper and on the local public radio station, as an open invitation to everyone in the Missoula and university communities to attend.

The memorial service at a local Catholic parish church began with the Calling Song by a well-known Native American singer and drummer. Two friends shared their memories of Barbara, and university officials spoke of her work at the university and her impact on them as a faculty member. The service included a Native American Honoring Song for those who have fallen in battle, as well as traditional Catholic liturgical readings for the dead and hymns by church singers. The priest spoke of how Barbara knew she would be buried in the land of her ancestors and believed, in the words of Chief Seattle, that "our ancestors are sacred, and their resting place is hallowed ground. So all the earth is sacred. There is no death, only a change of worlds."

The ceremonial potluck at the university afterward was a more striking symbolic evocation of Barbara's life, however, because it more seamlessly integrated a Native American tradition with the university community. The announcement of the potluck received substantial space in the local newspaper, so anyone who wanted to bring food would know how to participate. Everyone attending the memorial service was invited—perhaps 200 in all; perhaps 100 more, many of them Native American university students with their children, also came to the potluck.

Within the large ballroom at the university center, tables for eight were set up, covered with white cloth. It took an hour for everyone to come in and be seated and for the food to be readied, so people found tables with others they might know, talking and writing remembrances, on paper provided at each table, to be put in an album for Barbara's family. This time was quiet, formal, and unhurried.

When the meal was ready, some of Barbara's friends from her tribe explained the meaning of the traditional foods that had been brought to the potluck by her own people. The most significant traditional foods were a berry soup and elk tongue, prepared with broth, flour, sugar, and berries and cooked with "lots of prayers and love." These foods were "spiritual foods," and some of the food from this meal were to be taken to Barbara's grave by one of her brothers. So attendees were admonished not to take too much: "As you share this food with Barbara, don't waste it." In this way, it was made clear that the potluck was a communion meal with the person who had died. Although the memorial service in a Catholic church had not been a Mass, this potluck was transformed into a communion meal that included everyone who attended— Christian, Jewish, Native American, or nonbelievers in any religious tradition.

Barbara's friends at the potluck also spoke about visiting her in the weeks before she died. One said, "Barbara said she was scared, and I said, 'You don't have to be scared. Just pray for us when you pass over to the other side.'" Then an elder of Barbara's tribe, a man of seventy years, offered a prayer with great dignity—first in their native tongue and then in English—and invited everyone to "join in the meal and celebrate the gift we have been given of Barbara's life." The elders of Barbara's tribe and family members who were present were then served first, and the guests lined up at the buffet table. Our field notes conclude with these observations:

The potluck had as much power as the Memorial Service—was it the quietness of those leading it, their dignity, calmness? Those leading it had a sense of certainty, an assurance that there is a spirit world whose barriers are very permeable, especially in the ancestral grounds where the bodies of the dead are buried. The meal seemed as sacred, and more "real," than the memorial service. Even the University Center ballroom, hardly a hallowed place, seemed to have become another world for these hours, to which we were most welcome guests, as her friends, colleagues, and acquaintances (field notes, December 6, 1997).

Symbolic Interactions as Memorials and Rituals in the Subculture of the Dying

These symbolic interactions and events—dinners and potlucks, a visit to the home place—met two needs of those still living. They symbolized the continuity of life for the deceased person, by affirming that something connected with them—spirit, memory, values—would continue after their death. In addition, the symbolic interactions at these memorial events, particularly through the sharing of food, visibly reconnected the community of mourners with each other and especially with the family that had suffered the loss.

Continuity

Traditional religious funeral rituals or memorial services seemed to have little meaning for some of our participants and/or their families. What did prove meaningful was making a time of remembrance for gathered family and friends into a more personal experience of honoring the person who had died. Thus, Walt's family chose to have no service of any kind; yet the family believed that "the spirit goes on," and their time of private interment together, as well as the open house later, was a witness to their shared belief in the continuity of his spirit.

Sandy and Ralph planned a traditional church service for his memorial, with favorite hymns, a harp solo by the hospice volunteer who had visited them for more than a year, and a sermon by the minister, who related Ralph's faith that God would find some good work for him when he died and went to heaven. The memorial service was not a time for family and friends to speak about Ralph and what he cared about most. But Sandy found a way to bring in Ralph's values and his commitment to his land and the Swan Valley by insisting that the Missoula visitors all come out to see the homestead after the service. This visit seemed to mark the ceremonial return of Ralph's spirit to his land, as well as an assurance to those who knew them only in Missoula that Sandy would be all right—that she also was home and taken care of. This visit was unexpectedly moving at the time—and more so in retrospect.

The memorial tables at the services for Roberta and Dennis also served as symbols of their lives. Through photographs of children and grandchildren and symbols of favorite sports, work, and activities, these tables witnessed the continuity between their lives, now ended physically, and the lives of their families and friends.

The symbolic events that most powerfully created continuity for participants were the Thanksgiving banquet for Sharon and the potluck for Barbara. Both brought together the communities they had loved and guided; both involved a kind of direct participation and communal sharing that is very different from passive attendance at a memorial service. The banquet and the potluck assured the communities left behind that the spirit and the values of the person who had died would endure.

Social Networks Restored: The Symbolic Importance of Food

All of the events that families chose or created served a second cultural function: restoring the social networks that had been broken by the illness and then death. Death threatens the social connections in families and close friends, and one of the greatest needs at this time is an assurance that the social network, having been interrupted, will be reconnected. In spirit, the deceased also remains a member of this network. The caregivers, family, and friends who are brought together physically in this last symbolic interaction can understand that the hiatus in their own network is now officially ended and the social life for those remaining can resume, however slowly.

Eating together, for those still living, may have been the most powerful symbolic act to the researchers as participant-observers, although other participants did not particularly note its significance. Eating together helps assure those who remain of their own continued physical life and symbolically memorializes the person who died. All of the memorial services or gatherings had food—ranging from an afternoon coffee and cookies (for Sarah, Walt, and Kitty) to the lengthy ceremonial potluck and Thanksgiving dinner for Barbara and Sharon. Just as persons who are dying experience a "falling out of culture," so the survivors' fear of death—of falling out of culture and social life—is overcome by placing the individual's death in a context that allows them to turn away from death toward continued life (Seale 1998, 81).

Reaffirming the social network was particularly important for Dennis's family. He chose social isolation for his last months of life and was joined by his mother, father, and brother in this isolation during his last months. To a lesser extent, such isolation also was true for Ralph, who was separated from family and friends by the need to be near medical treatment in Missoula.

For Kitty, who had no family of her own, a simple memorial service at her church and a social gathering with refreshments afterward in the parish hall next door demonstrated the continuing social connections in her church family that had always sustained her—and to which she had contributed so much during her life.

The families of Roberta, Walt, and Sharon remained more connected to their own lives and social networks through the dying process. Nevertheless, the families found the memorial times helpful; in Sharon's case, Connie invited friends to the Thanksgiving dinner who were elderly and had limited mobility. Their presence helped reaffirm the continuing social connection among their shared faith community. In Barbara's case, the ceremonial potluck brought together several disparate networks: her large extended family, the local Native American community, the university colleagues, and many in the larger Missoula area, creating a new, visible community network.

Chapter 12

Some Directions for Understanding the End of Life

In this book, we show how certain characteristics and benefits of mainstream culture are modified when a person is declared incurably ill. Power and control, individual dignity, economic security, social networks, comfort, mobility, continuity, hope, and meaning can be diminished. Strategies that the study participants used to find alternative ways of retaining control, dignity, meaning, and so forth—despite their membership in the subculture of the dying—have framed the substance of our findings. As the preceding chapters demonstrate, these people exhibited diverse pathways to death; they found alternative methods of preserving as much as they could of the benefits of mainstream culture.

We make no claim that the findings of this study are broadly generalizable—at least, not in the way more controlled research may claim. Qualitative research must always offer such caveats. The study does suggest some directions for future research, however, as well as implications for community efforts to improve life at its very end. Despite the study participants' diverse pathways, enough similarities remain to allow us, in this chapter, to make some generalizations and to speculate about possible steps that might be taken to improve the lives of terminally ill persons. We also discuss the kinds of general indicators that might be useful for communities in determining if persons with terminal illnesses are likely to have support and quality of life during their last months.

Discontinuity

No realization can be more stark and shocking than that a person's physical continuity is about to end. Once this information was absorbed, the dying people in this study tended to seek out alternative avenues—or take comfort from existing means—of familial or spiritual continuity to replace the physical continuity that soon would cease.

This context of the human need for connection and continuity helps explain the importance of the need for and emphasis on continuity of care. Changes in doctors (Barbara and Roberta), nurses (Dennis), housekeepers (Dennis), and places where participants lived (Sarah) brought turmoil to these patients. To avoid problems such as these, communities must discover ways to preserve as much continuity of care as is humanly possible during the final months of life.

Our study demonstrates that terminally ill persons seek a transcendent continuity in their lives—just as they did when they were full-fledged members of the culture of the healthy. Although most of these participants believed in a life after death, they displayed a strong sense that their personal continuity also embraced things such as their children, their land, their writings, their tools, and their love. These connections brought visible comfort and peace. One can envision programs that help patients as well as caregivers recognize—and celebrate—such evidences of continuity in the midst of imminent discontinuity. One method is the "legacy book" of participants' stories and philosophy that we provided for each patient and their family (see chapter 9).

Diminished Control

The study also highlights differences among terminally ill participants with respect to their need to cling to power and control at the very time that such control becomes increasingly difficult to maintain. This need was most evident in the younger participants, for whom the normal cycle of life had not yet been fulfilled.

Possibly as a result of this need to hang on to some sense of control, the younger participants required more information about their illness and treatment than did the older ones. An old adage tells us that knowledge is power. Moreover, according to some people, 95 percent of successful medical treatment grows directly out of successful communication between physician and patient. This assertion is just as applicable for communication between a family caregiver and patient. Not all caregivers know what to expect of the person they care for, from the early stages to the final signals of death. For some caregivers, hospice provided such knowledge. The contrast was notable, however, in the nonhospice contexts. On the basis of our findings from this study, we would argue that information about how death happens, stage by stage, must become more readily and fully available to families—especially to family caregivers. Our findings support the value of processes that provide patients and caregivers with "anticipatory guidance" (Battaglia and Carey 1999; Green 1999) as they go through the various stages of a terminal illness.

The impact of diminished control over daily activities seemed to be heightened in the males in our study. Even when they were bedridden, they tried desperately to get outside with regularity (and sometimes succeeded), whereas our female participants were more content to remain indoors. To the extent that this gender difference is generalizable, it suggests that communities could mobilize to take housebound male patients for walks, rides, or other appropriate excursions. The participants who had who spent their lives among trees and rivers wanted to continue to see trees and rivers. Those who spent their lives in construction wanted to continue to watch local buildings being built.

Our study highlights the problem of finding support groups to provide knowledge (and resulting power) for patients with certain kinds of illnesses, as well as for their children—and for male as well as female caregivers. Although such groups exist for specialized illnesses (such as breast cancer), caregivers in our study had difficulty finding value in such groups when their own loved one's illness was different (even a different form of cancer—such as cervical rather than breast cancer). The absence of local support groups for children of parents with incurable illnesses also became clear. One obvious suggestion is for communities to develop and maintain more diverse and specialized forms of support groups or to develop a means of matching caregivers of newly diagnosed patients with caregivers who have been through the same illness. Even if terminally ill patients do not want to know more about their illness and its expected trajectory, or are not mentally competent, most caregivers need and want this kind of specific information.

Immobility

The problems that patients had simply in arranging to be transported from place to place and the problems their families had in arranging to be near them in their last days also were apparent in this study. Walt, Ralph, Sharon, Roberta, Mabel, and Kitty and their caregivers all experienced various kinds of difficulties with transportation.

Mabel is a case study of various unmet needs: the need for mobility and transportation to access distant family members, the need for respite care for her sole caregiver, the need for compensations for her failing vision, and the need to maintain contact with her community and reduce her isolation. Mabel was acutely aware of the cost of losing her mobility; over and over again, she brought up the topic of how little she got to see her closest family. One daughter lived in a nearby state; the others were all relatively closer. Her only living sister, as well as her nieces, nephews, and grandson, all lived in Missoula or nearby. Mabel often recycled the topic of not being able to "get out to see" her sister's granddaughter in Stevensville—twenty minutes away from Missoula. Bernice's son had built a home in Missoula, but as Mabel lamented, "I've never seen it yet." Because of Mabel's limited mobility (she was essentially wheel-chair bound), Bernice reported that she had been able to take Mabel out of their apartment only two times during the previous year—both times to go to the doctor's office. This minimal escape from the isolation of home may have met Mabel's medical needs, but as Mabel's constant laments about not being able to see her family indicate, it did not come close to meeting her emotional and social needs.

What can we make of the issue of the decreased mobility of the terminally ill? One might envision, for example, considerably more effort on the part of the larger society in providing drivers—possibly volunteers—with wheelchair-accessible vans and arranging for adjacent family sleeping and visiting quarters for patients who are in long-term care settings. As another response to the social needs such transportation would be designed to meet, one might suggest that physicians make home visits; this strategy would be an alternative to the profound discomfort evidenced by our study participants in their efforts to get to their doctors' offices. Something clearly is wrong when people who are dying have to make accommodations to suit the ease and comfort of people who are well.

Diminishing Social Networks

Repeated visits to participants who clearly were experiencing frequent pain and discomfort underlines the fact that pain appears to be less prominent or ravishing when there are social activities, particularly interesting visitors or even telephone calls, to focus the attention of terminally ill persons—even in their last months or weeks of life. For example, during some of our visits with Mabel, her sister called to talk to her. Even though just moments earlier Mabel had been describing to the researcher her pain and other physical complaints—telling her "tales of woe"—her conversation on the telephone was lively and free of complaints about her physical state. This simple attention given by others, and the chance to interact and take care of someone else, takes away the awareness of pain, if not its reality. In our visits with other participants—particularly Ralph and his partner Sandy, and Dennis and his mother Carrie—we found the caregivers depicting the patients' pain in ways that did not match the way these patients interacted with us during our time with them.

The terminally ill participants in this study addressed the problem of a naturally decreasing sphere of social networks accompanying old age and terminal illness in different ways. Dennis chose to depend on his mother/caregiver for his sole social support. Others, such as Walt, Sharon, and Ralph, kept open-door homes, welcoming new as well as old friends. We conclude that different people have different needs, and there can be no best way for everyone.

Perhaps more than anything else, studying just this small sample of caregivers revealed that once a caregiver is "selected" or otherwise identified, the rest of the family tends to return to their everyday lives—leaving all the work and expense to the one "selected" for this task. When the terminal phases last more than a few weeks, the constant and demanding work of caregiving is not often visible to others—even to other family members. Our study raises the issue of potential caregiver burnout, as well as the issue of the far-too-common isolation of the designated caregiver from other family members who might well be expected to carry their fair share of the care and expense. One can envision a caring community making good use of caregivers who have gained experience and demonstrated admirable competence, to become informal "coaches" of those who are just entering new caregiver territory. Perhaps more important, one can envision some sort of orientation and monitoring for entire families, including family members who will not become the designated caregiver, as a way of protecting the caregiver from burnout.

Declining Economic Security

Our study also made clear the importance of long and short range planning at the time—as well as before—a patient enters the designation of terminally ill. Families that planned ahead together—such as the families of Ralph, Walt, Roberta, and Sharon—seemed to have fewer crises, disruptions, and financial burdens to bear. Other families, such as Sarah's, Barbara's, and, to some degree, Sharon's, expressed greater financial concerns and were not well-prepared for the costs of an extended period of illness and dying. In some of these families, as in many others, most of the financial burden (as well as the caregiving burden) fell on one caregiver—often the adult child who lived closest. Such difficulties may stem from lifelong family dynamics and personality differences, which is all the more reason for health care systems and communities to provide financial planning programs, case management, and models of how financial burdens can be shared equitably, suited to the needs of families or individuals who are at the beginning stage of the terminal illness.

Patient Choice for Comfort

Perhaps because our study population was overbalanced with dying participants who chose home health care (with hospice help) over institutionalized care, we found an abundance of positive reactions to professional health care. Being able to stay in one's own home clearly was the study participants' idea of comfort (at least, as much comfort as possible under the circumstances).

Staying at home puts obvious stress, however, on those who provide the care-giving and medical treatment. For caregivers, it means constant dedication as well as time, energy, resources, and physical space. For those who provide medical treatment, it means trying to provide service and constant monitoring that is as good as might be expected at a nursing home or hospital.

Clearly, although participants who chose to spend their time at home derived great comfort from this decision, the choice came with certain costs to their caregivers. With regard to the three major participants in the experience of dying—patient, caregiver, and medical provider—giving preference to the patient's choice seems most humane and logical. This choice, of course, may not favor the needs of the caregiver or of those providing medical treatment. Giving preference to the medical provider would suggest that the patient be housed in a medical facility. This approach, of course, does not favor the patient—or, to a lesser extent, the caregiver. Curiously enough, there appears to be no choice that gives the preference to the caregiver.

Physicians, nurses, and helpers of all types received high praise from partic-ipants and their caregivers. The patients apparently were satisfied that they had been made as physically comfortable as could be expected. Our nonmedical observations confirmed that an enormous effort was made to ensure patients' comfort. The comfort of the caregivers—at the dis-preferred end of the stress point triad (patient, caregiver, medical provider)—was a different story. They finished their work exhausted and deprived of any social life or activities out-side the home. Some even felt guilty for not having done their jobs even better.

Obviously, communities and systems could identify resources and mobi-lize services to provide caregivers with guidance for and respite from their all-consuming and constant tasks. Moreover, just as careful planning led to improvements in economic security, it also contributed to patient comfort—again, as illustrated most clearly by the cases of Ralph and Walt but also by those of Sharon and Roberta.

Diminished Hope

Expectation of a good that is yet to be is problematic, at best, in the subculture of the dying. The younger participants (Barbara and Dennis) still hoped for remission, for new and experimental treatments, at least until a month before their deaths. Such hope was not as evident in the older participants, either because they were more ready to die or because they could not absorb the idea well enough to become hopeful of being cured. Instead, they found hope in other ways—including the transcendent hope for life and continuing connec-tion beyond death. Our study makes very clear that there is no single pathway to spiritual satisfaction at or near the end of life. Even our very small sample of nine participants found meaning through a variety of pathways besides the conventional ones offered by organized religions. Communities that are interested in improving the quality of life at life's end might consider recognizing and supporting a diversity of spiritual pathways.

Loss of Personal Growth

Death, by one definition, is the absence of continued growth as an organism. When it became apparent to our participants and their caregivers that the end was near, all expectation of future external growth or change appeared to be denied. If there was to be any growth at all, it would have to be internal: intellectual, emotional, relational, or spiritual. Although most of the study participants did not report great epiphanies or transcendent experiences, they all manifested some aspects of growth in the sense of completing important developmental tasks, as suggested by Byock (1996).

One younger participant grew intellectually by acquiring an understanding of his rare disease. Young or old, most participants exhibited some evidence of continued emotional and spiritual development even as their ends grew near. This finding suggests that the larger community should come to the aid of persons who are terminally ill by helping them understand their remaining opportunities for growth and taking on the role of sharers of wisdom. For younger patients who want to continue to grow intellectually, the medical profession might consider their role to be teaching as well as healing. For older patients, concerted efforts by clergy, social workers, and psychologists might support dying as a time of continuous emotional, relational, and spiritual development.

Loss of Dignity

The self-respect and dignity of the terminally ill patients obviously are assaulted by the threat of loss of physical life. There can be little dignity in having to wear diapers, in being bedridden, in exhibiting ugly body sores, or in being dependent on the constant care of others. Yet in spite of such indignities, our study participants preserved a semblance of dignity, albeit in quite different ways. Roberta maintained her regal presence, dressed as she always had, and continued to be the family matriarch. Dennis and Barbara maintained their dignity of mental powers by controlling the selection of pain medication that would permit them to stay lucid. Curiously, perhaps, Kitty and Mabel kept a sense of dignity by ignoring or even denying the existence of their illnesses. Ralph, Sharon, Walt, and Sarah preserved their habitual kindness, sense of humor, and pleasant dispositions through everything—a dignity of the highest order. In these efforts, the participants were aided by families who treated them with unfailing respect and recognized that dignity is accorded by allowing persons to have choices—in small things, if larger choices are not possible.

Communities should recognize and honor the inherent personal dignity of persons who are about to leave us through death—perhaps through rituals or ceremonies not yet even conceived. Although it may always be easier to see dignity in cultures other than one's own, one could do worse than to examine how American Indians convey respect and dignity for the person dying throughout the process.

Some Indicators of Quality Care for Communities

Since the inception of the Missoula Demonstration Project, many communities around the nation have called and asked for help in beginning their own community-based programs of care for persons who are dying. Many communities may want to begin by assessing their current level of care and patient satisfaction; few will have the kind of external resources that MDP has had, however, to conduct direct studies among persons who are terminally ill. A reasonable question to ask is what kinds of general indicators might be most useful—but would be more economically and less intrusive to collect than the qualitative data we report here.

One purpose of qualitative research is to identify the kinds of data that might be of value in larger-scale studies. This study has identified several empirical variables that may be correlated with the quality of care, dying, and death and could be collected through straightforward surveys or from existing records. Finding and documenting such indicators for the terminally ill would be a major contribution to a community's knowledge of the quality of care and the quality of life for persons who are dying.

The objective or quantitative indicators associated with "dying well" in this study were as follows:

- The length of time that a terminally ill person had some kind of recognized palliative care that was directed at the patient's comfort, including pain management and symptom relief (in Missoula, such care was always hospice care)

- The number of family members/friends who were directly involved with caregiving weekly

- The existence of a plan for care that explicitly acknowledged the terminal nature of the illness and was known to family and friends.

Although most of our participating families were providing home care, these indicators also may be applicable to patients whose care is provided in institutional settings such as a hospice house, hospital, or nursing home. These indicators are not meant to be exhaustive; we hope that other studies will identify additional variables that can be readily gathered.

These variables are not causal. They all reflect attitudes and choices made by the person dying and the availability of resources in the community itself. These indicators are simply "markers" of quality. They enable us to identify in very rough terms the situations in which dying is likely to go well for the individual and the family, as well as situations in which it is less likely to do so, without having to call up the dying person to ask them about their subjective state of comfort and satisfaction.

The length of time that the patient receives palliative care reflects the patient's decision to choose palliative care (on their own or on the encouragement and recommendation of a physician). Having the support of hospice-like, assertive palliative care (i.e., a team that includes medical, social, and spiritual assistance; effective pain management; support for the caregiver at home; and so forth)—as soon as a terminal diagnosis was given—for more than a few weeks before death was one indicator of the quality of the end-of-life experience. (In Missoula in 1997, palliative care by definition was care from the Missoula hospice; in other settings, and in future years in Missoula, additional forms of palliative care may be available.)

The choice of palliative care early in the trajectory toward death may function as an indicator that the patient already has accomplished some developmental tasks, such as accepting the finality of one's life. Whatever the reason for choosing such care, the choice of palliative care months, rather than a week or two, before death allows the extra support services to make a difference for the patient and family. The length of time receiving palliative care also indicates that the physician is able or willing to tell the patient and family that the condition is terminal months rather than days before death.

In situations in which the physician does not give a terminal diagnosis or the patient and family do not accept the diagnosis until much later in the trajectory, there simply is no time to institute measures that would provide physical and emotional comfort, improved quality of life, and the opportunity for completion of relationships and connection.

The number of individuals involved in regular care on a weekly basis, which may include family members or a combination of family and friends, indicates the strength of the caregiving system. A solitary caregiver, no matter how dedicated, cannot manage end-of-life care for very long without risking the patient's care and comfort or the caregiver's own health. Not surprisingly, the emotional, physical, and financial well-being of our primary caregivers correlated with how much help they got from others in the family, including family members who came from out of state to provide respite for a weekend on a regular basis and participated in care planning. In Ralph's situation, few family members were available, so Sandy simply recruited new acquaintances and extra hospice volunteers into an effective caregiving system. By contrast, Carrie tried to "do it all" for Dennis in a more isolated, rural area; as a result, Dennis had emotional difficulties at the end of life and a less satisfactory/ comfortable experience. Clearly, one caregiver should not try twenty-four-hour nursing care for months on end. Caregivers and those who work with them need to recognize the cumulative effects of a year or more of caregiving for someone who is dying, sometimes after years of caring for that person with a chronic illness.

The existence of an advanced care plan is defined by whether the patient, the family, and physicians or health care professionals have worked through a plan for the patient's care up to and including the patient's death. This plan need not always be written, but it requires something more than the patient's wish or demand (i.e., "I just want to stay at home") and more than a DNR order or living will—which are too limited for most end-of-life scenarios and leave out the family/caregiver role.

Part of a plan of care, given current medical interventions, should be a DPOA for health care. The DPOA allows a family member or trusted friend to act for the dying person during his or her last weeks of life. Modern medical care ensures that many individuals will experience an extended length of time when the body remains alive but mental cognizance and decision-making powers are diminished greatly. At this point, decisions will have to be made by someone else. As Roberta's case shows, the best plans to "keep Mom at home" cannot take into account all possible circumstances.

Table 12-1 lists the participants in this study along a continuum, from those with all three indicators of quality to those with the fewest. The ratings reflect the researchers' judgment, based on the accounts of patients and caregivers; they are intended to be suggestive of how other communities might look at their own end-of-life care, using more readily available data.

Looking at this array in relation to all that we learned about the study participants' end-of-life experience, the more objective or factual indicators appear to be correlated with study data that directly assess the quality of life and care for participants—in terms of their medical care, emotional and social outcomes, spiritual growth and meaning, caregiver stress, and caregiver experience of loss and grief after the patient's death as either natural and even healing or unresolved and devastating.

All three indicators may be important for a "good" outcome for the patient and the family/caregiver. Having only one—hospice care, a strong family team, or a plan—was not sufficient for the participants we studied. The families who perceived themselves as doing best—whom we also saw as coping well and even growing during this time, with less stress than others—had formed teams of family and friends to provide adequate help. And simply having a team of home caregivers was not sufficient; home caregivers needed weekly coaching and support from hospice's palliative care specialists in order to manage the physical, emotional, and spiritual demands of end-of-life care.

Table 12-1   Indicators of Quality of Care at the End of Life

Participant	Length of time in hospice care	Ratio of actual to potential family members giving care weekly	Advance care plan mutually agreed by patient and family	Rating of quality of care, dying, and death[a]
Walt	13 months	5 of 5	Yes	+ +
Ralph	16 months	1 of 1	Yes	+ +
Sharon	5 months	4 of 4	Yes	+ +
Roberta	6 months	4 of 6	Yes	+ +
Sarah	4 months	1 of 3	Yes	+
Dennis	0	1 of 4	No	+ −
Barbara	4 days	1 of 3	No	−
Kitty	7 months	no family	No	−
Mabel	18 months	1 of 3–4	Yes	−

[a]The ratings are as follows:

+ +   very good, from both dying person and caregiver perspectives

+   good, reflecting some caregiver distress but high patient satisfaction

+ −   mixed experience on part of both patient and caregiver

−   less than desirable from patient/caregiver's perspective

Both of these criteria seemed to be present in families that had had open discussions about planning for end-of-life care, with patient, spouse, and/or children all participating, well before the arrival of a terminal diagnosis.

Value of Study Experience to Ethnographic Researchers

Finally, we confess that we had a unique opportunity to see with the eyes of outsiders. When we have described our research to friends, the most common observation they have made to us has been, "It must be depressing to have to visit with dying people." We admit that we were a bit frightened during our first such visit; widely held stereotypes penetrate to all levels of society—even to us. We immediately realized, however, that this study was a special gift to us: a gift that energized us, taught us, and prepared us to face a similar future phase of our own lives.

Becoming friends with these participants was amazingly easy, which made our research goal of conversations, rather than interviews, a relatively simple task to accomplish. We attended the memorial services of those who died not as researchers but as bereaved friends of the family. On the basis of our experience, we believe that the community can demystify, even encourage, and then train lay persons to make regular visits to dying people. Such visits are not merely good deeds done for others. They can be integral parts of the continuous personal growth of the visitors themselves, as they were for us.

References

Ainsworth-Vaughn, N. 1998. *Claiming power in doctor-patient talk.* New York: Oxford Press.

Albert, S. M. 1990. The Dependent Elderly, Home Health Care, and Strategies of Household Adaptation. In *The home care experience,* edited by J. F. Gubrium and A. Sankar. Newbury Park, Calif.: Sage.

American Health Decisions. 1997. *The quest to die with dignity: An analysis of Americans' values, opinions and attitudes concerning end-of-life care.* Appleton, Wisc.: American Health Decisions.

Arno, P. S., C. Levine, and M. M. Memmot. 1999. The economic value of informal caregiving. *Health Affairs* 18, no. 2: 182–88.

Battaglia, A., and J. C. Carey. 1999. Health supervision and anticipatory guidance of individuals with Wolf-Hirschhorn syndrome. *American Journal of Medical Genetics.* 89, no. 2: 111–15.

Bernabei, R., G. Gambassi, K. Lapane, F. Landi, C. Gatsonis, R. Dunlop, L. Lipsitz, K. Steel, and V. Mor. 1998. Management of pain in elderly patients with cancer. *Journal of the American Medical Association* 279, no. 23: 1877–82.

Blandford, P. and Byock, I. 1999. *The demographics of death a rural western town: Contextualizing public data in preparation for a longitudinal community study of life's end.* Missoula, MT: Missoula Demonstration Project Working Paper.

Bluebond-Langner, M. 1996. *In the shadow of illness: Parents and siblings of the chronically ill child.* Princeton, N.J.: Princeton University Press.

Blumer, H. 1969. *Symbolic interactionism.* Englewood Cliffs, N.J.: Prentice-Hall.

Breitbart, W., B. D. Rosenfeld, and S. D. Passik. 1996. The undertreatment of pain in ambulatory AIDS patients. *Pain* 65: 243–49.

Byock, I. 1996. The nature of suffering and the nature of opportunity at the end of life. *Clinics in Geriatric Medicine* 12, no. 2: 237–52.

Caralis, P. V., B. Davis, K. Wright, and E. Marcial. 1993. The influence of ethnicity and race on the attitudes toward advance directives, life-prolonging treatments, and euthanasia. *Journal of Clinical Ethics* 4, no. 2: 155–65.

Cleeland, C. S., R. Gonin, and A. K. Hatfield. 1994. Pain and its treatment in outpatients with metastatic cancer. *New England Journal of Medicine*. 330, no. 9: 592–96.

Cleeland, C. S., R. Gonin, L. Baez, P. Loehrer, and K. J. Pandya. 1997. Pain and treatment of pain in minority patients with cancer: The Eastern Cooperative Oncology Group Minority Outpatient Pain Study. *Annals of Internal Medicine* 127, no. 9: 813–16.

Covinsky, K., L. Goldman, E. Cook, R. Oye, N. Desbiens, D. Reding, W. Fulkerson, A. Connors, J. Lynn, and R. Phillips. 1994. The impact of serious illness on patients' families. *Journal of the American Medical Association* 272, no. 23, 1839–44.

Danis, M., E. Mutran, J. Garrett, S. Stearns, R. Slifkin, L. Hanson, J. Williams, and L. Churchill. 1996. A prospective study of the impact of patient preferences on life-sustaining treatment and hospital cost. *Critical Care Medicine* 24, no. 11, 1811–17.

Davies, B., J. C. Reimer, P. Brown, and N. Martens. 1995. *Fading away: The experience of transition in families with terminal illness*. Amityville, N.Y.: Baywood Publishing.

Emanuel, E. J., D. L. Fairclough, J. Slutsman, H. Alpert, D. Baldwin, and L. L. Emanuel. 1999. Assistance from family members, friends, paid care givers, and volunteers in the care of terminally ill patients. *New England Journal of Medicine* 341, no. 13, 956–63.

Field, M. J. and C. K. Cassel, eds. 1997. *Approaching death: Improving care at the end of life*. Institute of Medicine, Committee on Care at the End of Life. Washington, D.C.: National Academy Press.

Fox, E., K. Landrum-McNiff, Z. Zhong, N. V. Dawson, A. W. Wu, J. Lynn (for the SUPPORT investigators). 1999. Evaluation of prognostic criteria for determining hospice eligibility in patients with advanced lung, heart or liver disease. *Journal of the American Medical Association* 282: 1638–45.

Frake, C. O. 1977. Plying frames can be dangerous: Some reflections on methodology in cognitive anthropology. *Quarterly Newsletter of the Institute for Comparative Human Development* 1, no. 3, 1–7.

Frank, A. W. 1995. *The wounded storyteller*. Chicago: University of Chicago Press.

Gallup International Institute. 1997. *Spiritual beliefs and the dying process: A report on a national survey* (conducted for Nathan Cummings Foundation). Princeton, N.J.: Gallup International Institute.

Glaser, B. G., and A. L. Strauss. 1964. Awareness contexts and social interactions. *American Sociological Review* 29: 669–79.

———. 1965. *Awareness of Dying*. Chicago: Aldine.

Green, K. 1999. Treatment strategies for adolescents with hemophilia: Opportunities to enhance development. *Adolescent Medicine* 10: 369–76.

Greenwald, M. 2000. *Voices of women: Perceptions and planning for long term care focus groups*. Executive Summary, prepared for U.S. Administration on Aging, U.S. Department of Health and Human Services. Washington, D.C.: Administration on Aging.

Gresham, G. E., M. Kelly-Hayes, P. A. Wolf, A. S. Beiser, C. S. Kase, and R. B. D'Agostino. 1998. Survival and functional status 20 or more years after first stroke: The Framingham Study. *Stroke* 29: 793–97.

Hanson, L. C., J. A. Earp, J. Garrett, M. Menon, and M. Danis. 1999. Community physicians who provide terminal care. *Archives of Internal Medicine* 159: 1133–38.

Harris, M. 1968. *The Rise of Anthropological Theory.* New York: Crowell.

Hines, S. C., J. J. Glover, J. L. Holley, A. S. Babrow, L. A. Badzek, and A. H. Moss. 1999. Dialysis patients' preferences for family-based advance care planning. *Annals of Internal Medicine* 130, no. 10: 825–28.

Hofmann, J. C. 1997. Patient preferences for communication with physicians about end-of-life decisions. *Annals of Internal Medicine* 127, no. 1: 1–11.

Kelly, M. M., and D. P. Corriveau. 1985. The Corriveau-Kelly death anxiety scale. *Omega* 31, no. 4: 311–15.

Knaus, W. A., J. Lynn, and J. Teno. 1995. A controlled trial to improve care for seriously ill hospitalized patients. *Journal of the American Medical Association* 274, no. 20: 1591–98.

Levine, C. 1999. The loneliness of the long-term care giver. *New England Journal of Medicine* 340, no. 20: 1587–90.

Malinowski, B. 1922. *Argonauts of the western Pacific.* London: Routledge.

McAdams, D. P. 1993. *The stories we live by: Personal myths and the making of the self.* New York: Morrow.

Mayer, D., L. Torma, K. Norris, and I. Byock. Forthcoming. Factor analysis of public knowledge and attitudes toward pain and pain management: Identifying targets for a community-based educational program. *American Journal of Nursing.*

Meshefedjian, G., J. McCusker, F. Bellavance, and M. Baumgarten. 1998. Factors associated with symptoms of depression among informal caregivers of demented elders in the community. *Gerontologist* 38, no. 2, 247–53.

National Alliance for Caregiving (NAC) and American Association of Retired Persons (AARP). 1997. *Family caregiving in the U.S.: Findings from a national survey.* Washington, D.C.: AARP.

Nuland, S. B. 1993. *How we die.* New York: Vintage Books, Random House.

Pound, L. 1936. American euphemisms for dying, death, and burial. *American Speech* (October).

Schulz, R., and M. T. Rau. 1985. Social support through the life course. In *Social support and health,* edited by S. Cohen and S. L. Syme. Orlando, Fla.: Academic Press.

Schulz, R., A. T. O'Brien, J. Bookwala, and K. Fleissner. 1995. Psychiatric and physical morbidity effects of demential caregiving: Prevalence, correlates and causes. *Gerontologist* 35, no. 6: 771–91.

Seale, C. F. 1998. *Constructing death: The sociology of dying and bereavement.* Cambridge: Cambridge University Press.

Seale, C. F., and J. Addington-Hall. 1994. Euthanasia: Why people want to die. *Social Science and Medicine* 40, no. 5: 581–87.

Silverman, P. R. 1999. *Never too young to know: Death in children's lives.* New York: Oxford University Press.

Silverman, M., and E. Huelsman. 1990. The dynamics of long-term familial caregiving. In *The home care experience*, edited by J. F. Gubrium and A. Sankar. Newbury Park, Calif.: Sage.

Spradley, J. P. 1979. *The ethnographic interview.* New York: Holt, Rinehart & Winston.

Staton, J., and R. Shuy. 1998. *Participants' perspectives on end-of-life care.* Report for Missoula Demonstration Project. Missoula, Mont.: Missoula Demonstration Project.

Stone, R. 1996. *The healing art of storytelling: A sacred journey of personal discovery.* New York: Hyperion.

Stuart, B., C. Alexander, C. Arenella, B. Kinszbrunner, R. Rousseau, M. Wohlfeiler, L. Herbst, D. Jones, S. Connor, T. Ryndes, C. Cody, and S. Buckley (Medical Guidelines Task Force, Standards, and Accreditation Committee). 1996. *Medical guidelines for determining prognosis in selected non-cancer diseases.* Alexandria, Va.: National Hospice and Palliative Care Organization.

Thomas, W. H. 1996. *Life worth living: How someone you love can still enjoy life in a nursing home.* Acton, Mass.: VanderWyk & Burnham.

Todd, K. H, N. Samaroo, and J. Hoffman. 1993. Ethnicity as a risk factor for inadequate emergency department analgesia. *Journal of the American Medical Association* 269: 1537–39.

Torma, L. 1999. Pain—the fifth vital sign. *Montana Nurses Association Pulse* 2: 16–17.

Trankel, M., and C. H. Asp. 1998. Community Survey on Death and Dying. Report for Missoula Demonstration Project.

Voelker, R. 1998. Two generations of data aid Framingham's focus on genes. *Journal of the American Medical Association* 279: 1245–46.

Wilson, P. W. F., R. B. D'Agostino, D. Levy, A. M. Belanger, H. Silbershatz, and W. B. Kannel. 1998. Prediction of coronary heart disease using risk factor categories. *Circulation* 97: 1837–47.

Contributors

Jana J. Staton, Ph.D., is a psychologist, educational researcher, and family therapist who works as a consultant on family and social programs for the state of Montana and the Missoula community. She has conducted research with grants from the National Institute of Education, Gallaudet University, and the U.S. Department of Education. She also was Director of Education for the American Association for Marriage and Family Therapy Foundation, where she developed a videotape-based training program for other professions that focused on communicating with families.

Roger W. Shuy, Ph.D., is a sociolinguist and distinguished research professor of linguistics emeritus at Georgetown University who now writes and consults out of his office in Montana. He has conducted research and program studies with grants from the National Science Foundation, the National Institute of Mental Health, the Ford Foundation, the Carnegie Corporation of New York, and the U.S. Department of Education. He is a co-founder and past president of the American Association of Applied Linguistics. His research and publications are in sociolinguistics, forensic linguistics, and applied linguistics.

Ira Byock, M.D., is a research professor in the department of philosophy and faculty member in the Practical Ethics Center at the University of Montana. He is a co-founder and principal investigator of the Missoula Demonstration Project, a community-based organization that is dedicated to the research and transformation of end-of-life experience locally, as a demonstration of what is possible nationally. He also is Director of the Palliative Care Service in Missoula. Dr. Byock serves as director for the Robert Wood Johnson Foundation national grant program, Promoting Excellence in End-of-Life Care, with offices at the University of Montana. He has published widely in the field of palliative care, with particular focus on the ethics of end-of-life care. His book, *Dying Well: The Prospect for Growth at the End of Life,* was published by Riverhead/Putnam in 1997. He also serves on the editorial boards of several professional publications, including the *Journal of Palliative Medicine.* His research interests include assessment of the subjective quality of life of people living with advanced, incurable illness and development of evidence-based, community models for caregiving, dying, and grieving.

The Missoula Demonstration Project Baseline Research

This appendix addresses the larger context for *A Few Months to Live*. This book is only a small part of the research and community service being carried out within the Missoula Demonstration Project (MDP).

Typically, clinical and sociological studies—including most end-of-life studies—have discrete, carefully defined boundaries. Standard research methodology dictates that questions to be studied should be carefully and prospectively defined. The research questions determine the types, quantities, and modes of data collection employed. Research findings are then reported in terms of facts and figures, in written articles with graphs, charts, and illustrations. This approach is a relatively confined means of conveying research results; it tends to omit the difficult question of larger community and cultural effects.

Attempting to describe something as broad as "society's approach to life's end" is tricky at best. Society is not a single, static entity. The dominant cultures and prominent subcultures provide for rich variations of attitude, values, and customs. Societies and communities have structural components, in the form of resources and services, processes ("the way things are done"), and formal and informal modes of social behavior. Consequently, communities and cultures are dynamic, complex, and constantly changing.

To capture the multitude of levels and the complexity of these interactions, one would need a three-dimensional hologram of an entire living community. Thinking about what movies are and can do—and giving our imagination free rein—we can envision what an ideal way of collecting data and reporting research might look like. Indeed, although the concept is far-fetched and financially out of reach, the technology of film offers a powerful analogy to explain the overarching design of the MDP's baseline, descriptive research.

How better to document and describe a society's, community's, and culture's attitudes, beliefs, customs, and ways of acting toward one another? With an unlimited amount of funds and expertise, we could create a series of films—each shot with lenses, filters, camera angles, film speeds, and exposures carefully chosen to fit the specific aspect of personal or community life under study.

A holographic cinema of this sort could provide sociologists and anthropologists with a powerful tool for studying and conveying the subjective experience of human beings. Much more of the tone and texture of a person's experience would be discernible through this medium. Editing options would enable an individualized "cut" of a holographic movie, based on the viewer's main interest. An ethicist might choose to see a version in which proportionately more time and attention was paid to communication between doctor and patient; a sociologist might select a version that emphasized family caregiving; a theologian would be particularly interested in issues of meaning and in whether and how spirituality was a source of strength or distress.

For the moment, at least, this all-encompassing, multidimensional holography-in-motion will remain in the realm of science fiction. The analogy remains conceptually valuable, however, as an idealized model for the MDP's descriptive research. In fact, we often have referred to the collective baseline research as a "high-definition snapshot" of life's end. That snapshot is the Community Profile. The Community Profile comprises twelve distinct studies, most of which have multiple components. Although the Community Profile is not a hologram, its component studies illuminate a wide range of aspects and perspectives, resulting in a picture that has depth and breadth. It can be viewed from a number of angles, each one contributing to a fuller understanding of the whole.

The Community Profile: The MDP's Baseline Research

The cross-sectional studies in the Community Profile focus on a period preceding any significant impact from the MDP's community engagement efforts. Five studies form the core of the Community Profile: the network and systems analysis, the community survey, the clinical experience study, the bereavement study, and the participants' perspectives on end-of-life care.

The network and systems analysis study is analogous to the view from 30,000 feet. It is an "environmental scan" that discerns the community's demographics and structural components that are relevant to end-of-life experience and care. The study describes the number and size of health care institutions and their relationships to one another, studied local funeral homes' patterns of practice, and explored how "connected" the providers of care perceived themselves to be to each other.

From the same height, but using a detailed mailed survey as a special filter to reveal the psychosocial landscape, the community survey on death and dying assesses prevailing attitudes, expectations, hopes, and fears of Missoula's population with regard to dying, death, caregiving, and grief. The same survey has been used in two demographically similar comparison communities in America's northwest.

Switching to "telephoto" and "macro" lenses of medical chart reviews and detailed, structured, family after-death interviews provided a close-up view of the medical experience of patients who died during 1996 and 1997. The clinical experience study employed a retrospective (after-death) design and drew from a sample from all 1996 and 1997 deaths in Missoula County. The MDP research team chose these years to avoid potential data contamination from MDP advocacy or community engagement intervention work that began in late 1997. The clinical experience study includes an after-death interview of a family member, a medical chart review, and a survey of the attending physician for each patient. This study has resulted in a wealth of interview data on 252 Missoula subjects; with the collaboration of all of the health care agencies in Missoula, the research team obtained medical chart data on the last year of life for 207 subjects. The data currently are being analyzed, and a report is being prepared.

Another change in lens "filters" represented by semi-structured interviews with family members in grief enabled the bereavement study to develop. Through qualitative analysis of transcribed responses to this open-ended interview format, this study documents the effects of a recent death on family members from their own perspective.

The fifth major baseline study initiated in 1997 was the participants' perspectives on end-of-life care (Staton and Shuy 1998). Drawing from a set of terminally ill persons who participated in an early pilot version of the clinical experience study, the participants' perspectives research offers an in-depth exploration of their experience with advanced illness and caregiving. This study, funded primarily by the Kornfeld Foundation, forms the basis for *A Few Months to Live*.

In addition to these core components of the Community Profile, targeted surveys have been conducted of physicians, nurses, faith community leaders, and focus groups, encompassing the full range of caring professions and people from all walks of life. These surveys contribute to the fullness of the Community Profile. When the Community Profile is complete, it will contain a richness of depth, complexity, and multidimensionality that will approach the idealized motion holograph.

The preliminary findings of the Community Profile are not surprising. The many problems associated with dying in America are present in Missoula as well: challenges of pain management, inconsistent respect for peoples' preferences for care, breakdowns in clinician-patient communication, financial stress, insufficient support for family caregivers, feelings of isolation and loneliness. Many Missoulians have little or no experience discussing death at home; more than half of the people surveyed said they rarely or never talked about death within their families while they were growing up (Trankel and Asp 1998).

Preliminary results from the Community Profile suggest that the quality of medical care at the end of life may be somewhat better in Missoula than nationally, at least in terms of communication with physicians and nurses and the treatment of pain. Missoula is no utopia, however. Health care for people with advanced illness remains fragmented and often poorly planned. Each ill patient and family has a sense of having to discover for themselves what services exist, and they often must struggle to obtain the help they need.

Indeed, in the picture that is developing from the Community Profile, Missoula looks more like the rest of America than different. The MDP has found—consistent with yet-to-be published national research—that most Missoulians want to die at home, although only a third of local residents actually do. We expect our families to care for us when we are dying, yet few of us have told our families what we would want, and fewer still have completed formal advance directive documents. Most of us are afraid of dying in pain, yet we are hesitant to take pain medication. Many of us (health care professionals and nonprofessionals alike) have misconceptions about pain medication: when analgesics should be used, side effects, development of tolerance, and risks of addiction—all of which are crucial elements in the quality of the dying experience (Mayer et al. 2000).

Like the personal experiences of dying, caregiving, and grieving that the MDP seeks to study, the MDP's research takes place in the real world. The best that the MDP can hope to do is to develop a picture that fairly represents the events and experiences on which it has focused, with a field of view that contains all relevant perspectives. In developing this snapshot, we are striving to present our findings in a straightforward, unbiased manner. If we are successful, the completed Community Profile will provide a clear overview of the topics and enable students, clinical colleagues, and researchers who require higher definition to focus on specific parts of the picture and find the information they need contained within.

Unlike movies, an obvious limitation of snapshots is that they represent a single point in time. In this case, that "point" is the years 1996–98. A longitudinal study would have been optimal; given the subject of dying and end-of-life care, however, such a study was not feasible. Dying persons die, and although families at times feel that caregiving responsibilities are endless, ultimately caregiving too comes to an end. The MDP plans a series of cross-sectional studies at roughly five-year intervals—approximating a longitudinal study. These studies will repeat key components of the Community Profile, documenting clinical, social, and cultural change—or lack of change—over time.

Continuous Quality Improvement in the Missoula Community

As extensive as its research efforts are, the MDP is more than a laboratory. The MDP seeks to engage multiple aspects of the community in ongoing efforts to improve the quality of life for dying persons and their families. A primary focus is improvement in professional and informal care. The MDP also seeks to foster new, culturally relevant ways of honoring the poignant, highly vulnerable, and tender time that surrounds life's end. All of these initiatives will be informed by evidence drawn from the Community Profile and related studies.

Over the next decade or more, the MDP will use its research findings to spark community forums, ongoing discussions, and programs of care that focus on how Missoula as a community can make things better. The MDP's strategy is not to impose a specific vision or set of values but to involve people throughout the community in defining what success would look like and working together to achieve it. This effort already involves the two local hospitals and every nursing home and home health provider in Missoula as active participants, along with many of Missoula's doctors and nurses, health care aides, social workers, and emergency medical technicians. In addition to health care professionals, the MDP's work involves ministers, faith community members, artists, writers, educators, and everyday people who are simply interested in becoming directly involved in end-of-life care.

The community engagement process already has yielded tangible results: The MDP's Pain Task Force has conducted conferences and workshops in which hundreds of area doctors, nurses, and pharmacists improved their knowledge and skills in pain control. State-of-the-art pain assessment tools and treatment protocols are now available in every health care setting in Missoula. St. Patrick Hospital recently added pain as a fifth "vital sign" (along with temperature, blood pressure, pulse, and respiration) to its computerized clinical flow sheets (Torma 1999). Similar efforts are underway in other health care settings. The Advance Care Planning Task Force developed "My Choices," a user-friendly form that combines a living will and a power of attorney for health care. Every local health care organization has endorsed its use—making Missoula the first city to have a consistent, community-wide document for communicating preferences regarding care.

The MDP's efforts go beyond issues regarding the direct provision of health care. The Faith Community Task Force is helping to expand the capacity of local ministers and congregations to support members who are confronting life's end and family members who are struggling to provide care. The MDP has convened conferences that have brought faith community leaders together for collaborative, in-depth exploration of these issues. The MDP's Life Stories Task Force has successfully raised local awareness of the precious nature of our collective memories. The task force was so successful, in fact, that a separate nonprofit community organization—Story Keepers, Inc.—has emerged to continue this nurturing work. As this book goes to press, plans are proceeding actively for new research initiatives, new task forces that focus on family caregiving and classroom education, and new avenues for volunteer training and services to local families.

The goal of the MDP's community initiatives is to build a community that accepts and integrates dying, grieving, and caregiving within the normal fabric of life. During an early strategic planning retreat, one MDP board member suggested that success for the MDP would be exemplified by a teenager on his way home from school who stops to check on the frail, elderly lady next door—not because someone told him to do so but because not doing so would feel unnatural. This criterion sets a high bar, but it reflects precisely the sort of cultural awareness and change in normative behaviors and social habits that we hope to achieve.

Particularity of place is an inherent limitation of the MDP's research and community innovations. Missoula is not a paradigm for all of America. No claims can be made that the information we derive, or the lessons we learn, will be directly applicable to communities elsewhere. In important ways, however, Missoula is typical of many American communities. The salient strengths and weaknesses of the American health care system are reflected in the experience of clinicians, patients, and families in Missoula. Missoula's culture is fairly homogeneous. The population is largely white, Anglo-Saxon, and Christian, although a close inspection reveals a diversity of ethnic, religious, and socioeconomic subcultures. Although current research documents important differences among religious and ethnic cultural approaches to death and dying, it also suggests that the subcultures are much more alike than they are different (Caralis et al. 1993; American Health Decisions 1997).

Across the spectrum of race, religion, and socioeconomic status, we all want ourselves and our loved ones to be well-treated for illness and comfort; to be cared for in a dignified manner; not to be abandoned; to be at home as long as practically possible; and to avoid being a physical, emotional, or financial burden to others (American Health Decisions 1997). Therefore, what the MDP learns about the things people value and experience as helpful or harmful in Missoula is likely to have relevance to others, if only as a point of departure for their own investigations and quality improvement efforts.

The Missoula Demonstration Project's research and community engagement activities reflect a commitment to act locally while integrating local and national perspectives. The MDP's efforts have importance far beyond the five valleys that make up Missoula County. The work already has attracted the attention of national media, leading foundations, academic institutions, and policymakers in Washington, D.C. The MDP has received numerous inquiries from community groups around the country seeking to replicate one or more aspects of Missoula's efforts. Researchers from a variety of institutions and distant states are using MDP surveys and data collection instruments and are contributing data for expanded comparative studies.

As baby boomers age and the number of people living with chronic illness or advanced old age soars, issues regarding dying and caring for those who are dying will remain at the forefront of our national priorities. Missoula's citizens have an opportunity to serve our nation simply by caring for one another locally in ways that combine medical excellence with compassionate and genuinely tender, loving care. We can build creative community models that ensure that people are comfortable and feel wanted, worthy, and dignified as they die.

Research Methodology for Studying Participants' Perspectives on the End of Life

This appendix describes the research methodology undergirding the findings presented in this book, including how participants were selected and how data were collected and analyzed. The fieldwork on which this book is based was carried out by Jana Staton and Roger Shuy. The third co-author, Ira Byock, also knew or had treated over half of the nine participants in his role as a hospice physician. The design of the study was a collaborative effort on the part of the three authors and other members of MDP's Research Committee at the time of its inception in 1997. Analysis of the transcripts and notes was conducted by Staton and Shuy.

Selection of Participants from Missoula

The population from which participants were selected included persons who were residents of Missoula County in 1997 or were receiving all of their medical care from Missoula health care facilities, even though they resided in nearby counties. A brief profile of Missoula's population, causes of illness, and death pathways provides a context for understanding the lives and deaths of the participants who became part of this study.

Missoula County's population is about 87,000 (1995 census estimate). About 8,900 (a little more than 10 percent) are over 65 years of age. In 1996—the last year for which we have complete statistics—555 deaths occurred among Missoula County residents, including sudden accidents and other illnesses for which the designation of "terminal" was never made. Excluding accidents and suicides, which average 10 percent of all deaths in Missoula each year, there are about 500 deaths from all kinds of illnesses—including, of course, those who die of old age, whatever their particular symptoms. Heart disease and stroke are the leading identified causes of death in Missoula, as elsewhere in the United States. Other common causes are cancers of all kinds and chronic obstructive pulmonary diseases (COPDs) such as emphysema. In the Missoula County statistics, about 100 deaths (20 percent of nonaccidental deaths) do not have a specific disease listed. These deaths appear to be attributed by attending physicians to the "natural causes" of old age.

The places where people live and die during their final days in Missoula are now fairly evenly distributed among hospitals (28 percent), home (28 percent), and nursing homes (27.5 percent); 10 percent of the deaths are reported as emergency room deaths or DOAs (roughly corresponding to the number of suicides and accidents), and an additional 6 percent are listed as "other."

The Missoula hospice program has been established for more than 20 years and now serves about 150 patients a year from Missoula County, many of them at home. The median length of service for hospice in the large sample from 1996 and 1997 in the MDP Clinical Experience Study was 52 days, whether at home or in the eight-bed Hospice House. Although this median length of service is three times the national length of service for hospice, it still reflects a pattern of patients and families choosing or being referred to hospice only days or weeks before death, even though hospice care is available and covered by Medicare or private insurance up to six months prior to death.

The MDP is particularly interested in the majority of this population who have (or whose family members have) some knowledge of their impending deaths and whose care, comfort, and personal experience might be affected by the community initiatives anticipated during the fifteen-year demonstration period. For the purposes of the Community Profile baseline research, we chose to study people with the most common terminal illnesses in Missoula: heart disease, cancer, and COPD. We excluded children and those whose deaths are either accidental or, if life-threatening, more likely to be treated at large medical centers in the larger cities of the Northwest.

The baseline research requirement that this study be completed before any interventions or community programs were initiated as a result of the MDP's efforts created certain compelling limitations. The research itself was bound by a one-year time period, during which time terminally ill persons had to be located and visited over the remainder of their lives—generally between three and six months.

How We Selected People to Participate

To identify Missoulians who were terminally ill, we systematically sought them out as follows. Potential participants were drawn from the larger sample of patients enrolled in the Pilot Clinical Profile of the MDP during a four-month period in 1997 (May through August). That sample came from referrals by physicians and health care institutions, including nursing homes, of patients in their care who were designated as terminally ill in accordance with the National Hospice Organization's General Guidelines for Determining Prognosis (Stuart et al. 1996). One of the consequences of asking physicians for referrals of patients who were "terminally ill" is that it excluded all patients who had thus far in their illness refused, or whose physicians refused, to accept this categorization.

The total number enrolled by the foregoing procedures during the four-month study Pilot Clinical Profile study was 102. To be referred on to our study, people had to be conscious and coherent enough to engage in some conversation, and they had to consent to participate. This requirement eliminated 19 of the 102 enrollees—because of closeness to death, dementia, and so forth (including almost all nursing home residents). An additional 58 of those enrolled in the Clinical Profile died within two weeks of enrollment, before we could contact them or their families. Eleven declined to participate in the initial Clinical Profile study, eliminating them effectively from the pool available to us. The pool of prospective participants available for this study, in short, was 14 of the original 102. Those 14 were asked by the Clinical Profile researcher if a different team of researchers could contact them to invite their participation in an ongoing, prospective research project, with the understanding that they could refuse consent after learning more about it.

In accordance with the protocol approved by the Missoula Joint Institutional Review Board, the research team sent an introductory letter and consent form to those referred from the Clinical Profile, then telephoned prospective participants or their caregivers to set up a preliminary meeting. During the preliminary meeting, the purpose and methods of the study were presented. In addition, a written consent form (included at the end of this Appendix) was given to prospective participants and caregivers. The consent form reiterated what the research team told them about the study's purpose, potential benefits, and assurances of confidentiality. The participants and the researchers then signed the consent form, and the researchers left a copy for the participants. Once agreement was secured, we sent each of the participants' physicians a letter explaining the study and indicating that their patients were willing to participate.

Two older males declined to be involved at all after we contacted them. One female's family caregiver was so skeptical about her involvement that we decided not to pursue the matter further. The family of another female in a nursing home agreed to meet with us and let us visit with the patient. During that meeting, we discovered that the family remained uncomfortable about their participation and that the patient also was incoherent and demented. We did not pursue their participation further. A third male was enrolled and visited twice but was so ill with a brain tumor that we could not gather useful information. Because he had no family members to provide additional information, we did not include him further in the study. Thus, we were left with nine people and their families as the focus of the research, all of whom consented without reservations.

Constraints

Any effort to obtain a terminally ill person's perspective faces several constraints, which reduce the numbers of individuals available. First, participants must have been diagnosed as terminal—often seriously reducing the time remaining for data gathering. Second, the need to get referrals from attending physicians places the physician in the position of a gatekeeper, able to screen in or screen out potential candidates. In addition, for the purposes of this research the individuals had to be coherent, feeling well enough to talk, and willing to participate—further reducing the available population. Although focusing on one disease might have been interesting for purposes of comparison, the selection criteria—applied to the small total population in Missoula County—made such a focus infeasible within the time period available. Ultimately, having a small cross-section of participants representing the major diseases that lead to terminal illness in Missoula proved equally desirable.

Although our participants were representative of the terminally ill population in Missoula in many ways, as a group they differed in one way from most of those dying in 1997. Seven of our nine participants (78 percent) chose hospice care—compared to only 18 percent of all patients dying in Missoula during 1996–97, according to the report of the MDP Clinical Experience Study (K. Norris, personal communication, 2000). Moreover, they chose hospice care early in the trajectory of their final illness: Participants in this study had hospice care for a median of 6.5 months prior to death. This high percentage of hospice patients in our study population occurred as an inadvertent result of the selection criteria. The physician, the dying person, and their family all had to recognize and accept that the person was terminally ill, or they would not be referred to our study in the first place. Those who accepted their condition much earlier than average, and chose palliative care, are thus unusual compared to the general population of those dying in Missoula in 1997.

In fact, there was no intent to select for hospice, and we had expected a more diverse range of caregiving support even in the small sample. We stress this point because other communities wishing to study prospectively the personal experience of people who are dying may encounter the same phenomenon.

Conducting a prospective study of people with a terminal diagnosis that requires patient and family consent and physician agreement to terminal status as criteria for participation will result in characteristics that are somewhat skewed relative to the population as a whole. In our study, the enrollment criteria resulted in a set of participants of whom the majority chose or accepted active palliative care early in their disease trajectory.

The other constraint inherent in the selection of this study population was that those with chronic diseases (e.g., chronic obstructive pulmonary disease [COPD] or congestive heart failure [CHF]) who were identified as terminal by their physicians were likely to live longer—sometimes far longer—than the predicted six months, even though they were seriously ill and had no prospect of recovery. (A high probability of dying within six months is the criterion for referral to palliative or hospice care; this criterion is based on cancer trajectories.) This difficulty was less well-understood or documented at the time of this study but has been verified with the large-scale SUPPORT data. The SUPPORT investigators conclude that "the goal of determining in advance—with a high degree of accuracy— which individual patients with COPD, CHF, or end-stage renal disease (ESRD) will die within 6 months is unrealistic" because of the nature of these chronic diseases (Fox et al. 1999, 1642). Invariably a majority (53–70 percent) will live longer than six months. "Many patients with COPD, CHF or ESRD never experience a time during which they are clearly dying of their disease" (Fox et al. 1999, 1638).

How the Data Were Collected

The data on which this study is based were derived from four sources: the terminally ill patients themselves, their caregivers, other noncaregivers or family friends, and supplementary materials. In addition to tape-recorded conversations, we also made field notes of each encounter with dying participants and their family members. We attended all of the memorial services that were held and made after-death visits to each caregiver. When appropriate and possible, we also made after-death visits with others who interacted with the study participants, such as clergy, social workers, and nurses.

On a few occasions, documents written by the participants were made available to us. In some cases, tape recordings of unrelated conversations were offered to us by the family. We also collected obituaries and other printed articles about our patients.

Data Collection Procedures

The data collection team, which comprised a male researcher (Roger Shuy) and a female researcher (Jana Staton), made initial visits together. After the first visit, we determined which one of us might appropriately make follow-up visits. Most often, we tried to match gender; among more elderly participants, their comfort with someone of their own gender seemed greater.

As professional researchers entering this type of setting, we realized that there was a strong possibility of a perceived asymmetry of knowledge and/ or status. We defused some of this perception by meeting the participants in their own settings—usually their homes, where they would have the most inherent power. We believe that this perception was further defused by the fact that our visits took the form of everyday conversations rather than interviews. In fact, after our first visits, our role changed from that of unfamiliar researchers to that of welcomed visitors. Unlike most doctor-patient communication, in which a doctor navigates between authority/expertise and the need to gain enough rapport to ensure effective cooperation and compliance, we defused any perceived role as experts by telling our patients and caregivers that we were there to listen and to learn from them. The fact that the data collectors were not medical professionals aided this effort considerably.

We tape recorded all visits, using a small, hand-held cassette recorder with a regular clip-on or lapel microphone. The lapel microphone greatly enhanced the quality of sound and ensured that the participants did not have to strain or talk loudly. Visits varied in length, depending on participants' energy and other circumstances; they averaged about 45 minutes. We made copies of each tape immediately after the visits. We then gave the copy to a tape transcriber, who made a written transcript of each visit. When the transcriber returned the tape and transcript, the researcher who did not make the visit reviewed the transcript and corrected it against the tape, using high-quality listening equipment. This procedure provided the opportunity for both researchers to listen to all material. The visiting researcher wrote field notes immediately after each visit.

We have followed standard procedures for ensuring the confidentiality of data on completion of the study, including storing tape recordings and transcripts in a locked area that is inaccessible to anyone but the researchers. The purpose of this study is not to reveal individual secrets or to be critical of particular health care services or individual providers. It is to describe, at a given point in time and in a given community, what went on in the experiences of nine dying persons and their caregivers—usually, but not always, their families.

Frequency of Visits

We began our visits in July 1997, as the referrals from the Pilot Clinical Profile began to provide us with names. In the first month we had only three or four patients; as the weeks went on, more were added. By mid-September, we had identified, gained consent from, and visited all nine participants more than once. We tried to make visits at least once every two weeks, sometimes more often and sometimes less frequently depending on participants' schedules, health, and comfort with having us as visitors. Follow-up visits offered the opportunity to determine any changes in perspectives and experiences of participants and caregivers and framed the iterative part of the research, enabling us to test, validate, and/or expand the information gathered in previous visits. We made a minimum of five visits to most participants before they died.

During this visitation period, we sometimes arranged separate visits with caregivers, again depending on their availability. In one case, where there was no other available caregiver to stay with the patient, one of us took the caregiver out for an hour's break to shop or just to have coffee while the other researcher sat and visited with her terminally ill husband. This procedure provided us with an opportunity to tape record both of them at the same time; it also provided the caregiver with respite and some variation in her daily routine.

After-Death Visits

We attended memorial services for the eight participants who died during the project and made at least one extensive after-death visit with each of the caregivers. We included the data from these encounters in the analysis.

Approach to Analysis

The study data are subjective in the best sense of that word: They record participants' attitudes, beliefs, values, and knowledge, regardless of whether these match the objective record. For example, one elderly woman professed not to know why she was ill, and her friends reported that her physician said that the cause of her illness was not known, other than that "she's older." These reports may not comport with the medical record; our purpose was to observe, record, and report the participants' experience, not the doctor's knowledge. We report some peoples' satisfaction with care, even when that care might not be deemed satisfactory on any quality assessment scale. We have refrained, however, from using or reporting some data concerning objective events or facts when there was some doubt about the factuality of what we were told (i.e., we could not verify the information, even through another family member).

The analysis was data-driven: The issues and themes that were significant to the patients and their families are the focus of the analysis. Just as we allowed our participants to introduce their own topics during our conversations with them, we also allowed the data—transcripts of visits and our notes of our observations and reactions during those visits—to suggest topics.

Although the study is data-driven, we do not suggest that we came to the study, or the analysis, as *tabula rasa*. We began the data collection with a set of potential topics or themes—drawn from literature, other MDP research projects, and our own personal and professional experience. At the beginning of the study, these themes provided the basis for the aforementioned "conversational starters" (see box, "Guide for Conversations with Participants"). In most cases, however, these topics were brought up independently by the patients and their caregivers themselves—which suggests that we had anticipated relatively accurately some of the things our participants wanted to talk about.

Guide for Conversations with Participants

General Quality of Life

Concerns:	What concerns you right now?
Troubles, problems:	What troubles you right now?
	When, where is this most troublesome?
	When does it get better?
Joys:	What brings you joy? Do others understand this?
Learning:	What are you learning from this experience?
	Have you talked with anyone about this?
Helpful:	What is *most* helpful right now to you, your family?
	What is *least* helpful right now to you, your family?
Family help, support:	Who helps you and your family now?
Regrets:	What would you have done differently in the past few years, knowing what you know now?
	Are there things you regret, that are left undone?
	Has anyone helped you deal with these?
Social, people:	Are you able to stay in touch with, see the people you care about most?

Fears:	What are your fears now? Have you shared these?
	—dying, finances, loss to family, being helpless
Goals, priorities:	What are your goals, priorities now, in the next few months?
	What would you like to be doing?

Specific Topic Probes

Medical care:	What's going well right now?
	Are you having difficulties with your medical care, providers?
	What would you change about your care if you could?
	What would you like to tell your doctors, nurses about your care that they don't seem to understand?
Pain and communication:	Is pain a problem for you now?
	What has the doctor/nurse done or said about it?
	Are you able to talk about it to him/her? to family?
	What helps you most when you're in pain?
	Do you find it difficult to express the amount, degree, kind of pain you have?
Care while dying:	What are your biggest concerns for your medical care when, if you get worse?
	What would you most like to have happen?
	Who have you talked to about this?
	Do you want to stay at home?
	How does your family see this?

Plans:	Have you made any plans for your care at the end/when you're dying?
	—Advance directive, Comfort One, DNR?
	Who talked with you about these?
	Does your family understand what you want?
Family:	Has your illness affected your family?
	Can you talk with them openly about dying, about what you want?
	Are there disagreements in your family about your care?
Finances:	Are you having financial hardship because of this illness?
	Are you worried about your family's finances after you die?
Communication:	What do you understand about your illness?
	Do you have unanswered questions about what's going on?
	Can you talk with your friends, family about your illness? Do they understand? want to talk?
	Do others understand what you're going through?
	Do others treat/talk to you differently? avoid you?
	Have you met, talked with others with your illness?
Spiritual, religious support:	What has been most helpful about what your church/pastor has done?
	What did you expect, need? Have these been met?
	Has someone talked with you about dying?
	What kinds of practical, emotional support?

Procedures for Transcript Analysis

1. We identified each transcript by date, as well as by a sequential code number, so that quotes could be located in the data. Our system was very simple: We used letters of the alphabet for the patients, and numbers in sequence to indicate which visit the transcript reflected. Field notes were identified by date and person visited.

2. We then identified every topic in each transcript, using the participant's own wording, and we indexed the topics. We speak of *indexing* rather than *coding* because indexing reflects whatever topics the person brought up, rather than fitting topics into categories developed *a priori*. If the person speaks about dogs and cats, the topic index uses "dogs and cats," rather than "satisfying activities." The index is thus more unique to the speaker, and retains the language of each. If the person says, "I feel so awful anymore. I don't know if I'm alive or dead," the indexing would use "feel awful," not "pain"—which is an interpretation.

   We decided not to use a predetermined coding system in our study. We agree with Ainsworth-Vaughn (1998) that coding for predetermined categories suffers from being an "either-or" approach. That is, when one codes data such as this, one makes an *a priori* decision that the coded item has one meaning and one function. Although such coding may appear to simplify the process of analysis, with naturalistic data such as these, it masks the norms of language use, in which there are multiple possible functions and messages in each utterance. Such coding also masks (or entirely ignores) the commonplace ambiguities found in everyday language use. In her study of conversation between physicians and patients, Ainsworth-Vaughn (1998) observes, "Coding cannot capture the multi-functionality and ambiguity with which speakers negotiate, leaving open multiple possible interpretations; and negotiation is central to medical encounters" (8).

3. The first step in indexing was for one set of transcripts from one family to be read independently by both analysts. We then compared our indexing, to ensure that the procedures for indexing topics were the same.

4. One analyst read and indexed topics from the complete set of transcripts from each participant and his/her caregivers and family. The transcripts were read in chronological sequence—that is, from the first visit through to the after-death visits with family members. Each topic was identified in the transcript and indexed in the margin. The topic identification is shown in italics, as the example on the following page illustrates:

| *Patient:* | I have a sister that just moved to Missoula, and another sister that was in Missoula for 5 years. She just moved, but she stops in and helps me when she can. | **Topic** *sister helps* |

Researcher: So you do have sisters that come and keep in touch with you emotionally . . . .

Patient: Oh yeah. I have strong family support.

5. All topics were then listed by page location on a face sheet for each separate transcript, so that all topics could be located by speaker, date, and page of transcript. A given topic, such as "not feeling comfortable" or various caregiver burdens, might be brought up many times by a given participant. Each occurrence, however repetitive, is indexed. The significance of repeated topics is that such recycling indicates the persistent strength of a participant's agenda and intentions, or the perceived importance of that topic. Because our conversations occurred in a relatively brief time frame relative to the participant's life and impending death, there was relatively little "change" in the conversational content over time. There was relatively more change in the concerns, attitudes, and topics of caregivers; the dated indexing allowed us to understand any changes that were occurring—primarily in the difference between what was shared prior to death and what emerged after death.

6. After all topics were indexed for a given participant and his/her family members who talked with us, a summary sheet was used to organize the topics by themes, developed from the initial conversational guides. By the time of the analysis, the MDP had created a set of broad domains of interest to guide all of the initial or baseline studies. These domains were themselves data-driven, emerging from the year-long dialogues within the MDP Research Committee that used preliminary data from the other contemporaneous studies, based on suggestions by the International Research Advisors.

The shared MDP domains used to organize the themes during the analysis framed the chapters for the report and ultimately for this book:

- Communication about Death and Dying
- Planning and Choices
- Professional Care and Doctor-Patient Communication

- Knowledge of Illness and Attitudes Toward Pain and Death

- Daily Life and Meaningful Activities

- Family Caregiving Experience

- Support and Lack of Support for Family Caregivers

- Personal Growth, Meaning, and Spirituality

- Final Days of Life

- Memorials at the End of Life

The final set of themes differed slightly for patients and their caregivers. The themes were further grouped to correspond to the MDP domains that had been developed as part of the Community Profile. The themes used in the analysis listed in the box, as an aid to other researchers who may be engaged in similar studies. Italicized headings are the original MDP domains that were developed by the MDP Research Committee and used across the various studies comprising the Community Profile. Themes that emerged from our conversations with participants are listed in boldface type.

We also provide a separate listing of the actual themes for analyzing the conversations with family caregivers; some of the themes necessarily differed from those for the dying person.

The use of domains and themes ensured that specific topics could be located and connected to other topics and that data from our study could be related to the domains of interest to the MDP, while retaining the particular and unique features of the individual participants.

For example, one of the participants owned a homestead ranch in a rural Montana county, with development rights entrusted to the Montana Land Reliance. Much of his conversation with us returned repeatedly to his excitement about the work of the Montana Land Reliance and his sense of continuity and closure in being able to preserve his family's land from future development. The topic, therefore, is "the land" and its preservation.

This topic—which was unique to transcripts of conversations with Ralph—is linked to other similarly unique topics in the lives of other participants, such as passing on a legacy of courage and bravery to children, giving away work tools, or providing for pets. All of these topics were grouped under the theme of "continuity of life" (our term). In turn, the theme of continuity falls within the domain of Personal Growth, Meaning, and Spirituality, which is one of the MDP's major areas of interest. Thus, the thematic summaries for each participant are uniform, whereas the topics reflect each individual's own unique circumstances.

Themes in Participant Conversations,
Organized in Relation to MDP Domains

Communication about Death/Death Attitudes
- **expectations**
- **openness/acceptance**
- **fears** (of planning ahead, burdens, unknown, judgment)
- **loss/control issues**
- **preparations for death** (other than Advance Directive, DNR)

Physical Symptoms and Management
- **pain** (severity and management)
- **other symptoms and management**
- **knowledge about/attitude toward illness**
- **satisfaction with symptom management**

Functioning
- **enjoyable activities**
- **degree of independence/dependence in daily living**
- **social context** (including interest in visitors)

Professional Caregiving (Medical)
- **continuity of health personnel**
- **communication with physician about diagnosis, prognosis**
- **Advance Directive, DNR, DPOA** (existence, patient/physician involvement and decisions)
- **satisfaction with doctors, hospice, nurses**

Family Experience
- **caregiving experience/activities**
- **stress** (physical, emotional, marital, social, financial)
- **importance/value to caregiver**
- **support for family from others**
- **economics** (effects on care; effects of illness on finances)

Personal Growth, Meaning, and Spirituality
- **continuity** (symbols of)
- **faith experience** (importance, support, beliefs)
- **desired support from community**
- **meaningful experiences/activities** (closure)
- **sense of peace, closure**
- **trust** (ability/willingness to accept dependence on others)

Bereavement
- **anticipatory grieving of patient**
- **regrets/last wishes**
- **losses, worries**

Themes in Caregiver Conversations, Organized in Relation to MDP Domains

Communication/Attitudes about Death of Loved One/Self

> expectations
> openness/acceptance of prognosis
> preparations for death (other than Advance Directive, DNR)
> openness of communication between caregiver and patient
> death of self

Physical Symptoms and Management

> symptoms most troublesome for caregiver
> knowledge about/attitude toward illness
> understanding/satisfaction with symptom management, palliative care
> difficulties in providing nursing care for symptoms

Functioning

> level of independence
> effects on family caregiver of dependency/caregiving

Professional Caregiving (Medical)

> continuity of health personnel
> communication with physician about diagnosis, prognosis
> Advance Directive, DNR, DPOA (existence, involvement in decisions)
> coordination, communication with/among professionals
> satisfaction with doctors, hospice, nurses

Family/Caregiver Experience

> caregiving experience/activities
> stress (physical, emotional, marital, social [move, work, etc.], financial)
> importance/value of experience to caregiver
> support from others
> economics (effects on care; effects of illness on finances)
> fears/worries/guilt

Personal Growth, Meaning, and Spirituality

> continuity (symbols of)
> faith experience (importance, support)
> desired support from community

Bereavement

> rituals of remembrance
> guilt
> physical status
> expectations of others
> changes and new life

7. Once the indexing was completed, the transcripts were re-read to begin the formal analysis of the *text*, *subtext*, and *context* of central issues. The patterns of communication in the conversations with participants are the observable *text*: what people say about a topic and how they actually say it. The *subtext* is the dynamics of meaning, relationship, beliefs, and values that underlie what is said. The analysis of the subtext draws on knowledge of all of the communication, references to topics already introduced, and the relationship (family, social, professional, etc.) between speakers. The understanding of the text and subtext was expanded by analyzing both in *context*—that is, the broader social environment within which any specific topic is discussed. The context in this case included knowledge of Missoula in 1997, its particular social and demographic factors, and the social history of the participants and their families.

The box below contains the text from the consent form that we used for all participants in this study.

Consent Form—Conversations with Study Participants Missoula Demonstration Project Community Profile, Part V: Participant Perspectives

Purpose of Our Study   Members of the Missoula Demonstration Project team want to improve the quality of life for people with progressive, life-limiting illnesses. To do so, we must first understand the experiences, feelings, beliefs, and concerns of patients with these diagnoses. We are conducting these conversations with you and others like you coping with a serious or chronic illnesses, so that you can discuss what's important to you right now, and share your views about your care and support.

Your Participation   We will schedule opportunities to talk with you whenever and wherever you are most comfortable. Together, we will decide the length of our conversations, and how often you would like us to come back. You can invite your family or friends to join us from time to time if you wish, as they are an important part of your life. We will make an audio-tape recording of our conversations with you, to ensure that we can remember the exact words you say. No one outside the research team will listen to these recordings, and whatever you say to us will be kept confidential, and will not be traced to you in any way.

Some Considerations   Participants often tell us that they benefit from having an opportunity to share their thoughts and describe their experiences to someone who is willing to listen. You may experience a similar benefit. However, talking with us may sometimes be an inconvenience or tiring for you, and you should tell us if this occurs. Also, you may experience some discomfort as you discuss any issues or difficulties you are having with family, caregivers, friends. You may stop these conversations at any time. If you should need assistance to deal with your feelings, we will provide you with the names of professional counselors who can help you.

We are not able to pay you for participation. However, you may find yourself telling stories about your life which you would like to save for future generations of your family. We will be glad to give you a copy of your audiotape for you to share with anyone you want.

We Assure Confidentiality   The tape recordings will not be played for anyone else. We will transcribe the conversations onto paper, and these will also remain confidential and will not be shared with other people. Your name will not appear anywhere on the typewritten pages, and only first names will be used for other people you may mention. If you ask us, we will delete from the transcript the names of any health professionals or institutions you may have mentioned in talking with us. The transcripts will be used for analysis only, and will then be locked away until they can be destroyed. This consent form will also be retained separately for five years, and then destroyed. You will not be identified by name or personal characteristics in any presentations or in any publications that might come from the analyzed information.

If you have any questions about this study at any time, you may call the Missoula Demonstration Project office at 728-6163, or Lola Goss at St. Patrick Hospital, at 329-5669.

Date:_____   _____

                                                              (Researcher)

I have read this consent form and I agree by signing or by orally stated consent to participate in the study. I have received a copy of this consent form.

Date:_____   _____

                                                              (Participant)

                      _____

                                                              (Family Participant)

Index